MANAGEMENT OF
LABORATORY
ANIMAL CARE
AND
USE PROGRAMS

MANAGEMENT OF
LABORATORY ANIMAL CARE AND USE PROGRAMS

Edited by
Mark A. Suckow
Fred A. Douglas
Robert H. Weichbrod

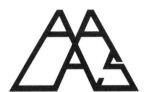

CRC PRESS

Boca Raton   London   New York   Washington, D.C.

Portions of *Managing a Nonprofit Organization* by Thomas A. Wolf (copyright © 1990 by Prentice-Hall Press) appear in Chapter 10. Reprinted with permission of Simon & Schuster, Inc.

Library of Congress Cataloging-in-Publication Data

Management of laboratory animal care and use programs / edited by Mark A. Suckow, Fred A. Douglas, Robert H. Weichbrod.
    p. cm.
   Includes bibliographical references (p.).
   ISBN 0-8493-2287-1 (alk. paper)
   1. Laboratory animals. 2. Biological laboratories—Management. I. Suckow, Mark A. II. Douglas, Fred A. III. Weichbrod, Robert H.

SF406 .M36 2001
636.088'5—dc21   2001043684

Visit the CRC Press Web site at www.crcpress.com

© 2002 by CRC Press LLC

No claim to original U.S. Government works
International Standard Book Number 0-8493-2287-1
Library of Congress Card Number 2001043684
Printed in the United States of America   5 6 7 8 9 0
Printed on acid-free paper

Preface

The use of animals remains integral to progress in biomedical research. As animal models, regulations, equipment, and financial issues have increased in complexity, so too has the art of management of laboratory animal care and use programs.

Management of Laboratory Animal Care and Use Programs is not meant to be an exhaustive review focused on the minutiae related to animal care. Instead, the book broadly addresses important concepts that the manager of a laboratory animal resource typically would need to provide effective direction and oversight to the operations of such a resource.

The book consists of 16 chapters written by individuals with substantial experience in the fields discussed. Pragmatic issues, such as financial management and regulatory compliance, are covered, as well as issues related to professional development and ethics, animal health, and public relations. All chapters are referenced to lead the reader toward additional sources of information, if desired. Readers are encouraged to consult multiple sources to obtain a broad perspective of management. In addition, the editors encourage qualified individuals to partake of management training opportunities, such as ILAM, and to obtain relevant certifications, such as the CMAR (Certified Manager, Animal Resources), for further professional development.

While application of the management principles described in this book may vary among facilities or even individual managers, it is the hope of the editors that the information presented might provide a starting point for those engaged in the management of all types of laboratory animal resources.

All royalties due the editors of *Management of Laboratory Animal Care and Use Programs* will be donated to the AALAS Foundation, Memphis, TN.

The Editors

Mark A. Suckow, D.V.M., Dipl. ACLAM, is the Director of the Freimann Life Science Center at the University of Notre Dame, where he is also an Associate Research Professor in the Department of Biological Sciences. In addition, Dr. Suckow is an Adjunct Associate Professor of Veterinary Pathobiology at Purdue University.

Dr. Suckow received his D.V.M. from the University of Wisconsin in 1987, and completed a postdoctoral residency program in laboratory animal medicine at the University of Michigan in 1990. He is a Diplomate of the American College of Laboratory Animal Medicine.

Dr. Suckow is an active member of the American Association for Laboratory Animal Science (AALAS) and has served as Chair of the Animal Technician Certification Board and of the Professional Development Coordinating Committee. He has published more than 50 scientific papers and chapters in books. His awards include the AALAS Young Investigator Award and the Excellence in Research Award from the American Society of Laboratory Animal Practitioners.

Fred A. Douglas, B.S., RLATG, is the Director of the Veterinary Laboratory Animal Care Unit in the School of Veterinary Medicine at Purdue University, where he has worked since 1982. In addition to directing the daily operation of the research animal resource, Mr. Douglas teaches in the Veterinary Technology Program at Purdue.

Mr. Douglas received his B.S. in Animal Science from the University of Nebraska in 1974. He is a Registered Laboratory Animal Technologist through the American Association for Laboratory Animal Science. He has been an active member of AALAS locally, regionally, and nationally. He has served as Chair of the Committee on Laboratory Animal Technicians, member of the Animal Technician Certification Board, Chair of the Institute for Laboratory Animal Management, and has contributed and reviewed articles for *Contemporary Topics in Laboratory Animal Science*. Mr. Douglas is also an active member of the Laboratory Animal Management Association (LAMA), and has served on the Board of Directors and as the President of that organization. He is currently the Editor-in-Chief of the *LAMA Review*.

Mr. Douglas has been recognized for his contributions to the field of laboratory animal management with such awards as the AALAS George R. Collins Award, the Purina Mills Animal Technician Award, the U. Kristina Stephens Award from LAMA, and the Charles River Medallion from LAMA.

Robert H. Weichbrod, Ph.D., M.B.A., RLATG, is the Manager of Scientific Activities (Southeast Region) for The Jackson Laboratory. Previous to this position, Dr. Weichbrod managed laboratory animal resources for the Department of Defense for 20 years. He has authored more than 50 scientific, managerial, and technical articles pertaining to programs involving the care and use of animals in biomedical research, training, and education.

Dr. Weichbrod received his B.S. in Zoology from the University of Maryland in 1976, his M.B.A. from Marymount University in 1988, and his Ph.D. in Public Administration and Policy from Walden University of Advanced Studies in 1993. His dissertation evaluating the use of laboratory animals in Department of Defense activities is a seminal work and has been cited during Congressional hearings on the topic. He earned his Laboratory Animal Technologist certification from AALAS in 1978 and was a charter class graduate from the AALAS Institute for Laboratory Animal Management in 1993.

Dr. Weichbrod holds academic appointments in Business Administration at Strayer University in Washington, D.C., and in Preventive Medicine and Biometrics at the Uniformed Services University of the Health Sciences in Bethesda, MD. He is a member of the Board of Regents for the Institute of Certified Professional Managers at James Madison University in Harrisonburg, VA. He was the founding Editor of the *LAMA Review* and has served on the Editorial Board of *Lab Animal* magazine since 1986. Dr. Weichbrod was President of AALAS in 2000 and has served as a member of the Association for Assessment and Accreditation of Laboratory Animal Care (AAALAC), International's Council on Accreditation since 1997.

Dr. Weichbrod's awards include the U. Kristina Stephens Award from LAMA, the AALAS George R. Collins Award, the Charles River Medallion, the Award of Excellence from the U.S. Secretary of Defense, and the Purina Mills Animal Technician Award.

The editors wish to thank Christine Andreasen, Nicole Brown, Omnese Campbell, Nicole Duffee, Chris Lyons, Dawn Vinson, and Tonia Walk for assistance and advice in the preparation of this publication.

Reviewers

The editors wish to thank the following individuals for serving as content reviewers:

James A. Alford, Jr., M.B.A.
Mary Ellenberger, D.V.M.
Robert E. Mueller II, Ph.D.
Ken Pyle, M.S., LATG
Dennis Stark, D.V.M., Ph.D.
Dennis Taff, M.B.A., M.S., LATG
Dawn Vinson, M.S.
Jan Wyrick Gnadt, D.V.M.

Contributors

James A. Alford, Jr., M.B.A.
Howard Hughes Medical Institute
Ann Arbor, MI

Lynn C. Anderson, D.V.M., Dipl. ACLAM
Merck and Co., Inc.
Rahway, NJ

Jacquie Calnan, M.P.A.
Americans for Medical Progress
Alexandria, VA

Fred A. Douglas, B.S., RLATG
Purdue University
West Lafayette, IN

Mary S. Freer, B.B.A.
University of Michigan
Ann Arbor, MI

Jan Wyrick Gnadt, D.V.M., Dipl. ACLAM
State University of New York
Stony Brook, NY

Janet C. Gonder, D.V.M., Ph.D.
Baxter Healthcare Corporation
Round Lake, IL

Gail A. Heidbrink, RLATG
Britz-Heidbrink, Inc.
Wheatland, WY

Bruce Kennedy, M.S., RLATG
California Institute of Technology
Pasadena, CA

Steven M. Kuhlman, V.M.D., Dipl. ACLAM
Pharmacia Corporation
Kalamazoo, MI

Stuart E. Leland, D.V.M., Dipl. ACLAM
Institute for Human Gene Therapy
University of Pennsylvania
Philadelphia, PA

Brent J. Martin, D.V.M., Dipl. ACLAM
Medical College of Ohio
Toledo, OH

Dennis B. Miller, RLATG
Medical College of Wisconsin
Milwaukee, WI

Robert E. Mueller II, Ph.D.
Bayer Corporation
Stillwell, KS

Christian E. Newcomer, V.M.D., Dipl. ACLAM
University of North Carolina
Chapel Hill, NC

Howard G. Rush, D.V.M., Dipl. ACLAM
University of Michigan
Ann Arbor, MI

Janet G. Skidmore, M.A.
Merck and Co., Inc.
Rahway, NJ

U. Kristina Stephens, M.A., RLATG
University of Georgia
Athens, GA

Mark A. Suckow, D.V.M., Dipl. ACLAM
University of Notre Dame
Notre Dame, IN

Farol N. Tomson, D.V.M., Dipl. ACLAM
University of Florida
Gainesville, FL

Catherine M. Vogelweid, D.V.M., Ph.D., Dipl. ACLAM
Indiana University School of Medicine
Indianapolis, IN

DeWayne H. Walker, D.V.M., Dipl. ACLAM
3M Corporation
St. Paul, MN

Patricia A. Ward, LATG
University of Michigan
Ann Arbor, MI

Acronyms and Expressions

The following acronyms and expressions are commonly used in the field of laboratory animal resource management and in this book.

AAALAC Association for Assessment and Accreditation of Laboratory Animal Care, International

AALAS The American Association for Laboratory Animal Science

ACLAM American College of Laboratory Animal Medicine; specialty board that certifies veterinarians as "Diplomate"

ADA Americans with Disabilities Act of 1992 (Public Law 101-336)

ALAT Assistant Laboratory Animal Technician, as certified by AALAS

ALF Animal Liberation Front; an underground animal rights organization

AWA (Animal Welfare Act; the "Act") Public Law 89-544, 94-279, and 99-198, which impact care and use of research animals in the United States

AWAR Animal Welfare Act Regulations; regulations promulgated by the USDA in response to Congressional mandate as written in the Animal Welfare Act

CITES Convention on International Trade in Endangered Species of Wild Fauna and Flora

CMAR Certified Manager, Animal Resources; certification offered to qualified individuals through AALAS and Institute of Certified Professional Managers

DEA Drug Enforcement Administration (United States)

EEO Equal Employment Opportunity Act of 1972 (Public Law 92-261)

FDA Food and Drug Administration (United States)

GLP Good Laboratory Practice; specific guidelines for testing as required by the FDA

Guide The *Guide for the Care and Use of Laboratory Animals*; published by ILAR

HEPA High Efficiency Particulate Air

IACUC   Institutional Animal Care and Use Committee

IATA   International Air Transport Association

ICPM   Institute of Certified Professional Managers

ILAM   The AALAS Institute of Laboratory Animal Management

ILAR   Institute of Laboratory Animal Resources of the National Research Council (United States)

IT   Information Technology

LAMA   Laboratory Animal Management Association

LAT   Laboratory Animal Technician, as certified by AALAS

LATG   Laboratory Animal Technologist, as certified by AALAS

LAWTE   Laboratory Animal Welfare Training Exchange

NIH   National Institutes of Health (United States)

OLAW   Office of Laboratory Animal Welfare, part of PHS

OPRR   Office of Protection from Research Risks, part of PHS

OSHA   Occupational Safety and Health Administration (United States)

PETA   People for the Ethical Treatment of Animals; an animal rights organization

PHS   Public Health Service (United States)

PPE   Personal Protective Equipment as it relates to occupational health

QA   Quality Assurance

QC   Quality Control

RLATG   Registered Laboratory Animal Technologist; indicates that individual holding the LATG certification has met continuing education requirements; also applies to ALAT (RALAT) and LAT (RLAT)

SOP   Standard Operating Procedure

SPF   Specific pathogen free; refers to content of disease-causing organisms of animals

Three Rs   Refers to "Reduction," "Replacement," and "Refinement" of animal use as proposed by Russell and Burch (*The Principles of Humane Experimental Techniques*, Methuen & Co., London, 1959)

TQM   Total Quality Management

USDA   United States Department of Agriculture; the USDA has promulgated
              regulations in response to the Animal Welfare Act

Contents

1 Management of People — A Most Valuable Resource

U. Kristina Stephens, M.A., RLATG

Before managers can organize effectively they must have a "vision," that is, they must be able to visualize what their organization will be doing in the near and distant future. The **"mission"** of the organization describes the larger purpose that gives meaning to the work performed. The **"mission statement"** explains why the organization exists, and it provides the overall framework and philosophy of the organization by broadly defining the organization's purpose. The "mission statement" identifies the organization's operating domain in terms of service and technology selections.

Human resources are central to any organization, and the manager as an individual and the staff members are very important parts of that organization. By organizing work efficiently, everyone can take pride in their work.

I.   ORGANIZING

The manager's own style of organization will depend on a number of factors, as stated in Susan Silver's book entitled *Organized To Be The Best!* (1). The manager's level of activity, whether one has any support staff, the image one wants to project, whether one deals face to face with the public, and the style one uses to work are all areas of importance. Silver further states that organization is a question of balance between the details and the "big picture." A quick and honest self-evaluation will reveal the areas on which the manager needs to focus. Organization will help save time and effort. For instance, organizing the weekly work-schedule for the facility together with the employee team can not only save time and effort, but also improve communication within the group.

II.   DESIRED QUALITIES OF EMPLOYEES AND SUPERVISORS

Two groups of laboratory animal technicians — a total of 150 technicians — participated in a survey in the early 1990s that dealt with desirable qualities for supervisors and employees in the laboratory animal science field (2).

The participants were asked to list 10 specific qualities that they would like to see in a technician. The qualities identified include the following.

A.   LABORATORY ANIMAL CARE EMPLOYEE QUALITIES RANKED HIGHEST

- Dependability
- Trustworthiness
- Truthfulness
- Sensitivity (caring) toward animals
- Good work habits
- Dedication
- Ambition
- Punctuality

B.   LABORATORY ANIMAL CARE EMPLOYEE QUALITIES RANKED HIGH

- Willingness to learn
- Willingness to help
- Sense of responsibility
- Consistent behavior
- Enthusiasm
- Friendliness
- Honesty
- Being a good role model

C.   LABORATORY ANIMAL CARE SUPERVISOR QUALITIES RANKED HIGHEST

- Truthfulness
- Honesty
- Fairness
- Dependability
- Openness to ideas expressed by others
- Non-manipulativeness
- Effective communicator
- Good organization capabilities
- Consistent behavior

D.   LABORATORY ANIMAL CARE SUPERVISOR QUALITIES RANKED HIGH

- Supportiveness
- Decisiveness
- Efficiency
- Compassion

In a recent discussion with a group of managers, the author found that the list of valued qualities has not changed markedly, but rather reflects a change in time and additional management concerns within the industry. In this regard, more current opinions of desired qualities include:

- Ability to get along with people
- A sense of compassion when working with animals
- A sense of importance of biomedical research
- Good communication skills
- Good manual dexterity
- Physical strength
- Dependability and integrity
- Having no substance abuse problems
- Willingness to participate in the organization's occupational health program, including related vaccinations

III. HIRING AND STAFFING

There are three critical aspects to hiring quality employees (3). First, there must be an effective recruitment program to provide a large group of candidates from which to choose. Second, the selection process should enable identification of the best candidate with a high degree of confidence. Third, the candidate of choice must be convinced to accept the offer of employment.

The staffing process starts by working in consort with the institutional human resources group regarding planning, recruitment, selection, and orientation of new hires. Selection of new employees ranks near the top of all supervisory responsibilities in terms of importance. One should carefully deliberate about selection of over-qualified people, because these individuals may easily become bored with routine tasks. Hiring the "right" person reduces the likelihood of motivational problems, personnel turnover, and persons with "difficult" personalities. The entire selection process can become a very expensive proposition both in time and money especially if the wrong individual is chosen.

There are several aspects for a manager to consider when hiring new staff members.

A. ASSISTANCE IN THE RECRUITMENT PROCESS

The manager can create a positive attitude within his/her group by providing opportunities for promotion from within the facility. One can solicit help from the staff in identifying candidates, making it a team effort. The manager can provide the employees with copies of the updated job description. Obtaining a list of technical or professional schools where potential candidates receive training and suggesting the best publications in which to place ads can assist human resources personnel in the recruitment effort. Arranging tours of the facility, participating in career-day programs, and accepting volunteers and offering summer internships can all generate interest in the field among qualified individuals.

B. WRITING A JOB DESCRIPTION

As a first step, one should evaluate the job description and the qualifications for the available position. When examining the tasks to be performed, the manager should make sure that *all* duties are thoroughly described. For instance, the term "Check" when requiring someone to "Check and feed the animals" requires further explanation.

As an example, a general job description for an Animal Resource Manager might be written as follows.

1. Perform overall management of facilities and animal care staff. Management includes:

   - Assignment and selection of animals for research projects, to include vendor selection
   - Supervision of staff and dealing with personnel-related issues
   - The training of personnel
   - The preparation and updating of original "Standard Operating Procedures"

2. Coordination of technical issues within the facilities, e.g., breeding colonies, occupational safety hazards, etc.
3. Developing facilities budgets and fee structure for services rendered.
4. Working with research staff to assist in coordination of work, grant applications, and protocol development.
5. Dedicated to meeting and exceeding research and animal care regulations set forth by federal governmental agencies and university agencies.
6. Working knowledge of accreditation process of the Association for Assessment and Accreditation of Laboratory Animal Care, International (AAALAC).
7. Candidate should have achieved AALAS certification at the technologist (LATG) level.
8. Graduate from the AALAS Institute of Laboratory Animal Management (ILAM) preferred.

C. REFINING INTERVIEWING TECHNIQUES

Prior to the interview, the applicant should receive several documents such as an updated copy of the job description, directions to the interview location, an offer, if any, for travel reimbursement, a brief agenda, a description of any testing procedures, and one of the manager's business cards with contact information. To prepare for the interview, the manager should (3):

- Familiarize him/herself with the position description
- Review the applications and résumés
- Note the positive features of the job

- Prepare a rating sheet for each applicant and provide copies to other individuals who will participate in the interview
- Schedule a time and place that will provide privacy and avoid interruptions
- Perhaps most importantly, review the questions to be utilized during the interview

The interviewee should have an opportunity to take a tour of the facilities, meet with other technicians, meet with principal investigators, and visit the human resources department.

D. THE INTERVIEWING PROCESS

An oft-raised question is "Who should conduct the interview?" The interviewer should be someone who has received special training in the skill of interviewing. The two most important characteristics of good interviewers are:

1. **Good communication skills** — especially with respect to asking the right questions.
2. **Enthusiasm** about the organization, the staff, the job, and the interviewees.

One or more of the candidate's future peers should be a member of the interviewing team. Peers can often spot people they would like to have or not have on their team.

The interviewer should make probing statements such as "Tell me about a problematic situation at work" and continue with such questions as "How did that happen?" "How did you react?" or "What did you do?"

In order to determine professional and technical competence related to duties and responsibilities as described in the job description, the interviewer could describe a hypothetical situation and then ask "What would you do?" Concerning measurement of the individual's motivation, the interviewer could ask "Did you ever go the extra mile?" and follow with further probing questions. Concerning teamwork, the interviewer could ask "Would you consider helping others, after you finished your own assigned work?"

Sensitive-issue questions should be handled delicately. The interviewer should avoid strong words such as "weakness" or "deficiency." Effective questions might include: "One of the areas of concern in our profession is the use of animals in research. How do you feel about the use of animals in research?" "Could you euthanize the animals you cared for at the end of the study?" "Could you collect samples and tissues from these animals?"

The interviewee may sometimes give clues of untruthfulness. The résumé may appear too good to be true, and his body language may give him away. Another clue may be if the information from the reference does not coincide with what the candidate tells the interviewer.

The interviewee can take several specific steps to improve interview behavior, conversation, and body language (4). One of the most intriguing interviews the author has experienced was conducted over the phone. In that case, there was no worry about being in an unfamiliar place at a certain time, what kind of clothes to wear, and other nuances such as body language. Instead, one only had to concentrate on answering the questions, and asking one's own probing questions, which served both the interviewer and the interviewee well.

It is advisable for the interviewee to prepare a résumé of his/her professional activities. The length of the résumé can be critical. The author was once told that a Nobel Prize winner had a one-page résumé describing his professional work. If he can do it, so can anyone. It is useful to prepare three different types of résumés: one that describes the entire career (20 pages); another that describes all management activities (1 page); and a third dealing with training activities (1 page). Peggy Schmidt offers several strong points in her book entitled *The New 90 Minute Résumé: For Job Hunters Who Want Top-Notch Results — Fast* (5). The reader is taken on an interactive trip by being asked to put together a fact sheet, develop a job target, compile a résumé, and then is provided with pointers on design of an effective résumé.

IV. LEGAL CONCERNS

The major thrust of relevant Federal and State legislation is to ensure that hiring, retention, and promotion decisions are made only on the basis of an employee's ability to perform the job. Important regulations follow.

A. AFFIRMATIVE ACTION (CIVIL RIGHTS ACT OF 1964) PUBLIC LAW 88-352

Organizations must establish objectives for hiring a certain percentage of women and racial minorities. These groups are to be given the same opportunity as Caucasian men, with the objective of having the same proportions of all groups as in the general labor market.

B. EQUAL EMPLOYMENT OPPORTUNITY ACT OF 1972, PUBLIC LAW 92-261

Managers must be aware of the legal requirements of the Equal Employment Opportunity (EEO) regulations and of their organizations' policies and practices. The manager must recognize and eliminate stereotyping and pre-conceptions of women and minorities and provide achievable expectations for all employees. A partial list of issues interdicted by the EEO Commission (3) includes:

1. Age, nationality, and marital status
2. Spouse's occupation or place of employment

3. Pregnancy or plans of pregnancy
4. Child or baby-sitting arrangements (the manager may ask whether there are problems in getting to work)
5. Military record, except as related to the job
6. Arrest record (the manager may ask whether the person has been convicted of a crime but not whether the person has been arrested)
7. Membership in organizations other than work-related ones
8. Religious affiliation
9. Questions asked only of members of a protected group (e.g., if the manager wants to ask women candidates if they can lift 50 pounds, the manager must ask male candidates that same question)

C. AMERICANS WITH DISABILITIES ACT OF 1992 (ADA) PUBLIC LAW 101-336

The legislative history of the ADA established intentions, as a national mandate, to open society to the disabled by ending discrimination in employment and most situations of everyday life.

The ADA protects individuals with physical and mental disabilities that limit major life activities. For clarification, a **disability** is defined as a physical or mental impairment, which substantially limits one or more major life activities. According to the law, people with disabilities who are otherwise qualified for a job may not be disqualified because they have difficulty in performing tasks that bear only a marginal relationship to a particular job. The ADA has a major impact on hiring and promotion. It requires that "**reasonable accommodations**" be made on behalf of physically or mentally challenged employees. The ADA defines a "reasonable accommodation" as "any change in the work environment or in the way things are customarily done that enables an individual with a disability to enjoy equal employment opportunities." Such accommodations may involve:

1. Physical — Installing ramps, re-positioning work stations, widening of doors, and installing grab bars in toilet stalls.
2. Other aspects — The accommodation requirement applies to all aspects of the employment experience, i.e., application for employment and work environment, including benefits. It may also involve deletion of certain non-essential tasks from the position descriptions.

A four-step process to determine a reasonable accommodation is as follows:

a. Analyze the particular job involved and determine its purpose and essential functions.
b. Consult with the individual about the precise job-related limitations and essential functions.

    c. In consultation with the individual, identify potential accommodations and assess their effectiveness with respect to essential job functions.

    d. Select the accommodation that is most appropriate for the individual and the employer.

D. THE AGE DISCRIMINATION IN EMPLOYMENT ACT OF 1967, PUBLIC LAW 90-202

The Act, amended in 1986, prohibits employers from placing an age limit on candidates for employment except for those occupations in which age is a realistic qualification (e.g., firefighter).

V. NEW EMPLOYEE ORIENTATION AND PERFORMANCE APPRAISAL

The organization's human resources group should provide information describing all the benefits, including insurance, sick leave, and allowed vacation days. A new employee must understand what he/she is expected to do and how well these tasks must be carried out. The new employee should be informed about working hours, length of the probation period, and what the performance standards are for the various tasks to be performed. The manager should keep a close eye on the new employee and should consider having weekly meetings to clear up any possible problem areas.

If position descriptions provide the "WHAT," then performance standards provide the "HOW WELL." Managers use performance standards to:

A. Facilitate the orientation of new employees

B. Enable the employees to assess their own performance

C. Provide a solid basis for performance appraisals, counseling, and disciplinary actions

D. Identify training and development needs

E. Avoid charges of discrimination and protect against grievance actions

When assigning tasks, the manager needs to maintain an account of expertise. Managers who maintain such an inventory of each employee's skills have an easier time organizing their staffs when time is short and specific work needs to be performed. Such an account of learned skills could include injection techniques, breeding techniques, and pre- and post-operative techniques. Cross training also helps when specific expertise is needed in certain areas. When assigning a task, it is advisable to allocate the entire task and to allow that individual to finish the task.

Each organization usually has its own evaluation forms and program. The manager should familiarize him/herself with the evaluation format and keep a running ledger for each individual to be evaluated. Strengths and weaknesses of each employee need to be documented in a fair and consistent manner.

VI. MOTIVATION AND MENTORING

Because the manager is often positioned in the center of the organization, it is important to understand what motivates one's self as well as the other staff members. Each human being fulfills his/her motivational needs in a very personal way. Specific motivations may change as alterations occur in lifestyles and needs. Poor morale within a work group lurks behind absenteeism, employee turnover, slowdowns, lower productivity, employee grievances, and transfers. A high morale results from an environment in which workers obtain satisfaction from their work and when the staff is motivated to excel in their assigned duties. This ultimately will lead to higher productivity (2).

The same 150 individuals responding to questions related to "Desired Qualities of Employees and Supervisors" responded to questions regarding motivational factors. Their responses are as follows.

A. MOTIVATIONAL FACTORS RANKED HIGHEST

- Taking care of animals and having stimulating work
- Being able to grow professionally and personally
- Having a chance to exercise independent thought
- Being treated with respect
- Being part of the team
- Working in a group that values honesty in communication

B. MOTIVATIONAL FACTORS RANKED AS SECONDARY

- Earning a higher salary
- Receiving better fringe benefits
- Maintaining job security
- Having flexible working hours

The technician groups responded strongly in agreement with Hertzberg's motivational factors theory, expressing needs of challenging, stimulating work, personal achievement, professional growth, and recognition (6). Several of Hertzberg's motivational factors, such as "development to do more" and "freedom to act" are in agreement with the technicians' responses. Hertzberg also developed a six-point list of motivational factors that seems in accord with the technician response (6). His points are as follows:

R	Recognition
A	Achievement
G	Growth of career
W	Work itself
A	Advancement
R	Responsibility

The most lasting motivation comes from the job itself. Management should develop several strategies to promote motivation by providing means of recognition, rewards, and support for career development. Other incentives that may provide powerful motivation are the creation of flextime, job-sharing, and part-time employment. Adding job-related educational and fun items to the work agenda may change a negative attitude to a positive one, perhaps by offering a site-visit to another laboratory animal facility, learning about a different species, learning a new technique, or by having the employee give a short informal presentation on a topic of interest.

C.   MENTORING

Mentorship involves providing guidance and widening the horizons of other individuals It can be an uplifting experience for all involved. Chip R. Bell offers advice regarding mentorship in his book entitled *Managers as Mentors: Building Partnerships for Learning* (7). He states that "passing along the wisdom" is essential. Several individuals, during the author's early career, helped her along. They were of different groups within the laboratory animal science field. Several were veterinarians, others were from the author's own peer group, and others were members of the vendor group.

Mentors need to have appreciation for the strengths of the protégé in order to further develop those strengths. Key characteristics of mentors include accessibility, being a good communicator, and having a high degree of integrity and commitment to the profession (8). The protégé should have a sense of team spirit with a professional vision. Ideally the protégé should be goal oriented rather than task oriented, and highly motivated.

Not all mentors are managers, but all effective managers should be mentors. The mentor should avoid patronizing remarks and train the protégé to think, not just do. A mentor can offer direction on how to be successful. Being a mentor takes time and effort. Mentors wear several hats by being teachers and guides. They share knowledge, which might have taken many years to acquire. Peers can become mentors to each other, but sometimes the roles may reverse over time.

Mentors need to have appreciation for the strengths of the protégé and build on those strengths.

VII. DIVERSITY

As reported in *Valuing Diversity: New Tools for a New Reality* by Lewis Brown-Griggs and Lente-Louise Louw, it is estimated that people of color, women, and immigrants constitute nearly 85% of the workforce in the United States (9).

Behavioral science researchers have discovered that 75% of the population is significantly different from any one individual (10). Most individuals think differently, make decisions differently, use time differently, communicate differently, handle emotions differently, manage stress differently, deal with conflicting opinions differently, and work at a different pace. If one can learn to work productively with all types of people, he/she will be more protective and efficient. Finding a common ground between individuals is very important.

There are four useful steps for one to enable him/herself to work with a diverse group:

Identify   Note your own style and identify the other individual's style.

Plan   Put together a plan.

Implement   Interact with the person face to face.

Evaluate   Look at the results of the interaction and note what went well and what did not work well.

It is a challenge for managers to find ways to effectively motivate and fully take advantage of the incredible creativity, energy, and skills of a diverse workforce. In the laboratory animal science field there are additional factors that may need to be examined. Specifically, various cultures that are represented among the work force today may have very diverse backgrounds in regards to religion and attitudes toward laboratory animals and animals in general.

VIII. DISCIPLINING, FIRING, AND DISCHARGING

Disciplining, firing, and discharging can be the hardest parts of being a manager. When carrying out the act of disciplining, the manager should make clear that discipline is not punishment, but that it is an effort to bump unsatisfactory performance up to an acceptable level while preserving the employee's perception of self-worth. The manager should make him/herself familiar with the organization's minor, more serious, and most serious infractions and the prescribed disciplinary action that should follow. Discipline should be fair, firm, and fast.

Many managers feel that it is all but impossible to fire anyone. However, if specific work standards are in place, and mandated procedures are followed, termination is not that difficult. All too often, managers foster problems by accepting unsatisfactory performance or behavior over a period of time, and by rating performance as satisfactory when it is not.

The prescribed procedure for personnel separations, both process and content, must be adhered to very carefully. Employers should provide employee handbooks that clearly state the organization's disciplinary policies. A clear position description, performance standards, and performance appraisal program should be made available to each employee. Without standards and documentation, the situation can become very difficult for the manager as well as for the organization.

For dismissal an employer must typically prove that:

A. There are specific work standards and policies, and that employees are repeatedly reminded about them.
B. What was alleged actually took place, involved the employee, and warrants the discharge.
C. Such behavior has not been condoned in the past, or that other workers have been discharged for similar offenses.
D. The sequence of progressive discipline followed prescribed policy and procedures.
E. The employee made no genuine effort to heed the previous warnings even though they had been informed as to the consequences.
F. The firing was based on behavior or results, not on discrimination, "whistle blowing" related to safety or regulatory compliance practices, military or jury duty, work compensation claims, or violation of "implied contract."

For example, in laboratory animal science, the manager needs to make sure that various animal handling techniques are mastered before the technician is given certain tasks to perform, and that the technician in question is aware of possible biohazardous conditions that may exist. The manager needs to act immediately if any inappropriate behavior is observed.

The manager must prepare him/herself emotionally and realize that the decision to terminate someone is a business decision. It is important for the manager to control his/her emotions before taking any action and to make sure that he/she has collected adequate data to support the termination.

REFERENCES

1. **Silver, S.**, *Organized To Be The Best! New Timesaving Ways to Simplify and Improve How You Work*, Adams-Hall Publishing, Los Angeles, 1991.
2. **Stephens, U.K.**, Technician survey responses: a discussion and application of motivational theories and desired qualities. *Contemp. Top.*, 31, 6, 1992.
3. **Umiker, W.**, *Management Skills for the New Health Care Supervisor*, 2nd ed., Aspen Publishers, Inc., Gaithersburg, MD, 1994.
4. **Schmidt, P.**, *The 90 Minute Interview Prep Book: Get Ready for a Winning Interview*, Peterson's, Princeton, NJ, 1996.
5. **Schmidt, P.**, *The New 90 Minute Résumé: For Job Hunters Who Want Top-Notch Results — Fast*, Peterson's, Princeton, NJ, 1996.
6. **Hertzberg, F.**, *Work and the Nature of Man*, World Press, Cleveland, 1966.
7. **Bell, C.R.**, *Managers as Mentors: Building Partnerships for Learning*, Berrett-Koehler Publishers, San Francisco, 1996.
8. **Suckow, M.A., Sharp, P.E., Alford, J.A., Lindsey, J.R., Maickel, R.P., and Ringler, D.H.**, Effective mentoring of laboratory animal science professionals, *Contemp. Top.*, 34, 6, 1995.

9. **Brown-Griggs, L. and Louw, L., Eds.**, *Valuing Diversity: New Tools for a New Reality*, McGraw-Hill, New York, 1995.
10. **Bolton, R. and Grover-Bolton, D.**, *People Styles at Work: Making Bad Relationships Good and Good Relationships Better*, AMACOM, American Management Association, New York, 1996.

2 Management of Education and Training Programs

Bruce W. Kennedy, M.S., RLATG

I. BACKGROUND

The role of the laboratory animal resource manager is constantly changing to keep pace with developments in biomedical technology. Depending upon the hat worn and the day of the week, the manager may discuss science with a principal investigator, explore repair options to a piece of equipment with a member of the physical plant, enter financial data into a new software package with an administrative assistant, lead technicians in a session on the proper restraint of a guinea pig, contribute to the design of a new facility, orient a new staff member, or address any of a multitude of facility-related issues. Being involved in each of the activities helps minimize errors, reduce accidents, and facilitate productivity in the vivarium.

The knowledge and skills needed to effectively run a laboratory animal resource are considerable. Acquiring such comprehensive knowledge involves training others and being trained oneself so that quality work will be performed efficiently. A primary task of a manager in any industry is to participate in training programs. This chapter focuses on many of the management issues that pertain to training as applied to a laboratory animal resource. Both the training that must be provided to others (e.g., technicians and investigators) as well as the manager's own training needs will be addressed.

Training is the exchange of information among parties. It is not simply placing facts in front of another person with the expectation that they will be learned. Instead, training is a package that combines knowledge, skills, and attitudes related to the information. The exchange is dependent upon the material, the trainer, and the trainees. Each of these components must be evaluated as part of the total package so that the training sessions will be effective. In short, the training should have the objectives of **performance** and **expectations**.

Communication is key for successful training. The effectiveness of communication, from transmission to reception, must be considered when training. Training is enhanced by 'doing,' not just seeing and listening. In other words, it is preferable that learning be active rather than passive. Training that involves some 'hands-on' experience (i.e., active) is generally far more effective in reaching the mind of the trainee. With active training, the brain must process and utilize the information presented, not just simply receive it via the eyes or ears. Techniques in laboratory animal technology can be demonstrated to reinforce the skill, so that which is described and shown by the trainer can be actively done by the trainee. Generally, this makes the process of training in specific techniques easier to deliver and evaluate. Presentation of factual material, on the other hand, often consists of delivery in a lecture format with the hope of retention. It can often be made more effective by employing training methods that involve presenting the material in ways that are less passive, with more active participation and mental exercises.

In many laboratory animal resource facilities, the supervisor or manager is certified as a Laboratory Animal Technologist (LATG) by the American Association for Laboratory Animal Science (AALAS). As such, many LATGs are involved in, and responsible for, the training within their institutions. The experience that the typical LATG has gained working in laboratory animal science is invaluable and worth sharing with colleagues in the discipline. It is important that LATGs also continue and maintain training for themselves. AALAS also offers a registry program for the accumulation of continuing education units and, in conjunction with the Laboratory Animal Management Association (LAMA), the **Certified Manager, Animal Resources (CMAR)** program.

Whether a trainer or trainee, those involved in training, particularly the laboratory animal resource manager, should subscribe to a set of **Training Principles**. As presented in Table 1, these rights and responsibilities, when understood and followed, will help ensure a more positive and effective training experience for all.

The laboratory animal resource manager who has responsibilities for training will have a litany of concerns for ensuring success of the program, including:

- Complying with federal and institutional regulations and policies that personnel using experimental animals be trained
- Maintaining training records
- Identifying opportunities for additional training
- Assisting personnel with their individual goals for training
- Obtaining training for oneself
- Employing novel training techniques to enhance the learning process
- Integrating and separating training with human resources issues
- Understanding that adults learn differently as individuals and differently compared to the ways children learn
- Creating the learning environment
- Determining what training needs to address
- Devising training materials
- Presenting training sessions
- Assessing the training received for both cost and effectiveness

TABLE 1. Training – Rights and Responsibilities

By recognizing what the job is as a trainer and what the expectations of those being trained (the learners) are, the overall effort will be more beneficial and productive. These rights and responsibilities apply whether the laboratory animal manager is training or learning.

Trainer	Learner
Be willing to conduct a training session.	Be ready to be trained.
Speak clearly.	Listen and be attentive.
Keep the training session moving and on course.	Don't side-track the session with inappropriate
Answer questions.	behavior and not-so-relevant questions.
Involve and inspire the learners.	Ask for more information and be willing to say
Know your training materials; don't apologize	"I don't understand."
for lack of preparation.	Participate in exercises and discussions; offer
Announce breaks and stay on schedule; respect	examples and describe how the material
the learner's time.	presented can be applied in your institution.
Organize the session; state the session's	Keep an open mind, yet disagree and state
objectives.	opinions and experiences to the contrary in a
Use examples for clarification and application to	courteous manner.
the work; support with data as necessary.	Maintain the schedule by arriving on time and by
Be adaptable to your audience.	adhering to allotted break time.
	Recognize that everyone has different training
	needs and we learn in individual ways.

A general overview of training management can be obtained elsewhere (1). The objective of this chapter is to provide the laboratory animal resource manager with tools and techniques to implement an effective training program.

II. A FEW BASIC CONCEPTS ABOUT TRAINING

A. THE PROCESS OF TRAINING

As mentioned earlier, training is a process to convey attitudes, skills, and knowledge about a particular subject. These components may also be termed the **ABC**s of learning: **A**ffective for attitude, **B**ehavioral for skills, and **C**ognitive for knowledge. If the three components are not in harmony, job execution may suffer. For example, an employee may have a stellar attitude (i.e., good affective qualities) when performing a task skillfully (i.e., the trained behavior), but may actually perform it opposite to what was intended because the knowledge was not properly passed on or gained (i.e., faulty cognition) during a training session.

The **affective** part of training deals with the way in which learning affects the participants' attitude toward the task. If the attitude of a trainee is initially negative about a training process, then the session and eventual outcome are probably doomed to failure. The training should impart positive attitudes about the process, such as the benefits of a gentle approach in handling animals, or complying with the laws regarding psychological enrichment of nonhuman primates. The importance of the training must be understood by the trainee in order to be appreciated, because it affects how the trainee will eventually perform. In some cases, there may be a need for remedial training to change an individual's attitude. For example, there may have been a change in institutional policy that requires that a staff member be retrained. The employee may feel that "I've always done it the other way; what's wrong with that?" The manager must understand that attitudes observed by trainees outside of the learning environment may play a role in training. For example, if safety is emphasized during training, but unsafe conditions exist and are tolerated within the facility, the trainee's attitude may deteriorate. The institution must demonstrate a positive attitude to reinforce what is taught.

The portion of learning termed **behavioral** relates to how skilled the trainee becomes as a result of participating in training. In this regard, skills that are technical in nature require utilization and repetition for proficiency. For example, if an employee is taught how to operate gas anaesthesia equipment and then is not given an opportunity to practice with it soon after, an animal on the operating table may feel pain or may not survive the surgery due to poorly developed skills (2). An administrative assistant responsible for completing protocol forms will do a better job with examples to practice, opportunities to use a computer, and someone experienced to evaluate the work on the first attempt. Thus, effective training means that the individual will 'behave' better, that is, be better prepared to do the job after practicing and developing skills.

The aspect labeled **cognitive** learning is the knowledge component, that is, the facts, figures, theories, and policies that dictate how the facilities are managed daily. Several examples include the cagewasher who understands the concept of pH is less likely to use an acidic soap solution inappropriately or unsafely; the animal care provider who has read the ILAR *Guide for the Care and Use of Laboratory Animals* and therefore knows cage space requirements will probably not overcrowd cages with too many animals; an investigator trained in donning protective clothing will be an asset in facility health maintenance; and the manager who studies psychology will be better equipped to deal with issues of human resources and to interact with colleagues. In other words, users who are armed with knowledge about the animal resource will help to ensure its proper operation.

Overall, the laboratory animal resource manager who understands the **ABC** learning concepts when conducting training will be more successful. Staff who understand both what must be done and why as a result of participating in training will apply that knowledge more effectively for the mission of the facility.

B.   ADVANTAGES OF TRAINING

Training offers several advantages, both **intrinsic and extrinsic**. The intrinsic values are those perceived as internal gains by the trainee, for example, an increased feeling of self-worth achieved through new knowledge and increased value to the employer. These tend to meet the psychological needs and desires of individuals. In contrast, extrinsic advantages are more material in nature; they are the benefits that can be quantified. For the employee, this may mean more money and for the employer, fewer errors in the work effort. In this way, then, both the employer and employee gain from training.

During training, the manager/trainer comes to know the staff better, how they learn, what motivates them, and what their interests are, resulting in improved personal relationships. Gaps in knowledge or misunderstandings about policies may be uncovered and then addressed so as to avoid errors. Trained, committed staff do a better and more efficient job when they are aware of their role and understand how to do their assignments. Management gains savings in time, effort, and money with a subsequent increase in productivity and a decrease in mistakes.

The employee derives personal satisfaction from training and a credential for possible promotion. With proficiency comes assignment of additional duties and opportunities. Improvement in morale and self-esteem are likely to result. Training can result in the trainee needing less direct supervision and enjoying more independence in executing job responsibilities.

Finally, the animals may benefit from training of personnel. The impact of untrained users (e.g., husbandry and research personnel) on elements such as recovery from surgery, collection of research data, and temperament of the animal may not be measurable in quantifiable terms, but is observed qualitatively (e.g., "she has a good way with those mice," and, conversely, "that primate always reacts negatively to him"). This concept about the subtle effects relates to the **3Rs principles of Russell and Burch** (3) to **reduce**, **refine**, and **replace** the use of animals. Training that is appropriately designed and assessed by laboratory animal resource management addresses these principles. This is particularly true when non-animal (*in vitro*) techniques are initially utilized as part of the training process.

C. THE NEED FOR TRAINING

The need for training can be attributed to several factors. Obviously, new and inexperienced employees need training in order to perform the jobs for which they were hired. Existing employees may need to be trained in new technology, new policies, new animal models, etc. Sometimes remedial training is needed so that everyone is performing a task in a similar and standardized manner; this would apply in the case of a person coming from another institution (or perhaps culture). Failure to train – or train effectively – can result in lost productivity, time, money, and animal lives.

Training needs to be evaluated for its purpose, that is, to establish the reason for taking the time and expending the effort to train in a busy laboratory animal resource facility. Is the material being offered on a 'need-to-know,' 'good-to-know,' or 'fun-to-know' basis? Training on regulatory issues falls into the category of need to know to keep the facility in compliance. Another example of need to know is the proper way to deliver an injection. A lecture on various cell types may be good to know for staff who are primarily cagewashers since this information may serve to prepare them for a job change or for cross-training purposes. When training on the nutritional requirements of laboratory animals, for example, some of the material can be presented as fun to know if it includes aspects of human nutrition, even though it may not be part of the curriculum. The personal perspective about the subject of nutrition can enhance the overall learning effort as a result.

It is important to establish a **learning environment** within the institution. One must remember to emphasize the importance of learning and training. One should consider these ideas and concepts:

- Is there a library of training materials? Is the staff allowed to check out training items to work with at home or within the institution?
- Does the institution support AALAS national and branch activities (e.g., meetings, workshops, seminars), by sending staff members to be trained and to participate in training?
- Does the institution have a training budget to cover expenses of training sessions, to purchase training materials, to provide economic incentives to pursue training, to pay for certification fees, etc.?
- Does the manager participate in training, both giving and receiving, so as to set a good example?
- Does the manager support requests by staff and suggest to staff opportunities for training?

A positive learning environment involves some cost and effort from management, but an atmosphere that is conducive to training can pay great dividends.

D. COST OF TRAINING

The costs associated with training are sometimes hard to gauge and therefore manage. The process of training costs money in terms of materials, expenses for off-site training, and loss of employee work time. However, the cost can be far greater if the employee is not trained to do the job properly and therefore mistakes, injury (to people or animals), or delays occur.

Some of the measurable (or tangible) components that figure into the cost of training include books and manuals, instrumentation, biomedical models, equipment to conduct 'wet' labs (e.g., animals, syringes, needles, etc.), travel expenses, registration fees, computers, and the trainer's salary. The manager may need to evaluate the cost of gathering staff members for a training session and any study time associated with learning the material.

With a limited budget, small amounts of money can be spent annually in order to develop a training library consisting of not only purchased items, but also items such as vendor donations, discarded caging, bones cleaned in the necropsy lab, etc. Inexpensive software can allow for in-house development of training materials that may lack the professional luster but do the job cost-effectively.

Some benefits to training are intangible. When fewer animals are 'lost' from gavage procedures after training, or employees get excited about a new surgical technique, or a faster, more efficient method for completing a task is developed, then the value of the expenditure can be calculated and realized. In practice, more emphasis is often placed on the consequences of inadequate training when mistakes are made.

A line item in the facility's budget for training attests to the institutional support and commitment for training. Such a commitment demonstrates the institution's interest in training and indicates tacit approval for training efforts.

III. UNDERSTANDING THE ADULT AS A LEARNER

Learning is a very personal and emotional process for the adult. It can be stressful if there are specific expectations that affect job security and that might influence the affective side of the individual. There may be bad memories from early childhood education. Mental acuity or the ability to receive, process, and store information might not be as good as it once was. Consideration by the manager/trainer of the various ways in which adults learn will promote a more successful training experience. The psychology of adult learning has been studied by social scientists such as Malcolm Knowles (known as the father of **andragogy** or the study of adult learning (4)) and Mel Silberman (5, 6).

Adults, as a group, learn differently than children. Traditionally, children are taught in a pedagogical fashion, that is, by listening to the teacher at the front of the classroom. In a busy laboratory animal resource, such a method has the potential to be less effective and lead to boredom. If lecture-style teaching was a 'turn-off' as a child, then an adult may be reluctant to return to the classroom without some other tangible benefit. Some principles about adult learners are that they tend to:

- Use their experience as a basis for learning
- Be self-directed in their learning
- Like immediate applicability of the training material
- Need to learn based upon their stage in life

A. MOTIVATION FOR LEARNING

Motivating adults to learn is different than for children. Adults have a greater "need to know" factor about what is being taught. Primarily, the adult learning process can be summed up as **WIIFM:** " What's in it for me?" The adult wants to know what he or she will gain by participating in training. Much has been made in management science of Abraham Maslow's theory about the hierarchy of human needs in the job environment (7), which purports that a person achieves personal survival, safety, affiliation, self-esteem and the esteem of others, and finally self-actualization, like climbing a ladder. This can certainly be applied to motivating adults to be effective learners. The adult learner will typically want to fulfill some basic needs, such as acquiring money for personal items, before wanting to learn for its inherent value. Table 2 summarizes many of the motivational factors with intrinsic and extrinsic value that may influence how and why an adult will commit to a learning experience.

These intrinsic and extrinsic factors must be carefully assessed in every group of adults. The laboratory animal resource manager should consider the following:

- Is the primary motivation that of money or personal growth? If a promotion with a large salary increase is involved, then the adult might be more inclined to learn effectively.
- Is the motivation that "The boss says so"? When management sees a need for training, the choice is taken away from the trainee.
- Are there external forces demanding that the work force be newly trained, even against some individual's willingness? If the company has been 'taken over,' for example, resulting in new policies, some employees may resent (the affective side of training) going to training sessions.
- Can the employee be motivated by some form of recognition, for example, a credential like AALAS technician certification or surgical research specialist certification by the Academy of Surgical Research (8)?

B.   LEARNING STYLE

In addition to knowing an individual adult's motivation for learning, it is helpful to assess learning style. For lengthy training programs, conducting a **learning styles assessment** could give both the trainer and trainees insight into how they learn. Taking the time in a class session at the beginning of a training program will not only accomplish this, but can also work well as an ice-breaker to establish rapport among the participants. There are several methods to evaluate learning style. One useful method simply divides people into three

---

TABLE 2. Motivating Factors in Training — What's in It for Me?

Intrinsic (internal value to the person)	Extrinsic (visible, demonstrable value to others)
Self-worth	More money
Pride	Praise
Self-satisfaction	Possible promotion
Recognition by peers	Will I be embarrassed if I fail?
Will I learn something interesting?	Certification (AALAS, AHT/RVT, surgical tech)
Knowledge that animals will receive better care	Opportunity for extracurricular activities like
Sense of increased safety	going away to a meeting
	Greater independence

groups as either predominantly **visual, auditory,** or **kinesthetic learners,** based on the trainees' preference to learn in one style over the others. As the groupings would suggest, individuals learn best in the environment that appeals to the appropriate sense. Visual learners would prefer watching a demonstration to learn something; auditory learners probably would enjoy listening to a lecture; and for the kinesthetic learner, participation in a hands-on wet lab would be appealing. Knowing that the class consists mostly of visual learners would mean minimizing lecture formats and using videotapes. The trainer can utilize this information to achieve the learning objectives.

Another learning assessment tool separates trainees into four learning groups based upon their personality style. The 'test' is reproduced in Figure 1. When completed, the students will have gained some insight into their learning style, labeled as **feeler, analyzer, observer,** or **organizer.**

Table 3 lists a few of the learning tools that would be appropriate. Characteristics of each style are given below:

1. The **feeling** learners are people oriented. They enjoy learning experiences that explore attitudes and emotions — the affective component.
2. The **analytical** learners do a lot of thinking, preferring the cognitive side of learning. They like to share ideas and concepts and participate in exercises where they analyze and evaluate.
3. The **observing** learners go with the flow, working in the comfort of groups. Although they act reserved, they are the supportive members of the team.
4. The **organized** learners are active training participants, doing the exercises and being expressive during them. These characteristics can make this type of learner useful to the trainer.

Certainly, no person should be limited to or characterized within any one group or label. Indeed, there is often crossover to other learning styles depending upon the situation. Still, it is revealing to understand how individuals, particularly adults, learn in dissimilar ways. The manager/trainer may need to accommodate these various ways of processing information and generate different methods of training for each.

All of these principles and concepts about adult learning can (and should) be used to the advantage of the manager engaged in training to create a more effective learning process.

TABLE 3. Effective Learning Approaches Based on Personality Style

Feeler	Analyzer	Observer	Organizer
Checklists	Lectures	Team games	Experimenting
Charts	Reading	Cooperative groups	Active learning
Hands-on examples	Writing reports	Visual thinkers	Brainstorming
Field trips	Panel discussions	Role players	Finding alternatives
How-to discussions	Forming hypotheses	Idea sharing	Doing case studies
	Working alone	Group discussions	Learning games

Figure 1. Personality test for learning style

Step 1. Rank all four responses to each question. Place a 1, 2, 3, or 4 in the space to the left of the response, with 1 being least like you to 4 being most like you. Use each number only once in each question.

A	B	C	D

1. I like instructors who

___ tell me exactly what is expected of me	___ make learning active and exciting	___ maintain a safe and supportive classroom	___ challenge me to think at higher level

2. I learn best when the material is

___ well organized	___ something I can do hands-on	___ about understanding and improving the human condition	___ intellectually challenging

3. A high priority in my life is to

___ keep my commitments	___ experience as much of life as possible	___ make a difference in the lives of others	___ understand how things work

4. Other people think of me as

___ dependable and loyal	___ dynamic and creative	___ caring and honest	___ intelligent and inventive

5. When I experience stress I would most likely

___ do something to help me feel more in control of my life	___ do something physical and daring	___ talk with a friend	___ go off by myself and think about my situation

6. I feel the greatest flaw someone can have is to be

___ irresponsible	___ unwilling to try new things	___ selfish and unkind to others	___ an illogical thinker

7. When solving a problem I prefer to

___ take immediate action	___ take a step-by-step approach	___ consider the impact on others	___ make sure I have all the facts

8. I learn best from activities in which I

___ take a leadership role	___ can remain uninvolved	___ am able to interact with others	___ can take my time

9. I prefer information to be presented in the following way

___ as bulleted points	___ in models such as flow charts	___ accompanied by examples	___ with detailed explanations

10. I am impressed by a trainer's

___ use of methods and activities	___ organization and control	___ personality and style	___ knowledge and expertise

Step 2. Add up the total points from each column above.

Total of As:	Total of Bs:	Total of Cs:	Total of Ds:
Organizer	Observer	Feeler	Analyzer

Step 3. Plot the totals for each category on the accompanying brain diagram.

Figure 1. (continued) Personality test for learning style

Step 4. Place an X on the appropriate number in each category for each score from step 2. Draw a line to connect the Xs. Then evaluate your "style" based upon the relative amounts of Feeler, Analyzer, Observer, or Organizer in the brain you have connected. Review the personality characteristics as they apply to the learning style. A higher score in one style suggests a tendency for that kind of learning. Relatively equal scores may mean there is no predominate learning style.

	Right Brain			Left Brain	
Feeler (below)					Analyzer (at left)
interpersonal		40			technical
emotional		36	A		scientific
caring		34			mathematical
sociable		32	N		dispassionate
giving		30			rational
spiritual		28	A		analytical
musical		26			logical
romantic		24	L		problem solving
feeling		22			theoretical
peacemaker		20	Y		intellectual
trusting		18			objective
adaptable		16	Z		quantitative
passionate		14			explicit
harmonious		12	E		realistic
idealistic		10			literal
talkative		8	R		precise
honest		6			formal
		4			
		2			

F E E L E R

40 36 34 32 30 28 26 24 22 20 18 16 14 12 10 8 6 4 2   2 4 6 8 10 12 14 16 18 20 22 24 26 28 30 32 34 36 40

O R G A N I Z E R

Observer (at right)		2		Organizer(above)
imaginative		4		systematic
adventuresome	O	6		administrative
open-minded		8		procedural
fast-paced	B	10		organized
metaphoric		12		conservative
original	S	14		confident
simultaneous		16		structured
visual	E	18		safekeeping
impulsive		20		disciplined
experimental	R	22		practical
risking		24		sequential
divergent	V	26		predictable
artistic		28		detailed
spatial	E	30		tactical
skillful		32		controlled
competitive	R	34		dependable
active		36		planning
		40		

IV. CONCEPTS OF A TRAINING PROGRAM — THE SIX "WS"

The manager of a laboratory animal resource is usually a significant member of the training effort within an institution regardless of its size. This does not mean that the manager necessarily must conduct all of the training. The manager is not always the best or most appropriate person to serve as the trainer. But clearly, the manager has the role and responsibility for ensuring that training occurs for the benefit of the resource. The manager is typically involved in obtaining institutional commitments, materials, and funds (9). The manager must demonstrate a commitment to training (see Table 1 for rights and responsibilities) and ensure that training will happen. The manager must decide how much training to conduct personally and how much to delegate. The role then essentially becomes one of coordination, planning, and scheduling training.

Development of a training program can be organized by answering a series of questions called the six **W**s. These are the questions of "why," "who," "what," "where," "when," and "how" about training. Formulating responses to them will help the manager establish the basis of a training session. Figure 2A is a form that can be completed while answering the six **W**s. It can be modified as needed. Figure 2B is the completed form as an example of a more hands-on, technical training session. Figure 2C is an example of a completed form for a 'dry' and fact-filled training session.

A. WHY DOES THIS TRAINING NEED TO OCCUR?

Knowing the primary goal for training will help define the training process. It is more than simply stating the need for training. Determining the overall objective of 'why train' will in turn define the kind of resources needed, who should do the training, and the final expectations of those who have been trained.

The trainer might think about each of these scenarios with its associated 'why' or objective as examples:

- Has a new investigator joined the group who will be doing different techniques with a new animal model? The objective could be twofold: to understand the biology and husbandry needs of this animal and to become proficient at the new techniques.
- Is the facility about to undergo an AAALAC site visit? The 'why' could be to provide information on regulations so that all personnel have a working knowledge of them.
- Has production, say in terms of cage washing, been showing a downward trend, possibly due to poorly trained new staff? Retraining everyone on all equipment and procedures may be the objective.
- Is the training for AALAS certification, principal investigator orientation, or IACUC member education? The objectives may depend upon the particular individuals undergoing training.

Sometimes the reason for training can be muddled with a **human relations (personnel) issue**. For example, Sally has been making mistakes while gavaging

Figure 2A. Form to systematically plan a training session

Title: _____

Audience (type and number): _____

Resources (people and things): _____

_____

What are the objectives? (what is to be learned)	What method could you use to present them? (lecture, demo, self-teach, worksheet, laboratory, computer, jigsaw, info seek)

Amount of time to present: _____

Any safety issues? _____

_____

Any logistical difficulties? _____

_____

How could you evaluate the learning process? _____

_____

What kind of documentation? _____

Figure 2B. Sample of a completed planning form for a training session
on a technique - injecting a mouse

Title: ___Proper SQ injection in a mouse___

Audience (type and number): ___Lab animal techs, research techs, PIs___

Resources (people and things): ___Experienced tech to teach, other experienced staff to assist in lab;___
___needles, syringes, saline, cull and live mice; videotape of someone doing the injection___

What are the objectives? (what is to be learned)	What method could you use to present them? (lecture, demo, self-teach, worksheet, laboratory, computer, jigsaw, info seek)
proper restraint of the mouse to satisfactorily hold the mouse	demonstration in a laboratory environment
fully inject the solution (saline or other)	observe tech, then practice
understand layers of the integumentary system	diagrams with cross section of skin; dissect layers of culled mouse
learn to create 'tent' of skin	observe tech, then practice
insert the needle adequately through the epidermis but not into the muscle	observe tech then practice skin insertion on a culled mouse

Amount of time to present: ___one hour, lecture and lab___

Any safety issues? ___proper handling of needles and their disposal, wear gloves___

Any logistical difficulties? ___observing technique of more than 10 trainees, location to hold the class___

How could you evaluate the learning process? ___inject dye to determine injection site, experienced___
___individual to observe technique___

What kind of documentation? ___sign-in sheet, certificate of attendance___

Figure 2C. Sample of a completed planning form for a training session on a fact-based or 'dry' subject - reviewing the ILAR *Guide*

Title: _What is the ILAR *Guide* all about?_

Audience (type and number): _new users (staff members, investigators, research techs)_

Resources (people and things): _IACUC member, facility veterinarian and/or manager_
1985 and 1996 versions of the *Guide*, question worksheet, animal study protocol

What are the objectives? (what is to be learned)	What method could you use to present them? (lecture, demo, self-teach, worksheet, laboratory, computer, jigsaw, info seek)
appreciate the purpose of the *Guide* in terms of research grants	lecture: explain the funding process and protocol approval by the IACUC in relationship to the *Guide*
appreciate the purpose of the *Guide* in terms of good lab animal care	lecture: describe the table of contents; explain the roles of ILAR, the NIH, the IACUC, inspections, etc.
use the *Guide* to obtain specific information	info seek: provide trainees a worksheet that asks questions from various pages of the *Guide*
put a copy of the *Guide* into everyone's hands	obtain sufficient copies and ask that trainees enter their name and office number on the inside cover (indicating 'ownership' of the book)
learn certain sections of the *Guide* well	jigsaw: divide chapters or sections of chapters among trainees; they train each other

Amount of time to present: _1 to 2 hours in a class room setting_

Any safety issues? _none_

Any logistical difficulties? _reading ability_

How could you evaluate the learning process? _answers to the worksheet, classroom participation_

What kind of documentation? _sign-in sheet, certificate of participation_ the rats. Is this because she no longer knows how to gavage (a training concern) or could it be because she is expected to gavage 50% more rats in the same amount of time, or that the rats are a different size than she has worked with before, or that she suffers from tendinitis (a possible ergonomic issue), making it more difficult for her to restrain the rats? All would be considered issues of management, but dealt with differently depending upon the perspective of training and human resource management.

The reason for training may hinge on **policy requirements**. Several regulatory agencies require that individuals involved in laboratory animal research be trained at the tasks they perform (see Table 4). The USDA's Animal Welfare Act and the Good Laboratory Practice regulations of the Food and Drug Administration and Environmental Protection Agency all mandate training. The National Institutes of Health (NIH) and the Association for Assessment and Accreditation of Laboratory Animal Care, International (AAALAC), while not putting forth laws, expect that personnel are properly trained. Internationally, various organizations have put forth training requirements, such as the working party report entitled **"FELASA Recommendations for The Education and Training of Persons Carrying Out Animal Experiments (Category B)"** (10). The requirements for training in countries of the European Union tend to be more stringent and compulsory than in the United States. Information on the training regulations of other countries can be reviewed through links at the Web site of the Animal Welfare Information Center (www.nal.usda.gov/awic/legislat/internat.htm) and IACUC.ORG (www.iacuc.org, look up "Documents — International," under "Documents").

B. WHO SHOULD HAVE TRAINING?

All persons who have any contact or impact on the care and use of laboratory animals should be provided training. Managers should have the vision that training goes beyond the technical issues provided to the husbandry staff and regulatory concerns given to investigative staff. Indeed, training should extend, for example, to administrative personnel who place orders for animals, physical plant workers who enter animal rooms to perform maintenance, security staff who monitor the facility, and human resources contacts who are involved in the unique personnel issues of the animal facility. All of these persons need to receive some aspect of training pertaining to their roles in the overall operation of the laboratory animal resource.

The laboratory animal resource manager is most likely to encounter people in the following roles during training situations:

- Animal facility personnel, including laboratory animal technicians, cagewashers, and veterinary technicians
- Research technicians, including those from the investigative staff
- Principal investigators (PIs), including graduate students, visiting and post-doctoral researchers, professional school students (veterinary or medical)

TABLE 4. Compilation of Laboratory Animal Training Requirements by Regulatory and Inspecting Bodies

Below are selected passages pertaining to the need for training of animal users from prominent documents that either regulate or influence the conduct of laboratory animal research. The word train and its variations have been underlined to reflect its relative importance.

- From the *ILAR Guide for the Care and Use of Laboratory Animals* (11):

  Personnel Qualifications and Training, p. 13: (Animal Welfare Regulations) and PHS Policy require institutions to ensure that people caring for or using animals are qualified to do so. The number and qualifications of personnel required to conduct and support an animal care and use program depend on several factors, including the type and size of institution, the administrative structure for providing adequate animal care, the characteristics of the physical plant, the number and species of animals maintained, and the nature of the research, testing, and educational activities.

  Personnel caring for animals should be appropriately trained (see Appendix A, "Technical and Professional Education"), and the institution should provide for formal or on-the-job training to facilitate effective implementation of the program and humane care and use of animals. According to the programmatic scope, personnel will be required with expertise in other disciplines, such as animal husbandry, administration, laboratory animal medicine and pathology, occupational health and safety, behavioral management, genetic management, and various other aspects of research support.

  There are a number of options for the training of technicians ...

  Occupational Health and Safety of Personnel, Personnel Training, p. 15: Investigators, technical personnel, trainees, and visiting investigators who perform animal anesthesia, surgery, or other experimental manipulations must be qualified through training or experience to accomplish these tasks in a humane and scientifically acceptable manner.

  Personnel should be trained regarding zoonoses, chemical safety, microbiologic, and physical hazards (including those related to radiation and allergies), unusual conditions or agents that might be part of experimental procedures ...

  Technical and Professional Education, pp. 100–101. (This section includes a listing of training aids of use to laboratory animal trainers and facility managers.)

- From the U.S. Government Principles for the Utilization and Care of Vertebrate Animals Used in Testing, Research, and Training (12):

  VIII. Investigators and other personnel shall be appropriately qualified and experienced for conducting procedures on living animals. Adequate arrangements shall be made for their in-service training, including the proper and humane care and use of laboratory animals.

- From the *Occupational Health and Safety in the Care and Use of Research Animals* (13):

  Education and Training, p. 114. Occupational health and safety objectives of an institution can be achieved only if employees know the hazards associated with their work activities; understand how the hazards are controlled through institutional policies, engineering controls, work practices, and personal protective equipment; and have sufficient skills to execute safe work practices proficiently. All that requires a multifaceted education and training effort that addresses the full range of health and safety issues related to the care and use of research animals. Approaches for providing an education and training effort depend on the size, resources, animal species, research activities, staff experience, and technical expertise of the institution.

The occupational health and safety goals of the institution and how they will be achieved, including precise guidance on regulatory-compliance strategies, are clearly communicated to all employees. This function is commonly carried out by the environmental health and safety staff through formal orientation, distribution of written guidelines, and periodic refresher training.

Supervisors in the animal care and research groups are actively involved in ensuring that their employees have acquired the necessary skills and attitudes to work safely. If deficiencies are present, on-the-job training supervised by an experienced employee is provided until appropriate standards of proficiency are demonstrated.

- From the Environmental Protection Agency (EPA) Good Laboratory Practice (GLP) Standards, EPA 40 CFR Part 792 Part III Toxic Substances Control Act (TSCA) and EPA 40 CFR Part 160 Part IV Federal Insecticide, Fungicide and Rodenticide Act (14,15):
  - TSCA section 792.29(a)/FIFRA section 160.29 (a) Each individual engaged in the conduct of or responsible for the supervision of a study shall have education, training, and experience, or combination thereof, to enable that individual to perform the assigned functions.
  - TSCA section 792.29(b)/FIFRA section 160.29 (b) Each testing facility shall maintain a current summary of training and experience and job description for each individual engaged in or supervising the conduct of a study.

- From the Food and Drug Administration (FDA) Good Laboratory Practice Standards, FDA 21CFR Part 58 (16):
  - 58.29(a) Each individual engaged in the conduct of or responsible for the supervision of a nonclinical laboratory study shall have education, training, and experience, or combination thereof, to enable that individual to perform the assigned functions.
  - 58.29(b) Each testing facility shall maintain a current summary of training and experience and job description for each individual engaged in or supervising the conduct of a nonclinical laboratory study.

- From the Animal and Plant Health Inspection Service, USDA, Subchapter A – Animal Welfare §2.32 Personal Qualifications (17):
  - (a) It shall be the responsibility of the research facility to ensure that all scientists, research technicians, animal technicians, and other personnel involved in animal care, treatment, and use are qualified to perform their duties. This responsibility shall be fulfilled in part through the provision of training and instruction to those personnel.
  - (b) Training and instruction shall be made available, and the qualifications of personnel reviewed, with sufficient frequency to fulfill the research facility's responsibilities under this section and §2.31.
  - (c) Training and instruction of personnel must include guidance in at least the following areas:
    1. Humane methods of animal maintenance and experimentation, including:
        (i) The basic needs of each species of animal;
        (ii) Proper handling and care for the various species of animals used by the facility;
        (iii) Proper pre-procedural and post-procedural care of animals; and
        (iv) Aseptic surgical methods and procedures;
    2. The concept, availability, and use of research or testing methods that limit the use of animals or minimize animal distress;
    3. Proper use of anesthetics, analgesics, and tranquilizers for any species of animals used by the facility;

4. Methods whereby deficiencies in animal care and treatment are reported, including deficiencies in animal care and treatment reported by any employee of the facility; ...

5. Utilization of services ... available to provide information;

(i)   On appropriate methods of animal care and use;

(ii) On alternatives to the use of live animals in research;

(iii) That could prevent unintended and unnecessary duplication of research involving animals; and

(iv) Regarding the intent and requirements of the Act.

- From the Council of Europe Convention, Article 26 (18):
  - Persons who carry out, take part in or supervise procedures on animals, or take care of animals used in procedures, shall have had appropriate education and <u>training.</u>

- From the Council of Europe Convention, Article 14 (19):
  - Persons who carry out experiments or take part in them ... including duties of a supervisory nature, shall have had appropriate education and <u>training</u>.

- Veterinarians
- IACUC members
- Physical plant personnel, including plumbers, electricians, and HVAC technicians
- Contract personnel doing tasks such as animal care, cagewash, and construction
- Equipment maintenance personnel

The various roles that individuals fulfill in a laboratory animal resource suggest that they will thereby demonstrate different aspects of the ABCs, that is, attitude, behavior, and cognition. When addressing trainees, the manager should evaluate these factors as a trainer. Factors of the trainees that need to be evaluated by facility trainers include the following:

1.   Age

Interest in the material, ability to learn, background knowledge, and other learning characteristics all may be influenced by the age of the participants in the training session. Differences in age become more important in longer training sessions. The younger person may have recently learned material relative to the training session and may come across as 'knowing-it-all.' Older trainees may have the attitude that 'you can't teach me anything.' A young trainer may not be received as well by the older trainee. If such situations arise, the trainer should utilize techniques of personnel management to smooth out the differences by recognizing and acknowledging the important contributions of all.

2.   Cultural or Socio-Economic Differences

Individuals growing up in an environment where learning was not emphasized may be a greater challenge to train. Different value systems about animals, and how they are used, may need to be addressed based upon the local culture and laws regulating their use. To some, a rat is vermin, so that person may not place high value on its welfare in the animal facility. Nevertheless, training to alleviate the pain suffered by a rat is just as important as for a nonhuman primate or dog. Similarly, customary housing practices with farm animals may not apply when it comes to their housing in a research facility, requiring a change in the mind-set of a farm hand working in the laboratory. As with the age factor, these differences may emerge more greatly in extended learning courses and, again, standard tools of personnel management may overcome such issues.

3. Gender Differences

There should be equal opportunity for all in the workplace. Training should not be gender-specific. Accommodating differences in physical stature may be necessary as it applies to executing the skill, but the attitude and knowledge components must be learned. It is important for the trainer to be conscious of not making gender-biased statements and use both pronouns 'he' and 'she' when giving examples.

4. Educational Levels

"OJT" or on-the-job training has been the traditional means for advancement in laboratory animal science. Individuals without benefit of a college education can still learn the material for the position in which they work. Sometimes the ability to learn or study may present itself as an issue, although special individual tutoring or extra homework assignments may help. In a training session encompassing individuals from high school to Ph.D. education, the trainer should be aware of the intimidation factor. This could inhibit the learning ability of some participants.

5. English as a Second Language (ESL)

Persons who do not understand English well may require a translator, a dictionary, or extra materials to be able to learn aspects of laboratory animal science. Study groups can be formed by grouping a more experienced, bilingual individual with the novice trainees. Use of handouts or lecture notes with vocabulary words and major points highlighted can benefit individuals whose first language is not English. The trainer should determine whether the human resources department offers ESL classes and bring such classes to the attention of trainees. Use of computer software to make rough translations of materials can be useful. The trainer should find out whether there are bilingual members within the institution who will help translate or perhaps will participate in training sessions. Given that laboratory animal science has specialized jargon, the interpreter may need some preparation before the training session.

6. **Disabilities**

The **Americans with Disabilities Act (ADA)** requires that reasonable accommodations be made for individuals with either physical or mental disabilities. Advances in the technology and development of electronic devices like computers (see the section in this chapter on computer-based training) have enabled many with disabilities to learn. Teaching and reading can be learned through the use of machines. Perhaps interpreters for the hearing impaired can be hired or are already available through the human resources department.

As a means of assessing the audience's existing knowledge, it may be appropriate to conduct a pre-quiz on the subject. Such a technique enables each trainee to determine what is already known and what is to be learned. In a sense, it can 'jump-start' the brain into retaining the major objectives and concepts of any training session. A well-constructed quiz can be used as an outline of the material for the presentation (perhaps a lecture). Further, another quiz after the presentation will assess what has been learned and is therefore part of the evaluation of the training process.

C. WHO SHOULD CONDUCT THE TRAINING?

The responsibility for training often falls on the manager, but it need not rest solely there. In larger facilities, there is a growing trend to employ a compliance officer (20) or quality control staff member, who plays a significant role in the conduct of training. Some institutions even have the fortune of establishing a training staff. Ultimately, however, someone must identify training requirements and enact programs to train staff.

For some topics, the trainer may not have enough skills or experience to do the best training job. Instead, it might be more appropriate to call in a guest instructor. Persons being trained might enjoy having a change of pace with a different trainer as well. While the charisma of the manager as an instructor could be helpful, objectivity could be an issue if the manager's responsibility is both training and evaluating the performance of an employee — particularly if the reason for the training is remedial or part of some disciplinary action. Therefore, other persons should be involved in training.

Personnel resources that can be tapped for training include other laboratory animal managers, principal investigators utilizing the vivarium, vendors to the business, the veterinary staff, science (biology, chemistry, computing, etc.) teachers from a local school, and members of the research lab (for example, to explain about techniques used in the laboratory). The facility manager should identify those on staff who can make the transition from being a passive trainee to a more actively involved trainer.

Professional training has become a business, even in the field of laboratory animal science. There are companies providing in-house training courses and training module design, much of the latter using electronic media. Whether training consultants should be hired is a decision that hinges on several factors in an institution including the cost, the reputation of the trainer(s) and company, the ability to do the training from within, and time commitments. Criteria such as very specific learning objectives, remedial training in case of absences or poor performance, writing and giving quizzes and/or tests, provision of training items like textbooks, audio-visual materials, and disposable supplies, and certification pass rates ought to be carefully evaluated and considered in the contract process. As with other contract processes in which the laboratory animal resource manager is involved, concerns for performance outcomes, completion rates, technical support, reliability of the products, and similar factors must be considered for training materials as well.

D.   WHAT CONSTITUTES THE TRAINING?

The process of determining the content of training is perhaps the most difficult. It is critical to convey all of the required information, but not so much that it becomes overwhelming and the important message is lost.

The trainer should begin by setting the objectives; that is, what the trainer expects the trainee should know at the conclusion of the training session. Often, it is best to phrase the objectives in the following way, using this chapter on training as an example.

The reader of this chapter on training will:
- Gain a basic understanding of the training process
- Be able to use the six "Ws" process to establish a training program
- Appreciate that adults learn differently than children
- Recognize that training can be accomplished using many tools other than traditional lecture
- Be aware that the laboratory animal resource manager has training options available

Note that the objectives begin with active verb forms, meaning there is action or activity associated with the item to be learned. Using verbs in this way tends to make the trainee receive the message more strongly and accept it as an instruction or directive.

Associated with each objective is the means by which it will be accomplished. For example, the objective to gain a basic understanding of the training process can be realized by reading specific material or by having a discussion. Figures 2B and 2C exhibit several objectives for laboratory animal topics and how they can be taught.

It may be necessary to create a schedule of learning topics (main points) with reading or preparation assignments, location of the session if it varies, and trainer. This is particularly useful for multiple sessions so that the participants know what to expect.

Preparation for a training session often follows the **3:1 rule**, that is 3 hours of preparation to 1 hour of presentation.

The decision of what to present will depend upon the specific laboratory animal resource. The laboratory animal resource manager has a significant role in helping to determine the specific objectives. For example, a nonhuman primate vivarium would necessarily address more detailed concepts about zoonoses and viruses, legislation specific to NHPs, and such compared to a facility housing only mice. Facts and procedures about water quality, treatment, and chemistry are in many ways more important to the general staff of a facility with mostly zebra fish aquaria than one with primarily dog runs. Some documents that will help to determine the curriculum are the table of contents of the ILAR *Guide*, the role delineation documents for animal technician training published by the Certification and Registry Board of AALAS, the syllabus *Education and Training in the Care and Use of Laboratory Animals: A Guide for Developing Institutional Programs* (21), and the guidelines published by the FELASA Working Group (10) on educating animal researchers. Collectively, these documents address the following issues which, in various degrees, can be included in a training program, depending upon the audience:

1. **Institutional policies**, including the ethics and responsibilities for the care and use of animals, qualifications of personnel involved, precautions and protections for animals and personnel, Institutional Animal Care and Use Committees, applicable laws and regulations, occupational health and hazards information, etc.
2. **Research and technology concepts**, including animal models, principles of animal usage, alternatives and *in vitro* procedures, record keeping, basic science, analytical and diagnostic techniques, research equipment and instruments, research methodology, etc.
3. **Animal husbandry** (dependent upon the species), including basic care, modes of housing, feed and nutrition, bedding, water, handling and restraint, cage and facility sanitation, environmental enrichment, breeding and genetics, identification, etc.
4. **Veterinary care**, including preventive medicine, treatments, individual animal and colony health management, recognition of normal health and behavior vs. disease and distress, surgery, anesthesia, analgesia, euthanasia, etc.
5. **Physical plant issues**, including safety and security, building construction, temperature and humidity controls, lighting, air quality, power and water sources, emergency response, maintenance, waste management, supply procurement, etc.

The manager who has not been involved extensively with training might find the process initially somewhat daunting. The thought will be 'Where to start?' There are fortunately many resources as described in this chapter and books like *The Corporate Trainer's Quick Reference* (22). Often, it is discovered that instructing practical or technique-based skills is easier than theoretical material. Of course, all of the material ultimately must be taught, so the innovative facility trainer/manager will challenge the training process to improve information transfer with each successive training session.

Teacher's guides can be obtained from many sources to help devise an outline for a presentation. AALAS offers the *Instructional Guide* for preparing lesson plans at the entering technician (ALAT) and experienced technician (LAT) levels. These can be used as a starting foundation and modified for other purposes. Other useful materials are those produced by **CURE (Connecticut United for Research Excellence, Inc.** (www.biorap.org), the **Kids4Research** partnership of organizations (www.kids4research.org), and the **Join Hands Educational Foundation** (www.joinhand.org), which have modules focusing on subjects such as cancer, AIDS, product safety, and allergies. While aimed at school-aged children, there are many useful charts, facts, and presentation tips that will appeal to adult learners in a laboratory animal facility. The pamphlets and brochures can be obtained for class distribution and incorporation into a training lesson, making the manager's job of identifying training needs and the process of training easier. In addition, they can bridge everyday life issues with the importance of the work done in the laboratory animal facility.

E.   WHERE SHOULD TRAINING BE GIVEN?

Ideally, it is easiest to conduct training within one's own animal facility. Of course, that is not always feasible, particularly if the information or needed equipment are unavailable there. It may be necessary to go to other animal facilities, academic institutions, vendor facilities, and such. The laboratory animal resource manager will be involved in making these arrangements.

Typically, an auditorium or break room is used as the location for training. One should consider other locations more appropriate for the material where the 'picture' of the situation is worth a thousand words. If the subject is cagewash operations, the crew could be brought to the cagewash facility while in operation and allowed to gown up with protective gear, observe a tunnel washer in use, examine temperature and pressure gauges, etc. For a session on necropsy, the trainer might make arrangements to prosect cull animals in the necropsy suite or a procedure room.

Evaluation needs to be made of potential confounding factors prior to a training session. Up-front planning to address logistical issues as follows can ensure the success of a training session:

- Audio-visual (AV) needs (e.g., slide, video, or computer projection; Internet connection; viewing surface)
- Wet lab set-up
- Distractions (e.g., noise, people or cart traffic)
- Safety (e.g., animal bites/scratches, chemicals, needles)
- Transportation of animals
- Size of the room
- Comfort of the room (e.g., chairs, lighting, temperature, ventilation)

- Availability of resources (e.g., equipment, supplies, animals)
- IACUC approval of animal procedures used in training exercises

F.   WHEN SHOULD TRAINING BE GIVEN?

Training is a continuous process; it is done as an investment in people for the future. The employee trained 20 years ago in laboratory animal technology, without any training since, will be woefully underskilled. Even employees satisfied with their positions within the facility still require training on personal safety issues, use of new equipment, the needs of a new study with different requirements, or changes in regulatory issues.

Training should be provided whenever necessary and required. Being spontaneous about training can be the most effective timing. While doing managerial rounds, an issue may arise on the spot which could be resolved by a short training session. This reinforces the need for quality effort all the time and demonstrates that the manager cares all the time, not just during an official training session.

Incorporating a portion of time in staff meetings for training has proven useful in some animal facilities. Since the staff are assembled anyway, it makes good use of the time.

It may be easier to plan time for training sessions for staff, whose schedules are more in control by management, than for investigators and other 'occasional' users of the facility. Everyone has a busy schedule, so providing sufficient advance notice about training is necessary.

Training may be held concurrently with events of the institution. For example, the new crop of graduate students at a university could receive training soon after the semester has started. Orientation sessions conducted for new employees may be a good opportunity to present training. (See Figure 3 for a sample form regarding compilation of a training history.)

A regularly scheduled training session may also be useful. For example, every Wednesday from 2 to 3 P.M. could be established as the formal training time. Staff will know to incorporate this slot into their workday. When scheduling a room, it is useful to obtain it for 30 minutes before and after. This allows time to set up and clean up, to evaluate the arrangement of the room (chairs, lighting, temperature, equipment) and make any changes, and to avoid being in someone else's time slot should the session run late.

Some licenses and credentials require periodic (e.g., annual) updates through refresher courses. The AALAS Registry program is an example, and requires completion of continuing education credits. Regulatory agencies may expect that personnel demonstrate that they have attended training sessions to maintain awareness of current trends. An institution must determine for itself whether sessions should be held every 3 months, once a year, or at some other regular interval.

Utilizing Web-based training may in some cases eliminate the need for establishing regularly scheduled classes, since they can be made available on an as-needed basis.

Figure 3. Sample form to compile a person's training history

This form was designed for use in the transgenic mouse facility of a university research program. It can be modified to suit the needs and objectives of other institutions.

Training Program Summary

Discuss each item. Concepts, as appropriate, are meant to be introduced, but not necessarily to completeness or competence (additional training may be necessary). Indicate in the blank, NA if not applicable, the initials of the trainer (staff or user), and trainee and date completed.

Name: _____

Initial Date:_____

Item	Staff employee	User of facility	Comment
Administrative			
access policies (key, keycard)			
barrier/conventional facilities			
PPE - personal protective equipment			
e-mail account			
medical evaluation			
supervisor and PIs			
identification card			
HR issues (check, etc.)			
general safety			
timekeeping			
weekend/holiday schedule			
SOPs			
training/in-house and level 1			
AALAS/certification			
Animal handling			
restraint			
animal health reports			
breeding			
transgenic terminology			
cage set-up (feed, water, bedding)			
mistreatment reporting			
regulatory issues			
OLAR and vet staff			

Figure 3. (continued) Sample form to compile a person's training history

Technique			
sentinel program			
ear punch identification			
ear tagging identification			
use of hoods			
technical service requests			
tail biopsy			
intra-peritoneal injection			
cardiac puncture			
euthanasia			
Equipment			
tunnel washer			
autoclave - big			
autoclave - small			
water softener			
chlorine dunk tank			
air lock			
water bottle filler			
steam generator			
light timers			
fax/copier machines			
Miscellaneous			

G. How Should the Training Be Presented?

The presentation of training material is dependent upon many factors. The main objective of training is to impart the attitudes, skills, and knowledge referred to earlier. How to accomplish this depends in large part upon who is being trained. Recognizing the characteristics of a group of adult learners will enable the manager/trainer to train more effectively.

Experienced managers will recognize the similarities to other aspects of their responsibilities in operating the animal resource, in that issues of training are to be identified, addressed, and then assessed as to their effectiveness. Some institutions have found a program of technical skills assessment to be a useful tool (2).

Overall, the major steps in the presentation of training are:

1. **First, the major training objective is identified**. This is a general statement of what the need is for training – in essence it is the first "**W**" or "why." For example, it is expected that 20 dog runs should be cleaned by an animal care provider in an hour's time. This has been determined by observation of experienced people utilizing the resources within that institution. Another objective might be that users of the facility are not complying with a policy at a satisfactory level. Note that the objective for similar tasks may vary by institution and expectations.

2. **Second, training standards are set**. This means preparing the standards, performance issues, and other criteria for training. In the first example above, it would mean reviewing how the runs are cleaned at the present time, considering that the steps and procedures may have changed. In the second example, it should be decided which users need to be trained. The trainer should evaluate why compliance is inadequate and how different affective and behavioral components of training can be implemented to improve efficacy.

3. **Third, the trainer should prepare** for the training session by fully identifying who will be trained, how they will be trained, and by whom. For the first example, will the kennel persons and the supervisor be involved? What training materials are necessary (e.g., dog run, SOP)? For the second, would new signs or a policy memo be as effective as assembling all the users?

4. **Fourth, the trainer should conduct** the training session and then evaluate effectiveness. Did the training session produce the results expected as identified in the first step? If not, then the trainer should re-evaluate and repeat those steps not completely fulfilled. Also, it should be determined whether the objectives are realistic.

Giving a lecture to staff (trainees) is often the default mode of training. Again, the relative advantages of active vs. passive learning should be considered. Words delivered passively may not be nearly as effective as viewing, observing, or being actively involved in a training session, particularly if there is immediate benefit for the trainee. Table 5 is a list of presentation ideas for training topics in the vivarium. *The Corporate Trainer's Quick Reference* (22) and the USDA's *Bibliography of Training Materials for Animal Facility Personnel* (23), although dated, are useful.

H.   Useful Resources, Methods, and Materials for Training

1.   Computer-Based Training

There is a variety of educational and training materials for laboratory animal science developed alongside computer technology. See the section pertaining to using computers later in this chapter for more information.

2.   Textbooks and Manuals

Standard textbooks can, of course, be used in training sessions for any discipline. In addition, a number of books specific to laboratory animal science have been published. Vendor catalogs (e.g., feed, caging, surgical instruments, animal models, equipment, etc.), equipment use manuals (e.g., cage washing machines, ventilated racks, anesthesia machines, etc.), and technical manuals are also useful and often are available at little or no charge.

3.   Audio-Visual Aids and Materials

Utilizing visual processes as part of the training session will enhance retention. The following may be useful in this regard:

  a. Actual items such as cages, syringes, anatomical models, synthetic representations.
  b. Slides, videotapes, remote video projection, overhead projectors. The trainer should be sure that the equipment is operational and that he/she knows how to use it. Inability to operate the equipment can be embarrassing and delay class time for everyone.
  c. Posters from government agencies, animal supply houses, or other sources to convey much information in a small space. Making use of a bulletin board or taping posters to the wall means the item will be seen many times; rotate them for variety.
  d. Computing equipment including CD-ROMs and network connections. Either included during a training session or made available for outside classroom work, training aids using computers can teach again and again.
  e. Writing boards and flip charts. The trainer might use such items to help interpret information during a training session. It is useful to include different colored pens as part of a training 'tool chest.' After using them in a real setting, it is worthwhile to critique one's own handwriting and size of lettering to assess effective communication.

4.   Puzzles and Games

The learning process can be made fun by using puzzles or games. Computer software is available to create crossword puzzles or word search games. Vocabulary words on a subject can be entered and the software generates the

TABLE 5. Ideas for Presenting Laboratory Animal Science Subject Matter (to be considered as appropriate to the audience)

- Basic concepts. For example, introduce metric units early in the course, then apply them to cage sizes, syringe volumes, dosage, animal weights, etc.
- Complete record-keeping forms in class as an exercise; everyone learns together and from one another and unclear concepts arise through discussion.
- Instead of reciting lecture notes, present information regarding regulatory documents by having class participants complete a worksheet that requires them to search through the document for the answers to questions.
- Use pH paper to teach concepts of acids and bases; test soaps, cage-wash waste water, acidified drinking water, etc.
- Invite vendors to teach about specialty topics like bedding and chemical safety, but avoid being brand-specific.
- Bring in samples of caging, bedding, feed, etc. to demonstrate differences.
- Conduct a field trip to visit another facility that houses animals that your facility does not have (be careful about being a vector of disease).
- Teach syringe handling, safety, and techniques by withdrawing saline (from expired bags) and injecting oranges or latex tubing.
- Use a stuffed animal to describe "rostral," "lateral," "ventral," etc. and to present anatomical concepts.
- Use handouts to help guide the training session and encourage people to write notes. If it comes out of the hand, it means something transferred through the brain.
- Begin each training session with a short quiz to test previously learned information.
- Quiz personnel in the vivarium hallway about what was taught in the last class. Look for "on the job" applications of recently taught material.
- Conduct a mock IACUC inspection of the facility.
- Utilize material from animal welfare or animal rights organizations in an exercise in understanding how public opinion about research with laboratory animals is influenced.
- Learn according to a subject or discipline approach
  example: instead of lecturing on anatomy and physiology, complete anatomy fill-in charts
  example: teach transgenic mouse handling along with genetics, aseptic technique, reproductive anatomy, and mating systems, etc.
  example: teach contamination control by discussing how an autoclave works, how to detect the presence of live organisms, fomites/vector, etc.
- Invite PIs to discuss their research, but with a focus on the animal perspective. Learn why the animal was chosen as the model. Discuss handling and restraint. The added benefit with this technique is the rapport built between husbandry/ technical staffs and the researchers.
- Create worksheets of word problems to practice metric unit conversions, dosage calculations, and other arithmetic-based lessons.
- Meet in cage wash to view machinery and demonstrate tasks to individuals who are primarily animal handlers.
- For the more advanced technician, such as LAT or LATG, create an exercise to design a facility.

game. Focusing on the actual words (vocabulary) will help those whose knowledge of English medical terms is limited. Several example puzzles for gastrointestinal physiology can be seen elsewhere (24). In a laboratory animal resource, a technician could be assigned the task to generate a puzzle by the manager.

5. Worksheets

Time spent by the trainer to create worksheets can pay dividends. Worksheets help organize the material into logical groupings; the major points are identified for the students. Effective worksheets generally take the form of a table with fill-in-the-blanks. For examples, see Figure 4 on rodent anatomy (p. 64), Figure 5 on anatomical systems (pp. 65–68), Figures 6A and 6B on protocol training (pp. 69–71), Figure 7 on euthanasia (p. 72), and Figure 8 on the ILAR *Guide* (p. 73). These figures represent different approaches to training using worksheets and they can be modified for individual use. Figures 4 and 5 utilize a blank table that is to be completed by the student who, in the process, is summarizing information. Figure 5 also incorporates illustrations (color, if possible) to add "interest" to learning and training, beyond just black and white text. Figures 6A and 6B are student and teacher versions of the worksheet, respectively, that standardize the information that any teacher in the same institution would provide to the students. The worksheet in Figure 7 is only the student version on another subject, but it is in a different format that includes subject headings (definitions, resources, and methods). Figure 8 is an example of an open-book worksheet, where the student searches a document, answers questions, and must cite the page where the answer was found. Worksheets can be presented during a training session or taken as homework.

6. Dry Labs

Instead of using 'real' equipment and animals, a dry lab can be employed. It is another form of virtual training. This avoids the complications of using animals, yet still prepares the student or trainee. Examples include use of a virtual rat to learn the hormonal regulation of GI function (25) and use of inanimate surgical models (8).

7. Jigsaw Learning Tool

This term applies to the process of separating material to be learned into portions, which are learned by individuals or groups. Like a jigsaw puzzle, there are many pieces which must be brought back together to create the whole. The participants reassemble and 'teach' their portions to one another. Disadvantages to this training technique are that some important information may be left out and it requires more time to learn and present. An application might be the study of an MSDS (material safety data sheet).

8.   Demonstrations

Seeing is often a more valuable way to learn than by just listening. Some subjects, such as installing a catheter, lend themselves better to a demonstration. Describing how to perform such a procedure probably will not convey the same image as watching someone hold the catheter, insert it into a latex tube, withdraw the stylet, etc. After viewing the demonstration, the learning process should be completed with actual practice.

Completion of forms is another exercise that is aided by demonstration. An animal health report or IACUC protocol form can be photocopied on transparency film (or used online if the capability exists). During the training session the form can be completed by a user (e.g., a technician or investigator) or the session leader.

9.   Case Study

The learning process can be truly enhanced by resolving an actual problem within the facility. Examples include redesigning an animal room for another purpose where new construction is involved, responding to the report following an inspection, or reviewing the health record of an animal from diagnosis through treatment. The issue can be presented, discussed, and resolved by the trainees.

10.   Lecture

Presenting a lecture is a tried-and-true format for presenting material. It is especially useful when certain and specific pieces of information must be communicated. It is, however, a passive learning method, which means the trainees are not as involved. Sometimes it is known as the 'talking head' method where the trainer is simply communicating but not embellishing the material. A lecture can be augmented with worksheets and other training devices as described here to make it more interesting and to increase retention of the material.

11.   Field Trip

A trip to another facility can be an effective training tool. The other facility could be a feed mill, cage manufacturing facility, animal vendor, or another laboratory animal facility. The facility manager should be cautious, however, of the potential for microbial cross-contamination between facilities.

12.   Symposium or Workshop

Sending staff to workshops can be very beneficial. The effort to develop the workshop is done by another group, lessening the load on at least one manager. The hosting institution may be well known for techniques and equipment unavailable at one's home facility.

13. Cooperative Learning

For some, group or cooperative learning can be effective. It is sometimes called the "buddy system." Two or more persons are involved in the learning process; sometimes one may be the senior person training others. Together they exchange or obtain information. In the buddy system, one may be teaching, observing and evaluating technique, and then counseling for improvement. In cooperative learning, members seek information and help one another along the way. The trainer needs to be careful about selection of the members based upon learning styles. Too many analyzers or feelers in one group may not yield expected results in terms of the learning process. The facility manager must evaluate that satisfactory training has occurred when cooperative learning is used.

14. *In Vitro* Methods and Models

In accordance with the 3Rs principles of Russel and Burch (3), use of alternative training techniques that do not use live animals is preferable. More and more models are being developed including the Koken® rat (Beltech LLC, Belmont, CA) or PVC rat (Micro-surgical Developments Foundation, info@microdel.nl), virtual labs on computer, preserved animal tissues, etc. Such items enable the trainee to practice what is learned, thereby fulfilling the behavioral and cognitive components of the **ABC**s of learning. Information on many of these items can be accessed on the LAWTE Web site (see reference 26 for a summary of alternative methods presented at the 1998 LAWTE meeting) or purchased from biological supply houses.

15. Vendor Materials

Several organizations, including AALAS, provide training materials for sale that can be used to augment training sessions. While AALAS does not maintain a library of educational materials for loan, it does provide for sale a variety of manuals and other printed material that is valuable for training. In addition, AALAS offers many tools for learning and teaching at its annual national membership meeting, where the learning resources center makes available audio-visual tapes, CD-ROMs, slide sets, and more for evaluation and review.

"Laboratory Animal Care Course," a correspondence course offered by PMI Feeds, Inc., consists of a notebook of written material and an exam that is sent to the vendor where it is graded. Those who successfully pass the course are awarded a certificate.

16. Professional Programs

Various organizations have training programs related to laboratory animal science. Periodically, these are announced on various list-serves such as CompMed and LAWTE. Some established ones are listed here.

a. Among the several veterinary technician programs, Delhi State University in New York offers many courses including a preparatory, week-long class for the

AALAS Laboratory Animal Technologist (LATG) certification examination. The resources at other veterinary technician programs might be made available if the program is approached with a well-thought idea.

b. Hahnemann University in Philadelphia has a master's-level program in laboratory animal science.

c. Veterinary schools have intern- and externships for persons interested in pursuing advanced knowledge in laboratory animal care, not only for veterinarians. For example, the Oregon Regional Primate Research Center accepts technicians in temporary capacities. The Armed Forces Institute of Pathology offers courses in pathology. Pharmaceutical firms sometimes accept students as interns and externs.

d. The Scientist's Center for Animal Welfare (SCAW), ARENA, PRIM&R, the Jackson Laboratory, and Charles River Laboratories all organize and host seminars pertinent to their areas of expertise.

I. COMMUNICATION IS AT THE HEART OF 'HOW' IN GOOD TRAINING SESSIONS.

The trainer can deliver information, but if it is not effectively received, then less-than-satisfactory results will be the outcome. There are three parts to the communication equation: the trainer's ability to present a training session, the transmission of the information, and the 'neural' ability of the trainee, which are looked at in turn below.

1. The Person Delivering the Information

The trainer must be able to effectively communicate the material. This involves vocal skills, including the volume, speed, pitch, and rhythm of delivery. Is the speaker monotone and thus not engaging? Does he pause too much with awkward silence or too many 'ums'? Does she vary the presentation to make it entertaining as well as a learning experience that conveys valuable information? Does the presentation seem rehearsed enough to demonstrate preparation and knowledge on the part of the presenter(s), but not so much that it is stilted and not responsive to the audience needs? Referring to Table 1 on training — rights and responsibilities, the trainer should speak clearly, effectively convey the material, and be enthusiastic. If the trainer is passive, simply reads passages of information, presents poorly, or is unable in any other way to communicate, the trainees lose. If the voice of the trainer is monotone, it could signal to the trainees that the material is not really all that important.

The trainer should also have a positive visual presence. Has the speaker dressed appropriately (e.g., scrubs for surgery training)? Does he move about in the training area? Does she express and gesture appropriately during delivery, making reasonable eye contact?

There is often fear associated with speaking before a group. Many call it having "butterflies in the stomach." The trick is to align those butterflies such that they "flitter" in the direction desired. Having a few butterflies is probably preferable to none at all, because the little 'edge' will avert complacency. There is nothing wrong with rehearsing a training presentation — before a mirror, among friends who can be constructively critical, in the empty training room the day before the actual session, etc. It may be helpful to join a speaking group such as Toastmasters, International to learn better speaking techniques and practice. Giving presentations with a public outreach group, animal related or not, is a less stressful means of gaining speaking experience. Another trick for dealing with presentation fear is to have props that can deflect attention from the speaker to the item in his hand.

Some speakers use cue cards or speak from overheads or slides in order to guide the presentation. Too much reliance on these 'crutches,' however, can detract from the main points of the presentation and there is the possibility of becoming more flustered if one loses his/her place.

The trainer is responsible for being organized in the presentation of the material. Props for the presentation should be laid out in some fashion, such as in the order they will be presented. It is important to be familiar with the objects — how they work or operate, how equipment is turned on and focused, etc.

2. The Transmission of the Information

The process of information getting to the trainee is called **transmission** and may be represented by a voice or sound, an object to view, or something to feel or sense. Like a crackling radio, the transmission can be interrupted. Background noise (e.g., cagewash, the animal, other persons, doors opening) can drown out the sound; too many people to train or small training objects can make seeing demonstrations more difficult; a looming deadline may decrease the attentiveness of trainers and trainees.

Related to communication are the presentation aids, that is, flip-charts, writing boards, slides, videotapes, overhead transparencies, objects, computer-generated images, etc. Because adults learn in different ways, the most effective means of information transmission will vary. Figure 9 (p. 74) summarizes the point that the same information can be presented by various methods, using text or images or some combination. A pie chart gives an almost instant understanding of the amount each of the factors influence. However, it is not as information intensive as the table and may be difficult to process for someone with visual impairments, including color blindness.

3. The Receiver, in This Case the Trainee or Student

Likewise for the trainer, the trainee should adhere to the training rights and responsibilities given in Table 1. Talking during training sessions can disrupt the transmission of material and distract the trainer. If disabled persons are involved in the training session, one should obtain appropriate accommodations. The Americans with Disabilities Act allows for sign language interpretation and purchase of equipment to aid in training. Sitting far away from the source of the information (e.g., the speaker, a video tape player, etc.) if hearing or visually impaired can be easily corrected by changing location. If language is a difficulty, one should ask for an interpreter or printed materials that can be reviewed and translated another time.

The manager with oversight of training programs should evaluate these features of communication that may influence the effectiveness of a training session.

V. COMPUTER-BASED TRAINING

The utilization of computing equipment, software resources, and the Internet for training is burgeoning. Known by the acronym **CBT**, computer-based training offers advantages to the laboratory animal science field as well. The laboratory animal worker must come to know a mouse not only as *Mus musculus*, but also as a piece of computing equipment. Increasing in both power and function with decreasing costs, computers are being used more and more in the vivarium. Besides being a research data collecting and facility management tool, they are being applied to training as well.

Among the CBT tools are Web sites and links to information, testing modules, question databases, CD-ROMs, virtual laboratories and training programs, hardware and software to help train, Web-based or online learning, and other electronic media that can be incorporated to tailor a local training program as needed. What follows is just a short list — browsing the Internet will lead the trainer to additional helpful CBT resources.

A. **The American Society for Training and Development** (ASTD) offers on its Web site, www.astd.org, a variety of computer-based training tools. It is oriented to training in the corporate world and does not address laboratory animal concerns specifically, but training hints can be obtained. There are demonstration copies of software to download and evaluate. It also includes an e-mail exchange on training issues. In addition, there are local chapters with membership meetings for the face-to-face interaction on subjects of training. The **International Society for Performance Improvement** (ISPI; www.ispi.org) is another professional organization with training as part of its mission statement. It is dedicated to improving productivity and performance in the workplace through human performance technology systems and its tools, many of which are training oriented.

B. **The Laboratory Animal Welfare Training Exchange (LAWTE)** Web site at www.lawte.org is specifically designed for training in laboratory animal technology. It includes links to training programs, question databases, vendors of software geared to laboratory animals, *in vitro* training aids, models of animal anatomy and physiology, and other training aids.

C. **The American Association for Laboratory Animal Science (AALAS)** has produced several CBT aids and is continually developing new ones. Some of its technician training manuals are available in CD-ROM disc versions with more images than the printed hard copy version for improved instructive purposes.

   The Web site www.iacuc.org, maintained by AALAS, contains links and references to training information oriented for the institutional animal care and use committee (IACUC). Its postings will help in training the IACUC with respect to laboratory animal regulations and can be especially useful for the non-affiliated IACUC member.

D. **The Web sites of universities** (UC Irvine, UC Davis, Florida State University, etc.) are good sources of information and ideas to train investigators (PIs) using the laboratory animal resource. When used as a centralized point to obtain facility policies and SOPs, documents, blank animal use protocols, record-keeping forms, etc., the training needs of PIs can be met. Some facilities are even using their sites to post training modules with quizzes that can be accessed at the convenience of the PI.

E. **The Norina database** (www.oslovet.veths.no/norina) hosts a tremendous volume of training and learning materials, especially alternatives, for laboratory animal science. It is a searchable online database of more than 3500 audiovisual aids and other alternatives to animal use from the Norwegian College of Veterinary Medicine.

F. **"Build your own training" software** packages enable the laboratory animal facility trainer/manager to tailor a training program to the needs of the individual vivarium. MicroMedium and Design-A-Course (www.b-and-a.com/dac/dacintro.htm) are two examples. They work like word processing packages where the course designer (perhaps the manager) inserts text, images, questions, and the like into the general framework of the program. The files created can be 'burned' onto a CD-ROM or run across the network. The trainee reviews the document and learns the specific information for the facility with the multimedia advantages of a computer rather than reading a stack of SOPs, reprints, and photocopied images. Similar to these, Microsoft® Powerpoint™ and Corel® Presentations™ software can be utilized and set up to run as a slide show.

G. **Interactive Media.** High speed communication lines have resulted in the development of interactive and **long distance tele-learning**. If a desired training program is not available locally, it could be obtained from another geographical area, saving the costs of travel and resolving scheduling concerns. For example, an animal technician in California can watch and learn from a demonstration of a technique in Illinois over phone lines. A professor in Florida can have chat-room-like classes online with students from 15 other states, utilizing text, images, and tests. For a hazardous bio-safety level 4 procedure inside a laboratory, investigators can watch remotely with a user-controlled video camera from afar, in a safe auditorium, in real time, allowing for immediate communication.

In a similar application, **virtual classrooms and universities** are being created using computer resources. Called Web-based or online learning, the field is relatively young and has tremendous potential for expansion and application. Virtual labs exist on the Internet, offering the experience to practice technique without actually utilizing animals or chemicals. An example from the journal *BioTechniques* demonstrates a polymerase chain reaction assay at www.attotron.com/cybertory/start.htm. AALAS has developed at www.aalasu.org its own online campus with numerous courses in laboratory animal technology and other disciplines that are useful for training laboratory animal personnel. A consortium of IACUCs at laboratory animal facilities in the Boston area have developed a Web-based program for training technicians and researchers with goals of collaboration, consistency, and efficient utilization of resources (27). Examples of online tutorials can be viewed at www.learn2.com.

Training can be assisted by other CBT technology. To accommodate provisions of the Americans with Disabilities Act (ADA) both hardware and software tools are available. For example, larger computer monitors can aid those with visual disabilities, making text and images more visible. Difficulties with reading can be addressed with software tools that read and speak printed text. A scanner 'reads' the text, which is then converted for speaking with a computer-synthesized voice. In some cases, the text can be translated into languages other than English. Software that creates crossword puzzles and word search games — even having laboratory animal technicians make the actual puzzle from scientific terms, converting them to clues and answers — provides additional ways of learning definitions and proper spelling.

Overall, CBT offers the laboratory animal trainer several advantages in developing and managing a training program. It means a bit more effort to design, create, and incorporate the products into traditional training courses, but the investment of time should prove worthwhile. Advantages include:

- Trainers have computing equipment and electronic media products to integrate into their traditional teaching methods.
- Adults are given the opportunity to accommodate their learning limitations or style (e.g., English as a second language, being older, advanced technology, learning disabilities)
- Alternative methods are offered for training various adult learners (e.g., investigators, research technicians, animal care providers) that include a patient and tolerant learning environment, own pace of learning for adults, and repetition of concepts from the 'machine.'

- Interesting and novel products are made available using new technology that is appealing to youthful and technology-oriented trainees.
- Consistent training can occur regardless of the session or instructor.
- There is accessibility to training materials that is independent of time (24 hours a day/7 days a week) or location (using a network or portable computing devices). Trainees can schedule their own learning time.
- It is cost effective because the same program can be repeated with fewer personnel and lower material costs after initial development.
- Training materials can be easily and quickly updated (on Web servers or CD-ROM writing devices).

VI. ASSESSMENT OF TRAINING

After the training session, an assessment or evaluation should be made. There are several parts to this effort, including documentation that training has occurred and then determining whether it was effective. After all, much effort goes into conducting training, thus the trainer and trainee need to know that the objectives were met and that meaningful information was exchanged. From the laboratory animal resource manager's perspective, it is imperative that trained personnel are caring for and handling the animals appropriately and that training objectives are met in a cost-effective manner.

A. THE LEARNING CURVE

The manager should be present during some of the training sessions to assess the material being presented and ask questions such as these: Was the learning curve too steep? Was too much information presented? Were participants paying attention or did they seem bored with the material? In multiple sessions, did the participants return time after time? Did they leave after the break? Should there have been more basic preparation for advanced material? For voluntary training sessions, could it have been described better so that it attracted the right mix of people? Was the style of presentation appropriate for the audience and the material that was taught? If the answers to these questions are less than satisfactory, then the course and its objectives need to be refined. The trainer should return to the steps of the six Ws, asking "why?" and "what?".

B. RECORDS

The trainee should obtain some kind of record that indicates he/she was trained. Often this is known as a CEU (continuing education unit) document. It should list the subject material, the location, the trainers or presenters (with a signature), the date, the amount of time, and the participant's name. Sometimes an equivalency of credit is given, like 0.2 CEUs as determined by an educational agency and may even be usable for college-level credit. For the manager, the CEU document will serve as evidence that the trainee did indeed receive the training.

A sign-in record (see Figure 10, p. 75) or attendance roster can also account for all persons participating in a training session. The original form can be filed chronologically by calendar year in a single file. This file can be reviewed or inspected as necessary to know what training occurred in a specific time period. Photocopies of this form can be filed in the individual's training file. Training received prior to the present position can be summarized and included as well. Thus, this file would represent a summary of the employee's 'lifetime' training.

It may be desirable to compile all of the training records and information into a large database maintained on a computer. It would then be relatively easy to determine when training needs to be updated, who in the facility has received a particular kind of training, who is competent at a particular procedure, etc. It may suffice to develop a simple table in a word processing or spreadsheet program.

The WIIFM principle (what's in it for me) can be applied to recognizing those who have participated in training. The manager might consider posting certificates of participation on a bulletin board, framing professional certifications and mounting them on the wall in the public area of the animal facility, or maintaining a grid of personnel and their more significant training activities. These measures can sometimes motivate others to be more participative in training and demonstrate the many avenues of training available within that institution. The grid has the advantages of pointing out deficits in training and making people aware of upcoming training (e.g., recurring training events, like annual primate biosafety training) opportunities. One potential disadvantage is that an atmosphere of resentment could arise toward those who frequently are recognized for participation in training.

C. FOLLOW-UP ON THE TRAINING

It is a waste of everyone's time and effort if staff are trained and then there is no chance to practice what has been learned. As soon as the training is given, there should be opportunity to put it to real use. The value of the training is underscored when it is immediately utilized.

After formal training sessions, the facility manager should meet with employees in hallways, animal rooms, cage wash, and procedure rooms to observe whether the training is being incorporated into daily activities. The manager's tool of "managing by wandering around" should be used to evaluate training. It is important to assess whether the goals and objectives presented during training are being utilized effectively. Both the employee and the employer have the responsibility to make training work. The manager needs to determine whether the training message was received by the staff, and if not, why not.

Such informal sessions offer more than just an evaluation of the employee and training. Efficiency of the task and utilization of resources can be evaluated. The personal attention accorded the employee can have mutual benefits to staff and management.

D. Quizzes and Tests

The tried and true method to determine whether something has been learned is to offer a set of written questions. Test-taking strategies therefore should be taught, as they teach critical thinking that is useful on the job. Generally, when faced with an issue to resolve, a person will draw upon experience, review what is known, discard obviously wrong options, and make a choice from the plausible remaining options. A similar mental process is engaged when answering exam questions. Whether essay, multiple choice, fill-in-the-blank, matching, etc., some learned information must be applied in determining the correct answer.

If one of the objectives of a training program is obtaining certification or licensure, it would behoove the training coordinator to include sessions on test-taking strategies. Similarly, for students who have not studied or are unaccustomed to studying, means and methods on how to study could be formally included in the course. AALAS has a *Study Guide for AALAS Technician Certification,* which includes a section on computerized testing.

One should always strive to write "good" questions, but even a "bad" question can be used as a learning tool. A good question provides just enough information that the answer is not a give-away. It avoids the use of double negatives (e.g., "which of the following is not?" type questions). A multiple choice question has the 'stem' and several choices, all but one of which are distractors. See the article (29) on validating exams for animal handlers for more insights into writing questions.

There are many sources of questions in laboratory animal technology. AALAS has developed workbooks for the technician manuals and for several documents used in the field (e.g., ILAR *Guide for the Care and Use of Laboratory Animals*; GLP regulations). Established training programs usually keep a bank of questions, quizzes, and tests used over the years. The University of Texas at Austin has made available a question database at its Web site accessible by link through the LAWTE Web page.

The technique of evaluation by written questions may not always be the most satisfactory or appropriate to assess knowledge in certain situations. Other methods to consider include:

1. For an investigator, a lab practical – with live animals, animal models, or instrumentation — to demonstrate proficiency with a technique may be more appropriate. The premise is, "The student has learned 'on paper' and now needs to demonstrate proficiency." To be equitable, a

list of criteria to be demonstrated by the test-taker needs to be pre-established. For example, for a test on cardiac puncture technique, familiarity and proficiency with several aspects of the procedure should be demonstrated, including the purpose, how to anesthetize the animal, safe needle use, quantity of blood to be taken, and the extent of hemolysis in the sample.

2. The proper completion of an IACUC animal use proposal may be the assessment tool when training a group of animal researchers.

3. Adequate cage cleaning and room sanitation done by the husbandry technician within an expected amount of time shows that the primary aspects of the job were learned.

Test anxiety is just one obstacle to successfully demonstrating knowledge, skill, and ability. Therefore, if the ultimate goal is to prepare students for an exam, the trainer should make that part of the course. The trainer should include regular quizzes (the added benefit here is that students keep up with their studying), perhaps at the beginning of each class session. Also, one might have tests that are reviews of accumulated material (mid-terms and finals). Students can 'grade' their own tests or exchange papers. It is important to allow for plenty of discussion, since the aim is for people to learn the material and apply it on the job. Often, much more is learned by the students during test review, when the more important points are brought out.

E.   PERFORMANCE REVIEW

Training should be considered to be part of an employee's achievement ladder. Gaining additional skills and knowledge means that employees are likely to progress within the organization; he/she will be qualified for a promotion and his/her new skills may enable the organization to offer a new service to the investigators. When regarded as the "resident expert," there might be a new-found sense of pride and personal satisfaction. Possibly, this skill can be shared with others in the laboratory animal science community, at an AALAS branch workshop for example, so that the arm of training reaches out to others.

Training is important enough to fulfilling job duties that it should be a part of every employee's performance review (see Reference 2 for how a skills assessment program was implemented in one animal facility). The manager might include training as one of the many factors for which the staff member is to be evaluated. For entry-level employees, the criterion could be participation in weekly training sessions. For the more advanced, it may be achieving one's AALAS certification. For senior personnel, serving as a trainer as well as obtaining training could be included.

When it appears that training is not working, an evaluation of all the components must be made, including training materials, trainers, communication, time factors, personal commitment, learning abilities, review of the ABCs (affect, behavior, cognition), individual or groups of trainees, and so on. It may be necessary to have remedial training for certain individuals. There is an aspect to training called **re-entry**, which focuses on the trainee being able to apply what has been learned in class effectively at the workplace as he/she comes back to work after training. The manager with oversight of training will need to explore each of these perspectives to keep the training on track.

F. 'OUTSIDE' EVALUATION

Regulatory and accrediting organizations will review the training conducted within a laboratory animal resource (29). Evaluations of several facets may be made, including a review of the training topics presented, who has participated in the training programs, the training monitoring process, documentation of animal user qualifications, training of IACUC members, and whether or not animal users have been instructed in the importance of the reduction, refinement, and replacement of animals (the 3Rs).

An institution's training program should be organized and prepared to allow for such an evaluation by an outside agency. A format such as that presented in Figures 3 and 10 may be useful.

VII. TRAINING THE LABORATORY ANIMAL RESOURCE MANAGER

To stay abreast of developments in the field of laboratory animal technology (and its related disciplines), the laboratory animal resource manager must take time for personal training. Scientific knowledge continues to advance and the animal facility, led by the manager, must keep up in order to provide the research staff with services.

A. CYCLE OF LEARNING

A simple four-step process will help the manager address his/her own learning cycle. The manager should:

1. Assess needs: In what areas is training needed? Is there a need to take a short day course or a longer semester course? Can it be self-taught, taken online, or obtained at another institution? How much money and time will it cost?
2. Design or choose a program that is suitable. Will it require travel to the course? How much time to commit? How much depth of material is necessary?

3. Facilitate own goals: Is the course being taken because the boss has mandated it? Will motivation to learn be increased because it is a personal choice? Will it be applicable in other facets of the job and life?

4. Evaluate what was learned and begin the cycle again: How much was gained by taking the course? Would it be recommended it to others? Was it cost effective, meaning amount learned vs. money and effort expended? Can one practice and utilize what was learned? What more needs to be learned to be more accomplished with the material or technique?

B.   OPTIONS FOR PERSONAL TRAINING

Obviously, attendance at AALAS and Laboratory Animal Management Association (LAMA) functions is a good way to obtain current information and continuing education in the laboratory animal science field. There are other training avenues to pursue:

1. Working toward a degree
2. Taking courses at community colleges
3. Attending seminars from professional organizations such as the Society of Quality Assurance and American Management Association
4. Attending workshops offered by recognized training organizations

It is also important to read journals, not just on management, but any other subject that relates to day-to-day functions of the facility. For example:

1. Many business magazines have short articles on management topics that can be read easily while traveling to meetings.
2. The *LAMA Review* is a good compilation of management subjects. The manager could read the article and evaluate it for how it can (or maybe does not) apply to his resource facility.
3. Regular and timely review of *Contemporary Topics* from AALAS. Reading at least one article in each issue will provide bits of knowledge.
4. Review of journals pertaining to the discipline of training, such as *Training*.
5. Reading the bulletins issued by vendors and suppliers to the animal resource.

To train to be a better manager, one might read books by renowned management authors like Ken Blanchard (*The One-Minute Manager* (30), *Managing by Values* (31)) and Peter Drucker (*Management: Tasks, Responsibilities, Practices* (32)) as well as other books on management and supervision (1). Even books about sports and coaching can provide the laboratory animal resource manager with insights and analogies to situations in the vivarium.

Training the manager to train is a concept for which various 'train the trainer' programs are founded. Viewing oneself while conducting a training session can be very insightful. The best technique for this is with a video camera. It can be viewed later (in the privacy of one's office). Others can contribute constructive criticism about distracting mannerisms, awkward pauses or "ums" while speaking, clarity of the presentation, use of the props, etc. Participation in public outreach programs can give opportunities to practice presentation skills. Speaking about "animal research" at a local civic club or school program is usually less fact-based and more entertaining, so one can focus on how to present.

Another source of information for the manager of a laboratory animal resource includes a variety of computerized listserves that deliver to one's electronic mail account. Examples include:

1. CompMed for issues pertaining to laboratory animal science and medicine. Announcements of meetings — around the world, nationally, and locally where information on lab animal training can be obtained — are often placed on this Web site. Contact national AALAS at www.aalas.org for more information about signing up.
2. LAWTE (Laboratory Animal Welfare Training Exchange) is an organization with the mission of assisting those involved in training laboratory animal science professionals. The Web site at www.lawte.org provides an abundance of training information, sources for training tools, and announcements of the group's meetings and activities.
3. LAMA (the Laboratory Animal Management Association) hosts both a Web page (www.lama-online.org) and e-mail service (LabAnimalManagers @egroups.com) to provide managers with information to better do their jobs.
4. The Transgenic List Web Site (www.lists.man.ac.uk/mailman/listinfo/ transgenic-list) and *Primate Newsletter* (www.brown.edu/Research/Primate) are but two of many specialized electronic services for getting information on particular animal models and usage from a research point of view. Available are archives of previously posted information, FAQs (frequently asked questions), protocols and procedures, and links to related Web sites.
5. AALAS sponsors the Web site www.iacuc.org, which includes training materials specifically oriented to laboratory animal care and use committee members.

Various organizations provide training for individuals in the sciences and can serve as resources. For example, the Industry Initiatives for Science and Math Education (IISME; www.iisme.org), founded by San Francisco Bay Area industries in partnership with the University of California at Berkeley, offer teachers opportunities in industry to learn technology and bring it back to the classroom. The American Physiological Society has a program for teachers to work in the laboratories of physiologists. Teachers from such programs could have a component during their externships working with the manager of the laboratory animal resource, contributing their experience and talent to its training program.

The laboratory animal resource manager should be involved with professional activities. Contacts made with colleagues and peers lead to discussions that train the manager in an informal way. Activities could involve volunteering on a committee, participating in a training workshop, writing and submitting articles for newsletters or journals, etc. The manager might participate in the writing and development of a research paper for publication and learn more of the scientific process and concerns of a research group. When the manager becomes either the trainer or trainee, additional insights into the process of learning are realized. The investment to produce good training materials and sessions pays great dividends not only for the trainees, but also for the manager/trainer.

The manager should be credited with efforts in continuing education by submitting paperwork to the AALAS registry. After achieving technician certification at any of the levels, this program recognizes those who pursue additional training by maintaining a database at the national AALAS office. Persons who meet the requirements may then include an 'R' for registered before their certification level (e.g., RLATG). This distinction will let others know that the individual has continued in various training programs.

Recently inaugurated is a program to credit the laboratory animal resource manager with a credential for having experience and knowledge in animal resources management. This program, called **CMAR** for Certified Manager, Animal Resources, is the result of a tri-party agreement among AALAS, LAMA, and the Institute of Certified Professional Managers (ICPM). Consisting of four modules, the manager studies subjects about human resources, fiscal management, and labor regulations, as well as laboratory animal management.

VIII. TRAINING MANAGEMENT CASE STUDIES

It may be valuable to review these exercises taken from actual circumstances in laboratory animal facilities. Try first to apply your knowledge of training and management to the issue, then read about possible approaches.

A. TRAINING OF NEW PERSONNEL

The manager of a laboratory animal resource decides to fire John because of poor performance, but asks that he stay on until a new employee (Susie) can be hired and John can train her. *What is wrong with this scenario?*

An often-used management tool is to train by the buddy system. Susie will learn all that John knows but the problem is this will include his poor methods and probably his bad attitude, too. Even if letting John go means the manager will be short-handed — and it will be an additional burden to have someone else train Susie — the training of Susie will be more effective when done by someone other than John.

B. TRAINING OF A NEW EMPLOYEE

Robert arrives for his first day of work at the vivarium. The training coordinator greets Robert and sets him up in the library or break room with a stack of SOPs and AALAS training manuals. "Look at these," she says, "and I'll be back in a few hours to check on you." *What is wrong with this scenario?*

All of Robert's enthusiasm and energy are now directed at black print and white paper. What he needs is to tour the facility; observe what others are doing; establish relationships with people; find out where the restrooms, supplies, and other important items are located; see how the traffic patterns work; etc. It is likely to be boring and mundane for the new employee to just sit and absorb training material without being actively involved.

C. CROSS-TRAINING

Often, resource managers feel that they must know the many details of the jobs performed by their staff members. Thus, for example, if the cagewash supervisor takes a week's vacation, it is likely that the manager would fill in. To prepare for the absence, the manager writes abundant notes to cover every potential task that might occur in an attempt to self-train quickly. *What is wrong with this scenario?*

Indeed, the manager should have a simple or elementary understanding of the work being performed by the people in the department, but it is not reasonable to expect managers to know everything. To accommodate absences of staff, be sure to have them cross-trained in different jobs so that they can easily substitute. This relieves the manager of having to 'know it all.' The concept of teamwork means everyone will pitch in.

D. MISTAKES

Errors are creeping into work. Veterinary treatments have a high incidence of poor clinical outcome. Investigators are complaining about technical services. All these mistakes must be the result of bad training. *What is wrong with these scenarios?*

Training is only an aspect of getting people to do their jobs. The manager must evaluate the problem and decide in what way training has contributed to the mistakes and how it can be utilized to repair and avoid them. The fact that mistakes occur can be seen positively, in that they point out some kind of deficiency in the training process. If they seldom occurred before, perhaps it was the people involved who managed on their own to overcome the error. Some of the best lessons are learned from mistakes and the laboratory animal facility manager must be skillful with human resources tools to recover and benefit from them.

E. MEMORIZATION

"We talked about it in class, therefore the techs should have learned it." "Why does Dr. Brown keep giving me these protocols with mistakes in them?" *What is wrong with these scenarios?*

Retention of material can be very difficult when there is so much information to know, not only in the laboratory animal facility, but also generally in life. The trainer can provide flash cards to help teach facts. Protocols and other forms can be completed with sample input as examples of what is desired. Trainers can teach memorization skills for word or fact association. Sometimes knowing the information is not so important as knowing where to find it. For example, isn't it better to be able to apply space requirements from tables in the ILAR *Guide* vs. learning and then forgetting what the exact numbers are? "Cheat sheets" posted in the animal facility or on an institutional Web site can provide detailed factual information that users need but cannot always remember.

F. HOMEWORK

"How do you expect me to pass the certification exam?" "Most of us barely have time to get our work done, let alone go to class." "When am I supposed to study?" *What is wrong with this scenario?*

It would appear that the institution has not made enough of a commitment to training. Inasmuch as the training will benefit both the employer and employee, mechanisms must be devised so that the employee can study some on the job and be motivated enough to spend some personal time as well. Suggestions include giving homework assignments, making training items available for check-out, and holding break- and lunch-time study sessions. The 'downside' of assigning homework is whether personal time spent on work-related tasks is to be compensated; that is a local issue that will need to be addressed but can be eased if presented from the standpoint that the technician will benefit by investing personal time and doing homework.

G. DIFFICULT LEARNERS

In almost every learning situation, there will be an individual who is a challenge. The manager and/or training coordinator must take steps to deal with such individuals so as to avert interruptions in the training program. By attempting to assess what the difficult learner really needs, the trainer can resolve the problem. For example, the "dominator," who interrupts the flow of the session, can be interrupted courteously by asking for input from others or may need to be counseled privately as a human resources issue; the "talker," who disrupts by holding side conversations, can be asked questions of the last topic covered or asked to review what was covered; the "know-it-all," who is the presumed expert with experience, can be involved in the discussion so as to give credit for expertise or can be tempered by the trainer providing the perspective that the training is for the good of all the trainees; the "non-participant," who simply sits through sessions, can be asked simple questions repeatedly on subjects for which it is known he knows something about and he can feel good about answering; and the "negator," who complains about everything, can be turned around by asking the others to help solve the problems as a class exercise.

H. So Much Training To Do

A small biotech firm hires an experienced LATG as a working supervisor/ manager. Business is good and the vivarium staff is growing. There are more records to review, husbandry staff to hire and train, and animal protocols with new technical procedures to support. The supervisor is stretched thin and worries about the future. *What is wrong with this scenario?*

More help is necessary; without it, animal care and research projects could suffer. The supervisor should approach management about hiring a facility trainer. The responsibilities would include develop and implement a training plan for each position in accordance with Standard Operating Procedures; provide ongoing technical training for animal husbandry, safety procedures and facility-specific requirements; develop computerized technical training modules, slide presentations, and videos; provide AALAS certification classes; develop and maintain a database of all training received by each employee; and annually review and directly observe each employee to ensure that all maintain their technical competence and that research requirements are not disrupted.

IX. SUMMARY

This chapter presents many of the basic concepts related to training in laboratory animal technology. Much of it is a 'how-to' on conducting training, although it is not meant to be an all-inclusive treatise on managing training efforts. The manager who trains will have to follow the 'links' of training to other helpful resources.

Training should be both rewarding and challenging. The process of training in laboratory animal technology can be enhanced by incorporating some of the different ideas and concepts discussed here, in addition to the traditional lecture-style of information presentation.

Confucius said, "I hear and I forget, I see and I remember, I do and I understand." It follows then that, as applied to training, an individual will learn better by being involved in the learning process. More than just speaking and delivering information, if the trainees are participating (doing), then more will be gained (understanding). When the resource manager coordinates the opportunities for training and empowers the participants, they will be more knowledgeable and able to do a better job with the laboratory animals they use.

Figure 4. Worksheet for rodent taxonomy and species characteristics

	Mus	Rattus	Mesocricetus	Cavia	Meriones
Kingdom			Animalia		
Phylum			Chordata		
Class			Mammalia		
Order			Rodentia		
Family					
Genus	*Mus*	*Rattus*	*Mesocricetus*	*Cavia*	*Meriones*
Species	*musculus*	*norvegicus*	*auratus*	*porcellus*	*unguiculatus*
Research uses					
Caging					
Handling/ restraint					
Physiological data					
Sexing/ breeding					
Characteristics					

Figure 5. Worksheet for Anatomy

Note the use of a different font and animal images for variety in training.

Anatomy Overview

the body is a machine with pumps, hydraulics, electricity, waste mechanisms, heat generators, communication devices, etc.

use a medical dictionary
use models of animals

differences among animal types
        mammals
        birds
        fish
        unicellular animals

terminology
        -itis
        -ology (histology, the study of cells)
        -ectomy

cell
 nucleus
 different types

tissue
organ
system

gross anatomy - overall

internal anatomy - necropsy, autopsy

cavities
        thoracic, pleural
        abdominal, peritoneal

Figure 5. (continued) Worksheet for Anatomy

Diagram parts of the animal body

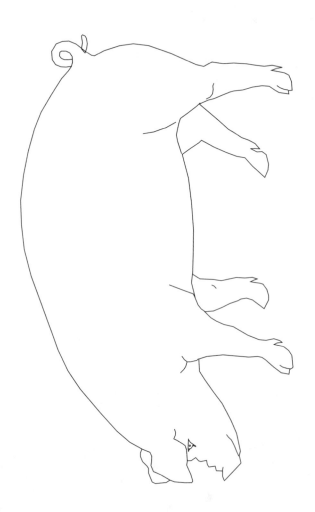

Figure 5. (continued) Worksheet for Anatomy

system (give name)	organs in this system	cell types	functions of the system	disease or conditions	terminology (-ology, -itis)

Figure 5. (continued) Worksheet for Anatomy

system (give name)	organs in this system	cell types	functions of the system	disease or conditions	terminology (-ology, -itis)

Figure 6A. Worksheet for a "Protocol" training session

(trainee's version)

Define what a protocol is.

List at least five components of a protocol.

For how long is a protocol valid?

Who approves the protocol?

Roles of animal-related organizations: What does the abbreviation stand for and what does the group do in terms of protocols?

USDA

NIH

AAALAC

IACUC

OLAR (or institutional equivalent)

Figure 6B. Worksheet for a "Protocol" training session

(trainer's version)

Materials needed:

For trainer :	appropriate pages of ALAT Manual
	ILAR *Guide*
	blank and completed institutional protocols
	animal users handbook or equivalent
	animal cage card
For trainees:	pages of ALAT Manual
	blank protocol
	worksheet

Define what a protocol is.

A description of how a research project will be conducted. Specifies what will be done. Fairly general, but with liberal interpretation.

The protocol helps to (1) track research projects, (2) comply with regulations, and (3) deal with the ethics of animal research. For the PIs, it helps them to organize the project.

List at least five components of a protocol.

Title. Approval date. Signatures (PI and IACUC). Safety factors (biological and chemical hazards). Euthanasia/pain and distress issues. Participants and their training. Purpose of study. Research procedures. Species and how many animals. Alternatives considered. Other items depending upon the institution and extent of work. Maybe attachments (surgery, transgenic work).

Why must a protocol be completed?

Federal law (Animal Welfare Act/USDA); funding and compliance with laws like the NIH; protection of institute policy. To assure appropriate animal care. To minimize duplication and unnecessary animals use (3Rs). To approve the use of animals used in research, testing, and education.

For how long is a protocol valid?

Institutional dependent. Often, three years with annual renewals at the second and third years.

Who writes the protocol?

The principal investigator and associates complete the protocol form.

Who approves the protocol?

The IACUC after a review process. The IACUC consists of a staff veterinarian, a lay person not associated with institution (often a member of the clergy or a "pet" person), other knowledge-able scientist. The committee chair signs the protocol, indicating approval, with an approval date. There is often an expiration date, which would indicate the protocol is out of date.

Significant changes to a protocol must be submitted to the IACUC for approval. Examples include the addition of personnel, additional animals to be used, changes in research procedures involving the animal, different alleviation of pain and/or suffering.

<u>**Figure 6B. (continued)** Worksheet for a "Protocol" training session</u>

(trainer's version)

Using protocols in the laboratory animal facility...

Records PI name and protocol number on cage cards to identify specific animals. Gives knowledge that Dr. So-and-so is permitted to do work with animals and on a specific project. Allows for tracking of information (veterinary treatments, cost accounting, etc.); both a husbandry and management benefit; shared knowledge for other staff members.

Roles of animal-related organizations: What does the abbreviation stand for and what does the group do in terms of protocols?

USDA - United States Department of Agriculture

NIH - the National Institutes of Health

AAALAC - Association for the Assessment and Accreditation of Laboratory Animal Care, International

IACUC - Institutional Animal Care and Use Committee

OLAR (or institutional equivalent) - Office of Laboratory Animal Resources

Exercises

complete a blank protocol with hypothetical information
use worksheet for note taking or as a quiz

Figure 7. Worksheet for a "Euthanasia" training session

Definitions
euthanasia

pain

perception of pain

Regulations behind euthanasia

Resources
NIH *Principal Investigator's Handbook* (or equivalent institutional handbook with materials on euthanasia)

AALAS training and instructional manuals

2000 Report of the AVMA Panel on Euthanasia

Methods
detecting death

safety factors

by animal

by method

"acceptable" and "unacceptable" techniques

Figure 8. Worksheet for the ILAR *Guide*

Open book worksheet: Provide the page number where found and the answer to each of these questions.

According to the *Guide*, why is pain a stressor?

How much space does a 25 g mouse need?

What does the *Guide* say about bedding changes?

Name two things in which personnel working in a laboratory animal facility should be trained.

What characteristics should the wall of a laboratory animal facility possess?

What is the *Guide's* definition of euthanasia?

What does the *Guide* say about emergency veterinary care?

What is the highest recommended temperature for a room housing rabbits?

What temperature range of water is recommended for effective disinfection of animal caging?

Figure 9. The three channels of delivery in communication

The same information can be delivered or 'transmitted' in many different ways. This figure demonstrates two things: (1) the three channels or factors that constitute delivery of information and (2) two methods in which that information can be presented.

The table (below, left) conveys more information about factors of communication and probably appeals more to the analytical learner, but it would take longer to mentally process and absorb all the information. In contrast, the pie chart (below, right) provides a concise, visual presentation of the same information which satisfies the visual learner, although it may not be as detailed and complete. Further, if it were in color, it could be difficult for the visually impaired to interpret, so using a variety of hatched fill-lines might be preferred.

There are many valid ways to transmit information. The manager who trains should adopt methods that are most suitable for the particular situation.

Three Channels of Delivery		
Factor		Portion of Total Communication Effort
verbal	using words that engage both parties	7%
vocal	the presence of voice, its quality and signals	38%
visual	the behavior and overall presence of the speaker	55%

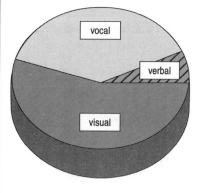

Three Channels of Delivery

Figure 10. Sample form to document a training session

Record of Training

(attach other information as appropriate; file original form in facility file and copies in individual employee's training file)

Title of training program:	
Date(s):	
Length of session:	
Trainer(s):	
Trainer's affiliation:	
Location:	
Outline of content:	

Method of presentation (circle all that apply):   videotape   discussion
          lecture   audiotape   slides   panel   demonstration
          other (describe):

Employees' names (printed)	Employees' signatures

Supervisor's signature and date:
(verifying above information)

REFERENCES

1. **Plunkett, W.R.**, *Supervision: The Direction of People at Work*, 6th ed., Allyn & Bacon, Boston, 1992.
2. **Edgar, K.S.**, Establishing a "Technical skills assessment program": Applying performance standards to job training, *Lab Anim.*, 28, 38, 1999.
3. **Russell, W.M.S. and Burch R.L.**, *Principles of Humane Experimental Techniques*, Methuen and Co., London, 1959.
4. **Lee, C.**, The adult learner: neglected no more, *Training*, 47, March 1998.
5. **Silberman, M.**, *101 Ways to Make Training Active*, Pfeiffer & Co., San Francisco, 1995.
6. **Silberman, M.**, *Active Training*, Lexington Books, Lanham, MD, 1990.
7. **Maslow, A.H.**, *Hierarchy of Needs from Motivation and Personality*, Harper & Row, New York, 1954.
8. **Dennis, M.B.**, Alternative training methods II: Incorporating inanimate surgical models, *Lab Anim.*, 28, 32, 1999.
9. **Shepherd, M.J.**, Meeting large regulatory requirements in small institutions, *Lab Anim.*, 25, 35, 1996.
10. **FELASA working group: T. Nevalainen, I. Dontas, A. Forslid, B.R. Howard, V. Klusa, H.P. Käsermann, E. Melloni, K. Nebendahl, F.R. Stafleu, P. Vergara, and J. Verstegen**, FELASA recommendations for the education and training of persons carrying out animal experiments (Category B), *Lab. Anim.*, 34, 229, 2000.
11. **Committee to Revise the *Guide for the Care and Use of Laboratory Animals***, *Guide for the Care and Use of Laboratory Animals*, National Research Council, National Academy Press, Washington, D.C., 1996.
12. **IRAC** (Interagency Research Animal Committee), U.S. Government Principles for the Utilization and Care of Vertebrate Animals Used in Testing, Research, and Training. Federal Register, May 20, 1985, Office of Science and Technology, Washington, D.C., 1985.
13. **National Research Council**, *Occupational Health and Safety in the Care and Use of Research Animals*, National Academy Press, Washington, D.C., 1997.
14. **Code of Federal Regulations, Environmental Protection Agency, Good Laboratory Practice Standards, EPA 40 CFR Part 792 Part III**, Toxic Substances Control Act, 1989.
15. **Code of Federal Regulations, Environmental Protection Agency, Good Laboratory Practice Standards, EPA 40 CFR Part 160 Part IV**, Federal Insecticide, Fungicide and Rodenticide Act, 1989.
16. **Code of Federal Regulations, Food and Drug Administration, Good Laboratory Practice for Nonclinical Laboratory Studies, FDA 21 CFR Part 58**, 1978 as amended.
17. **Code of Federal Regulations, USDA, Title 9 (Animal and Animal Products), Subchapter A – Animal Welfare**, Washington, D.C., 1985.
18. **Council of Europe, European Convention for the Protection of the Vertebrate Animals used for Experimental and Other Scientific Purposes, Article 26**, Strasbourg, 1986.
19. **Official Journal of the European Council, Legislation, Article 14**, Strasbourg, 1986.
20. **Sutherland, D.L. and Russell, D.R.**, Evolution of a training program built on employee involvement, *Lab Anim.*, 25, 41, 1996.

21. **Committee on Educational Programs in Laboratory Animal Science**, *Education and Training in the Care and Use of Laboratory Animals: A Guide for Developing Institutional Programs*, Institute of Laboratory Animal Resources, Commission on Life Sciences, National Research Council, Washington, D.C., 1991.

22. **Moss, G.**, *The Corporate Trainer's Quick Reference*, originally published as *The Trainer's Handbook*, Kogan Page, London, U.K., 1991.

23. **Kreger, M.D.**, Training Materials for Animal Facility Personnel: AWIC Quick Bibliography Series, 95-08, National Agricultural Library, Beltsville, MD, 1995.

24. **Bailey, C.M., Hsu, C.T., and DiCarlo, S.E.**, Educational puzzles for understanding gastrointestinal physiology, *Advances in Physiology Education,* 21, S1, 1999.

25. **Hsu, C.T., Bailey, C.M., and DiCarlo, S.E.**, "Virtual Rat": A tool for understanding hormonal regulation of gastrointestinal function, *Advances in Physiology Education*, 21, S23, 1999.

26. **Duffee, N.**, Alternative training methods I: Proceedings of the 1998 LAWTE meeting, *Lab Anim.,* 28, 24, 1999.

27. **Cody, C., Braun, M., and LaMorte, W.W.**, The Boston IACUC Consortium: A collaborative effort responds to training needs, *Lab Anim.*, 29, 39, 2000.

28. **Waraczynski, M., Urven, L., and Busse, R.T.**, Revising and validating an animal handler's certification exam, *Lab Anim.*, 29, 55, 2000.

29. **Slauter, E.**, Evaluation of a training program: a USDA perspective, *Lab Anim.*, 29, 25, 2000.

30. **Blanchard, K.**, *The One-Minute Manager*, William Morrow, New York, 1982.

31. **Blanchard, K. and O'Connor, M.**, *Managing by Values*, Berrett-Koehler, San Francisco, 1997.

32. **Drucker, P.**, *Management: Tasks, Responsibilities, Practices*, Harper & Row, New York, 1974.

3 Personal Leadership Skills

Fred A. Douglas, B.S., RLATG and Dennis B. Miller, RLATG

Individuals involved in the management of a laboratory animal resource play a crucial in responsible animal care and use. Because a good program of animal care and use is multi-faceted, the routine of the laboratory animal manager/administrator has the potential to be extremely busy. Responsibilities include, but are not limited to, animal procurement, husbandry, regulatory compliance, personnel management, teaching, and administration. Depending on the size of the facility and/or number of investigators, the pace can be overwhelming, particularly to the novice.

Managing the pace is a key factor in effective management. To do this effectively requires leadership. In this regard, leadership is best accomplished through following a sound set of principles. These principles, referred to as **personal leadership**, provide the framework with which to lead the program.

I.   LEADERSHIP DEFINED

Leadership engenders influence. Before the laboratory animal resource manager can influence others, he must be able to influence himself. Good personal leadership skills allow the laboratory animal resource manager to maximize his or her abilities in the performance of specific duties. Stephen Covey, in his popular book, *The Seven Habits of Highly Effective People*, spells out three "habits" that he calls personal leadership skills (1). They are:

- Being proactive
- Beginning with the end in mind
- Putting first things first

For the manager these skills translate into managing goals, time, self, and the journey called the "career." This chapter will explore insights into the personal application of these skills by the laboratory animal resource manager in the research facility environment.

II.   PERSONAL LEADERSHIP SKILL #1 — MANAGING GOALS

The first foundational skill for the laboratory animal resource manager is management of goals. Goals are important to the manager's leadership, so much so that international leadership expert John Maxwell defines success in terms of the "progressive realization of a predetermined goal" (2). Goals are a powerful influence; without them, the facility may experience poor operational methodology, less-than-optimal productivity, unclear direction, and loss of personnel potential. Without personal goals the manager may move from job to job, course to course, career to career, and wonder why he or she feels so unfulfilled in life. With goals come focus and direction. They provide guidance in the decision-making process. If the manager finds him/herself with competing priorities, he/she need only to open his/her list of goals for the year/month/ week and determine which of them will receive the attention. Goals offer a yardstick to measure performance by the management, animal care, and the research technical staff as well as by the facility and institution. Every manager should have personal as well as facility goals that influence daily activities. Examples might include to achieve a particular certification, attendance at courses that will enhance one's professional growth, publication of an article in a professional journal, development of a strategic plan for the animal resource, or updating a certain number of standard operating procedures annually.

Managing goals effectively requires that they be contextual, organized, disseminated, and maintained by a system of accountability.

A. CONTEXTUAL MANAGEMENT OF GOALS

A common mistake made by many managers is the practice of developing goals "in a vacuum"; that is, setting goals with no specific direction. Bob Shank calls this mistake "the error of viewing goals as the guiding force" (3). Put another way, one should avoid setting goals simply for the sake of setting goals. Goals should be the end point of a process, not the beginning point. To achieve this, goals should be developed contextually. For example, if a new manager in the field writes down as a goal to become certified as a Laboratory Animal Technologist (LATG) within the year, it is obvious that this goal is not achievable since 6 years of experience are normally required to sit for the examination. The context of being a newcomer to the field will prevent him from achieving his/her goal. If, on the other hand, a manager sets a goal for the animal resource to become accredited by the Association for the Assessment and Accreditation of Laboratory Animal Care, International, and the institution has spent the past couple of years preparing toward this end, he/she has identified a goal that is well within the context of the present situation.

A well-managed research facility will develop the framework for relevant goals. This framework or process consists of several elements:

- The institution's mission statement
- Vision statement
- Goal statements

1.   Mission Statements

Mission statements are common in most institutions. Often, they are displayed in some public place within hallways and offices. **The mission statement defines the reason that the institution exists.** A good mission statement taps into the intellectual side of the institution and answers three questions: (1) What function does this research facility perform? (2) For whom does the organization perform this function? and (3) How does the facility go about performing this function? To be effective the mission statement must be simple, accurate, believable, dynamic, and enduring. An example of a research facility mission statement might be, "To provide professional animal care, appropriate housing, and technical support for the research and teaching efforts of the institution and to strive always to improve the responsible care and use of laboratory animals." Simply put, this mission statement declares that the facility exists to take care of laboratory animals in a professional manner.

2.   Vision Statements

Vision statements extend the mission statement and declare a preferred future. **They answer the question, "What does the carrying out of the mission of the research facility look like"?** Vision statements access the emotional side of personnel. They describe things as they *can be*. The vision statement allows goals to be meaningfully set. Vision statements should be bigger than life, inspiring, clear to the employee, futuristic, and empowering. The vision statement of the research facility whose mission statement was earlier expressed might read like this:

- The research unit exists to support the teaching and research efforts of the School. *Our desire is to touch tomorrow's career field leaders today.*
- Our animal care program is managed and operated in such manner as to *provide a benchmark for all institutional programs nationwide.*
- Our animal care staff *are international leaders* in their field as evidenced by their participation in research projects, refereed journal articles, seminars, book chapters, and professional organizations. By this vision statement the employees of this facility are inspired to be "locally minded and globally committed."

Once an institution or facility has committed to paper its mission and vision statements, the animal care staff may develop effective goals to supervise the daily operation. These goals may touch on such areas as husbandry SOPs, in-house inspections, equipment procurement, and development of training programs.

B. MANAGEMENT THROUGH GOAL STATEMENTS

It is extremely important that goal statements be properly developed and formatted. Common mistakes made in writing goals include development in isolation, lack of clarity, and incompleteness. Goals should be developed by as many members of the research facility staff as possible. Goals should be developed by all who will be working toward achievement of the goals — management, supervisory personnel, and animal care staff. Dynamic goals that motivate a staff are those for which the staff has had a vital role in the development process. A good management practice to achieve this is for the entire staff to annually review the facility's strategic plan, including the mission statement, vision statement, and goals. Based on this review, the goals should be discussed and agreed upon for the upcoming year.

In many cases, goals thwart success because they are not clear or are incomplete. Meaningful, appropriately formatted goals clarify the focus so as to maximize their achievement. A good acronym for goal setting is **S.M.A.R.T.** The S stands for **"specific."** Goals should never be written in general terms. The specificity of a goal statement adds clarity and enhances its ability to be accomplished. The specificity of a goal tells an employee exactly what is expected of him. The M refers to **"measurable."** Goal statements should be written in terms that are concrete and objective. A goal of "doing all of my mouse rooms daily" is not as clear as "I will care for 500 mice per hour daily." A goal written in this manner allows the progress of performance to be monitored effectively. The A is for **"achievable."** Goals must carry with them the hope that one can accomplish the task. A goal to be "the outstanding animal care technician in the local branch of AALAS" may or may not be achievable depending on a number of factors. However, a goal by an animal caretaker to "care for all the animals assigned to him/her on a daily basis" is within the realm of accomplishment. R stands for **"relevant."** Writing articles for refereed journals is probably not reasonable for a junior animal care technician working in the cagewash area as opposed to learning the maintenance policies and procedures for the operation of key equipment. A relevant goal for a manager might be to train his animal care supervisors on the operation of new software being used by the facility. The T stands for **"time-bound."** A well-written goal will have a time frame attached to it. The manager may write a goal of having all performance evaluations accomplished "by December 31st each year." This gives the goal a target for completion. S.M.A.R.T. goals eliminate most, if not all, of the common problems associated with poorly written goals.

C. DISSEMINATION OF GOALS

Once goals have passed through the mind, finger tips, and onto paper they must be communicated. For goals to contribute to the overall effectiveness of the animal care program, they must be shared with all who are vital players in the process. This includes everyone vertically and horizontally within the chain of authority. Dissemination can be accomplished by a number of means — electronically, hard copy, or verbally at staff meetings. Preference should be given to meetings. A meeting, whatever the format, provides an opportunity for those concerned to raise questions, to clarify the intent of the goal, and to understand the expected outcome.

D. ACCOUNTABILITY

Managers who are serious about goals will develop and utilize a system of accountability for goal management. The system may take any number of approaches — routine personal reviews of goals and progress, a formal checklist turned in to the boss, or informal staff gatherings designed to discuss the progress made to date. Key areas to consider in the area of accountability are to be sure that all parties understand the accountability system, the focus/intent of the goals, the time frame, and what is expected of each player. If the individual maintaining the accountability is unclear about how the system works, he/she will be hampered in the performance of his/her responsibilities. Similarly, if he/she does not understand the focus/intent of the goals, his/her feedback has potential to be seriously flawed. One key factor in the success of the accountability system is the relationship between the two parties. The one responsible for overseeing accountability must be committed to the success of the individual being held accountable. This environment will promote honesty and trust in the process and facilitate success in reaching the goals.

III. PERSONAL LEADERSHIP SKILL #2 — MANAGING TIME

Two of the most precious resources that a laboratory animal resource manager/administrator has are the people who work for him/her and the time that each day offers for his/her utilization. Given the fast-paced, ever-changing world of research and regulation, it is imperative that the manager be effective in his/her use of time. Three basic facts of time management sharpen the focus of this all-important skill. First, the manager must always remember that the quantity of time cannot be changed. Each day is 24 hours long, and what sets apart the great from the not-so-great manager is how those 24 hours are used.

Second, it is critical for the manager to come to grips with the fact that one will not get everything done in a day's time and sometimes not even in a week's or month's time.

Third, the wise manager is the one who appreciates the gift of a lifetime, in other words, that he/she is not eternal. The manager who affirms this reality will be the one who applies discipline with respect to time management. Conquering the art of time management requires the following:

- Understanding the **goal of time management**
- Mastering the **skill of time management**
- Shifting the **paradigm of time management**
- Choosing the right **tools for time management**
- Properly applying the fundamentals of time management by **living the system**

Each of these aspects warrants some discussion.

A.   GOALS OF TIME MANAGEMENT

Historically, time management books, seminars, and workshops have concentrated on developing the efficiency of the reader or attendee. In other words, the foundational assumption was that the individual was a procastinator, a waster of time, or lacked understanding with respect to efficiency. In the current research climate, even if a manager were fairly efficient and applied the principles of time management, there would be no guarantee that he/she would leave work a satisfied individual or that his/her work effort would make an impact on the animal care program. This raises the question, "What should be the goal for the good use of one's time?" The goal of time management is really threefold.

The first goal and highest priority of time management should be **"effectiveness."** The proper aim of time management is getting the most important things done. Accepting the fact that not everything can be accomplished in a day establishes the importance of doing the most important things. As Covey puts it, "You can be a hard working individual but if you are in the wrong jungle your time and effort are wasted" (1). If the manager is working hard at developing policies and procedures for the facility when he/she is short-staffed, the priorities are awry. The best policies and procedures in the world will not compensate for the lack of adequate numbers of well-trained staff. The institution's mission statement and vision statement can provide guidance for the research facility manager in defining effectiveness.

The second fundamental goal of time management is **"balance."** Balance has to do with maintenance and development. One may have the best cagewash machine in the world, but if it is not maintained and upgraded in a timely fashion, its usefulness will be diminished. The manager who fails to take time to maintain his/her personal and professional life will likewise note the law of diminishing returns in his/her work output and influence. To accomplish this, the manager must create a balance within his/her life. Some have called this concept the "well-rounded square." This concept views each individual as being made up of physical, intellectual, emotional, and spiritual sides. Efforts to stimulate and develop new facets in each of these realms will keep the manager fresh and creative in his/her work. For example, reading a book every month can bring the individual into contact with new ideas to try in the workplace. Daily physical exercise can maintain the body in a state of readiness for extra stresses and strains that might be experienced while working at the facility. Meeting people outside of the workplace can sharpen interpersonal skills. Meditating on inspirational literature can be refreshing to the individual's spiritual side.

The third and final goal of time management is **"efficiency."** Most managers attend time management events in order to increase the pace of output. The smart manager, however, is the one who increases output within the framework of effectiveness and balance. This enhances the work effort by ensuring that the manager is getting the most important things done. There are many ways and means to improve efficiency. One method is for the manager to improve frequently used skills. For example, if the job requires a great amount of reading, completion of a speed-reading course might help improve efficiency. Another means to increase efficiency is through **synergizing**. Synergizing means performing several activities simultaneously. For example, some managers read junk mail while reviewing incoming voice mail; others take along an employee on an errand to discuss concerns that affect the employee.

Efficiency can also be improved through **organizing and categorizing**. Some managers have difficulty in tracking critical events and deadlines. Maintaining a "tickler file" with information on important upcoming and ongoing efforts and deadlines can resolve this problem and save precious time for the manager to do other important duties.

B.   THE SKILL OF TIME MANAGEMENT

If the highest goal of time management is effectiveness, then it is imperative that the manager know how to prioritize. If the manager is adept at determining the most important things to do on a daily basis, the program of animal care will help to accomplish the aims of those it is serving. In this regard, the **Pareto principle** is extremely helpful. This principle encourages the manager to work smart. Simply stated, the Pareto principle says, *"20% of one's priorities will give one 80% of one's productiveness, if one spends all one's resources on the top 20% of one's priorities."* For the manager, the priorities are resources such as time, people, equipment, and finances. Some examples of the Pareto principle applied are:

- 20% of the manager's time will produce 80% of his/her results.
- 20% of a manager's staff will produce 80% of the facility's work effort.
- 20% of the faculty of the institution will be involved in 80% of the research effort.
- 20% of the leadership will make 80% of the decisions within the organization.

To master this skill, then, the smart manager will determine who or what are the top 20% of his/her priorities and focus his/her attention on them.

C.   THE PARADIGM OF TIME MANAGEMENT

Typically, people manage time "by the seat of their pants." The plan for the day is often made over a cup of coffee at breakfast or in the shower before leaving for work. This style leads to "management by crisis." To bring effectiveness, balance, and efficiency to the forefront, the manager needs to change his/her paradigm. Rather than thinking in terms of "one day at a time," it is much better to think of a week at a time, a month at a time, or even a year at a time. For example, in a military battle the point of view of the general is much different from that of the private. The general typically has view of the entire battlefield. He/she is able to bring the right resources in the right quantities to the right point at the right time. The private only sees that portion of the field that he/she is occupying and is only concerned with what lies directly in front of him/her. Those who manage time by thinking over the coffee cup are like the private and those who manage their time by considering longer blocks are like the general. The latter are able to do the right things at the right time and in the right manner.

D.   TOOLS OF TIME MANAGEMENT

Just as having the right software program is essential to manage cost analysis in a research facility, having the right tool is critical to assist in good time management. The purchase of a time management system which enhances the ability of the manager to follow the above mentioned principles is important. There are many fine time management systems available, and a thorough review of their strengths and weaknesses should be conducted before any purchase is made. The system selected should have some of the following attributes:

Context — The system should enable the user to think and plan time within the context of the goals that have been set. As discussed above, setting the right goals is critical.

Balance — The system should promote the balance that the user seeks to achieve. The system should assist the users to center their time around the roles that they have identified.

Personal — The system should be designed in such a way as to promote flexibility for the user. The system should allow the user to customize the kit to fit his/her particular personality.

E.   LIVING THE SYSTEM

Time management properly executed is a system. The system involves knowledge and application of a process based on that knowledge. The system's foundation consists of a mission statement, vision statement, and goals based on those statements. Stephen Covey describes how to develop a personal mission and vision statement with accompanying goals (1). This should be the starting place for the manager. Once these are developed the following system may be utilized routinely to accomplish effective time management.

The first order is balance. In order to achieve balance the manager needs to identify the roles that he/she currently plays out in his/her daily routine. Some examples are manager, teacher/trainer, compliance officer, spouse, community service advocate, and volunteer for professional organizations.

Next, the manager needs to identify annual goals for each role. For example, the manager might set a goal to fully train all of the animal care staff in the facility standard operating procedures. Another goal might be to present a seminar at a professional meeting. These goals will be effective since they are based on the framework of a well-thought out mission and vision.

Next, on a weekly basis the manager should identify specific activities that need to be performed which will support the accomplishment of the goals. Typically, there may be as many as eight to ten activities for each role. Examples of activities might include ordering of animals and supplies, conducting performance reviews of employees, or meeting with an investigator to discuss issues of concern. Of the activities identified, one should decide which two or three are the most important, and then devote particular attention to those activities. This is the Pareto principle at work.

Next, the manager should link each activity to a day/time that it will be approached. A good rule of thumb with respect to time is to double whatever amount that one thinks that it will take to do the job. For example, if it is thought that a meeting will take 1 hour, then the manager should plan for 2 hours.

The final step is the execution of the plan. This requires commitment to keep on schedule and to accomplish the most important things during scheduled times. As one anonymous individual has said, "The amateur performs when he feels like it but the professional performs when he doesn't feel like it." There must be a commitment to being a "professional" time manager.

The strength of this system is that the responsibility is tempered by flexibility. Should a particular planned event fall through, a simple consultation of the weekly plan gives opportunity to move the scheduled task to another time slot in the week. Effectiveness is not lost. Balance is not lost. Rather, good management is enhanced and good leadership is maintained.

IV.   PERSONAL LEADERSHIP SKILL #3 — MANAGING SELF

Although Covey advocates "being proactive," it really has to do with **"managing self"** (1). Being an effective leader in a laboratory animal resource facility requires such qualities as initiative, integrity, discipline, and thoroughness. In a fast-paced program of animal care and use, these qualities are often tested to the limit. The manager's character is vital to the effectiveness of the program.

Many in the workplace feel that there is little correlation between private behavior and public performance. However, recent events such as school violence, workplace violence, and political corruption point out that this may not be the case. One's private values likely affect one's actions. Those private values are defined as **character**. Therefore, the determination and development of character of the manager is of utmost importance.

Performance rises and falls on character. Many leadership experts feel that character is the primary quality of an effective manager/leader (4). Character strength creates influence and begets leadership. Character is the driving force behind actions. Character qualities such as initiative, integrity, discretion, and patience result in productive work.

A hypothetical daily routine of a manager highlights the importance of character. A faculty member seeking advice must be assured that the information has been thoroughly researched and is the best available. Thoroughness assures that this is so. Regulatory compliance in a research facility is often a battleground. In some situations, it is a test of an investigator's research goals vs. the requirements of a regulatory mandate. In other instances, it is the view of the investigator vs. the perspective of the attending veterinarian. In these cases, the integrity of the manager can be severely tested as he/she may find him/herself caught in the middle of issues or concerns.

The development of the manager's character is a process. Ideally, it arises from a meaningful interaction with a mentor. Animal care technicians who demonstrate promise for future leadership should be identified early in their careers and coached/counseled with attention paid to knowledge, skills, and character. A good program of mentoring should identify ideal attributes that will serve the budding facility leader in his future endeavors. These qualities should be incorporated into training and coaching sessions that involve daily work routines and special projects, and they should be discussed at the annual performance review.

Character training programs have been developed as organizations recognize the value of such efforts. These may be located by searching the Web or through business magazines. Some companies have developed and implemented character-based training programs for mentoring their own employees. One such example is Kimray, Inc., an oil and petroleum equipment supply company. Within 1 year of establishing the program, employee morale and productivity increased, while worker compensation costs were reduced by 80%. The program developed by Kimray, *Character First®* (5), is being marketed to institutions, schools, and cities. The program consists of materials sent monthly to the facility which highlight a "character quality of the month" and provide topics for discussion and ideas for application.

V.   CAREER MANAGEMENT

Most managers would never consider building an animal resource facility without a plan. Indeed, vacations, social activities, even trips to the shopping mall are all usually planned in advance. Yet, many managers do not have a career plan and instead aimlessly move from one job to another. Whether one is beginning a career, planning a career change, or evaluating a current career, a plan to guide one's professional life is useful.

Three basic steps to prepare a career plan have been suggested (6). First, it is important to assess one's skills, values, and interests. Second, one should research job opportunities. Third, the educational and job pathways that will lead to the desired position should be identified. These same steps can be used for guidance throughout the career.

We begin to discover and assess our skills, values, and interests when we are very young. Our interests are addressed when our parents ask, "What do you want to be when you grow up?" As we move through our working lives, it is important to periodically assess interests, since they may change. Many people choose a career based on an interest developed early in life and then fail to reassess their current interests over time. Failure to consider current interests could lead to dissatisfaction with one's career.

When choosing and managing a career, consideration of skills and personal values are as important as identifying areas of interest. One may wish to be an opera singer, but if one cannot carry a tune, other career choices may be more appropriate. Although this appears to be a simple concept, many people find themselves in jobs in which their skills do not match the requirements of the position. In this regard, it is critical that an honest evaluation of skills be conducted.

Assessment of values is also a key aspect of making a correct career decision. Questions such as "What's important to me?" "What's going to make me feel good about myself?" and "At the end of the day and ultimately at the end of my lifetime of work, what do I wish to have accomplished?" should be answered. Assessment of personal values is particularly important when choosing a career in laboratory animal science because of the moral and ethical issues related to the use of animals in research. If one's personal values do not fit the values of the profession, then a less-than-fulfilling career may lie ahead. To be truly happy, one should learn about oneself and choose a job that provides fulfillment day in and day out. It has been said that "Doing the work you love means living your philosophy" (7). In other words, one should put one's values to work by determining that his/her career and work will reflect the true nature and identity of the person.

When developing a career plan, it is important to learn as much as possible about the vocation of interest and opportunities within that field. One should find out everything there is to know about a particular field and the career path options that exist. Libraries are a logical place to begin researching career opportunities. In addition, one should talk to people in the field of interest or even arrange to volunteer in a work environment within the field. Professional associations such as the American Association for Laboratory Animal Science often have useful career information in both printed and electronic formats.

Continuing education is a critical aspect of career development in several ways. First, it provides individuals with additional knowledge and skills that allow professional development. Second, it stimulates thought as learned ideas are put into practice. Third, it may illuminate professional opportunities that one had not previously considered. As we learn, we discover skills, likes and dislikes, and identify abilities. As we learn, we discover new areas of interest and opportunity. The educational process should never cease; lifelong learning is increasingly necessary for success.

A career in laboratory animal science can be a wonderful and fulfilling opportunity. The professional happiness and success of a laboratory animal resource manager is dependent on joining the needs of the scientific community with individual talents. As the Greek philosopher Aristotle said, "When your talents and the needs of the world cross, there lies your vocation." Career management is one management tool that one must never stop using.

REFERENCES

1. **Covey, S.**, *The Seven Habits of Highly Effective People*, Simon & Schuster, New York, 1989.
2. **Maxwell, J.**, *Developing the Leader within You*, Thomas Nelson Publishers, Nashville, 1993.
3. **Shank, B.**, *Total Life Management*, Multnomah Press, Sisters, OR, 1990.
4. **Maxwell, J.**, *Developing the Leaders around You*, Thomas Nelson Publishers, Nashville, 1995.
5. *Character First!*®, Kimray, Inc., www.kimray.com, Oklahoma City.
6. **Mitchell, J.S.**, *The College Board Guide to Jobs and Career Planning*, College Entrance Examination Board, New York, 1994.
7. **Boldt, L.G.**, *How to Find the Work You Love*, Penguin Arkana, New York, 1996.

4 Bioethics and Laboratory Animal Research

Jan Wyrick Gnadt, D.V.M., Dipl. ACLAM
and Stuart E. Leland, D.V.M., Dipl. ACLAM

This chapter summarizes the history of moral issues surrounding the use of laboratory animals in research, provides an introduction to moral theories for animal protection, identifies some specific ethical concerns commonly found in laboratory animal facilities, and reviews practical methods for managing and resolving ethical concerns.

The first part of this chapter provides a historical perspective leading to the development of the major theories utilized to frame the current debate involving animal use and protection. Understanding these theories provides an outline for thinking and developing concepts about moral commitment to animal welfare. Developing a personal ethic (an ethos), in the context of an historical perspective, will assist the manager in defining root issues and understanding the structure upon which arguments emanate and are measured. In general, the concepts of morality and ethics are personal and the development of an ethos requires knowledge, introspection, logic, and consistency.

The second part of this chapter focuses on ethical concerns in the laboratory animal resource. The laws and regulations that govern animal use are reviewed. Public perception about the use of animals, and how these perceptions affect research personnel in the workplace, are discussed. Common ethical concerns are examined in terms of their potential positive and negative effects on research personnel and animals. Specific questions are raised, in relation to each ethical concern, in an effort to sensitize the reader to the complexity of these issues and also to serve as a guide for policy decision making. Finally, there is a discussion about basic managerial techniques and skills. It is a goal of this chapter to assist the animal resource manager, who serves a pivotal administrative role in the laboratory animal resource, in gaining the knowledge, expertise, and confidence necessary to identify and address bioethical issues.

I. INTRODUCTION

Morals are those prevailing beliefs of right and wrong that are so deep-seated in a society that they form a community standard. **Morality** refers to the body of these beliefs and includes standards of acceptable behavior and rules of conduct. For some individuals, but not all, morality is used as a basis for the argument that all humans have rights. Ethics is the science of morality involving principles of right and wrong behavior. The *science* of **bioethics**, that branch of ethical theory which deals with biological research and medicine, dates back to the 1800s when the British Parliament passed laws aimed at preventing cruelty to animals (1).

Although ethics evolve over time, bioethics languished for centuries as society tackled more pressing and basic questions of ethics. However, in the last 40 years, with scientific advances resulting from molecular applications, the use of animals in research has increased steadily. This has thrust the field of bioethics into the limelight as society discusses such issues as gene therapy, xenotransplantation, cloning, and *in utero* manipulation. To understand the core principles behind the debate on the use of animals in research, it is useful to understand the historical progression of bioethical theory as well as case law, which has influenced societal attitudes regarding animal-based research.

II. HISTORY

At the center of the bioethics debate is whether or not nonhuman animals are, or should be, considered part of the human moral community (2). A broader ethical question, with major ramifications on bioethics, is whether or not morality confers rights. Can moral standing or obligation towards someone, or something, be used to imply that the thing has a right?

Some individuals, including animal rightists, believe that morals confer rights. According to these individuals, the presence of universal morals, such as to tell the truth, respect privacy, and protect confidential information confer an equivalent "universal right." Also included in this argument are morals for codes of conduct including do not kill, cause pain, maim, or deprive of goods. Animal rightists argue that these morals apply to human conduct concerning nonhuman species and, therefore, nonhuman species have a right to such treatment. Thus, the possession of morals by one species transcends species barriers and confers inalienable rights to another, unrelated species. The term **animal rightist** emanates from the belief by some individuals that humans have a universal moral obligation to animals and therefore, animals have rights. Unfortunately, for the majority of individuals, the relationship between morals, or moral obligation, and rights is not so defined (3).

To further examine whether nonhuman animals have moral standing in the human moral community, one must ask whether nonhuman animals have morals. If they have morals, they must have the capacity to make moral judgements about the conduct or behavior of one in their own species (2). How is this judgement communicated and implemented? Only through such actions can a societal standard of conduct and behavior, or morality, develop. This is an important dilemma because, if nonhuman animals do not have moral standing, then some may argue that humans bear no responsibility for their welfare.

Membership in the human moral community has, historically, been based on two properties: being human and the ability to reason. But what does it mean to be human? To address this question, a number of underlying issues concerning the nature of nonhuman animals have been discussed relevant to their moral standing. One issue is the level and type of mental activity that occurs in nonhuman animals and about the ethical significance of this mental activity. Philosophers on one end of the spectrum argue that nonhuman animals lack all mental capacity, including feeling and consciousness.

This philosophy was best articulated by Descartes (1596–1650), who argued that nonhuman animals do not have the capacity to feel pain and are in fact *automata* that act "mechanically, like a clock" (4). He further reasoned that because they lacked language and abstract reasoning, they therefore lacked a mind. Descartes absolved humans from any crime or guilt in killing, eating, or experimenting on nonhuman animals.

On the other end of the spectrum was Hume (1711–1776), who argued that, through life experiences, nonhuman animals gain understanding, which is used to infer consequences and therefore suggestive of a form of reasoning. In his *A Treatise of Human Nature*, Hume discussed sympathy, cooperative schemes, love, and pride in nonhuman animals as analogous to human capacities (5).

In the middle of the spectrum lay other philosophers, including Aristotle (384–322 B.C.) and later, Kant (1724–1804). They concluded that nonhuman animals have minds and may experience pain, but the pain they experienced was not a matter of moral concern. Furthermore, if humans inflicted the pain, it was not a form of cruelty. They believed that nonhuman animals lack the ability to reason, and therefore could not belong to a moral community.

What does it mean to have the ability to reason or to rationalize? Ethologists and psychologists study behavior, intelligence and adaptation by first acknowledging that nonhuman animals exhibit understanding, intention, thought, imagination, and communication. By attributing such capacities to nonhuman animals, some may argue that they have reasoning capacities similar to humans. Therefore, the argument continues, they are deserving of whatever protection humans enjoy by virtue of having the same properties (2). The truth is, however, that very little is understood about the mental capacities of nonhuman animals. Observation of behavior does not yield adequate understanding of whether the nonhuman animal really has certain mental states or is just acting as if it had such states. Using human language to describe behaviors, mannerisms, and expressions in our nonhuman animal species can cloud our ability to objectify their actual meaning.

Darwin (1809–1882) argued against the hypotheses that major cognitive or reasoning differences existed between the species. He theorized that human biological and psychological structure, function, and behavior evolved along a spectrum of processes that existed elsewhere, though perhaps to a lesser degree, in nonhuman species (6). This severely undermined the previously held belief that humans were the only species to act rationally and thus deserved unique and sole moral consideration. The debate over the ability of nonhuman animals to reason remains fervent. Unfortunately, until this is settled, or until moral philosophers redefine membership in the human moral community, the ability to determine if nonhuman animals have moral standing remains inconclusive at best, and perhaps impossible.

III. STANDING

The centerpiece of moral philosophy is to justify a moral position or standing. Because some morals are universal, this is intuitive in many cases. For example, nobody needs to justify the moral position of the value of life. The justification is more difficult, however, when it comes to our use of nonhuman animals in food production, hunting, sport, recreation, religious sacrifice, or research. **Standing** refers to one's position within a community in the estimation of others. The term standing has profound meaning when it comes to discussing legal rights, for an entity cannot be the beneficiary of rights unless it has standing in the eyes of the court (7). Historically, nonhuman animals have not had legal standing in the British or American legal systems. However, recently, in a potentially landmark decision, a Washington, D.C. appellate court held that an individual, funded by the Animal Legal Defense Fund, had legal standing to represent nonhuman primates and sue the USDA (8).

Moral standing refers to whether an entity is the kind of entity to which moral principles can be applied. If one were to attribute moral standing to nonhuman animals, it would suggest that the nonhuman animals have relevance similar to that of human beings. A mainstream moral philosophical viewpoint is that if nonhuman animals have the capacity for understanding, intention, and suffering, or have desires or preferences, then these morally significant properties themselves confer some degree of moral standing. But, do these properties alone confer standing for nonhuman animals? If so, how much standing do they have? Much of the discussion about standing has centered on the criteria for being a person. What is it that distinguishes a person from a non-person? An entity not fitting the definition of a person would lack moral standing and could not possess rights.

A summary of cognitive conditions necessary to qualify as a person has been developed by several philosophers and includes the following:

- Self-consciousness
- Capacity to engage in purposeful sequences of action
- Capacity to understand reasons for acting
- Capacity to communicate with other persons through language
- Capacity to make moral judgements
- Ability to reason

Most philosophers believe that more than one of the above cognitive conditions are required to be a person. Using the above cognitive conditions, nonhuman animals may not be able to qualify for significant moral standing. If, however, one considers less demanding cognitive conditions including intention, understanding, desire, preferences, suffering, and having beliefs, then nonhuman animals would likely acquire a significant degree of moral protection. Cavalieri and Singer deny that there are *morally* significant cognitive differences between healthy humans and nonhumans (9). Others have suggested the consideration of noncognitive properties, such as those of sensation, perception, and emotion, when determining which nonhuman animals deserve moral standing (10).

A frequently used word in discussions of moral standing, popularized by Peter Singer, is **speciesism** (11). A **speciesist** believes that the interests of members of the species *Homo sapien* are to be favored over the interests of members of any other species. Singer believes that one cannot use species membership as the sole determining factor as to whether, and to what degree, an entity enjoys moral standing or moral rights. He argues that one must establish morally relevant differences between species in order to justify differences in treatment or moral standing. The term has been co-opted by groups favoring moral standing and rights for nonhuman animals who suggest that *speciesists* fail to respect the lives and right of animals merely because they are nonhuman. The animal rightists are quick to discredit their opponents by labeling them *speciesists* without acknowledging the intense ethical and philosophical history and debate involved in developing this philosophy. Thus, the majority of individuals working to establish a nonhuman animal ethic develop some aspect of speciesism and conclude that nonhuman animals do not have the same standing as humans. Speciesism is a commonly held belief and should not carry negative connotations.

IV. MORAL PHILOSOPHIES

There are a number of moral philosophies that have played, and continue to play, a significant role in the discussion of nonhuman animals and ethics. Knowledge of these philosophies is vital for reflective study in nonhuman animal ethics and much of the current debate relies on the terminology, arguments, priorities, and conclusions elaborated in these theories.

A. UTILITARIAN THEORY

Utilitarian theories are the most widely discussed philosophies in the development of ethical issues about nonhuman animal use. Utilitarianism is rooted in the concept of cost-benefit analysis. An action or practice is right if it leads either to the greatest possible good consequences or to the least possible bad consequences for all affected parties. The majority of the American public rely on principles established in utilitarian theory to support much of their ethics, including those surrounding nonhuman animal use (12). Four conditions are necessary for a theory to qualify as utilitarian:

- **Each action is considered on the basis of the balance it achieves between positive and negative consequences**. If only negative consequences are possible, the correct action should result in the least negative of these consequences. Positive consequences are measured by the second condition, the standard of goodness.
- **The standard of goodness states that the goodness or badness of a consequence is measured by items that count as primary goods**. Primary goods, such as living without pain and distress or living without physical boundaries, are prioritized differently by individual utilitarians. For one utilitarian, the priorities generally remain constant; however, each utilitarian may have different concepts about what constitutes a primary good.
- **Actions are morally right or wrong according to their consequences, rather than by virtue of any intrinsic moral features these actions may have**. Thus, fidelity, trust, altruism, and friendship have little moralistic value to the utilitarian other than the consequences resulting from upholding or failing to uphold the standard.
- **All parties affected by an action must receive impartial consideration**.

Not all utilitarians give equal weight to these conditions, especially the standard of goodness and impartiality clauses, since both of these depend upon one's perspective. For example, research may be beneficial and therefore be judged "good" for the human recipient, but not necessarily for the animals in the experimental protocol. Although much research affects nonhuman animals in a positive manner, the impartiality of this argument is debatable. Therefore, individual utilitarians may develop different recommendations based on different weights given to the above conditions.

One of the pioneering utilitarians was Jeremy Bentham (1748–1832). He argued that nonhuman animals, like humans, have the capacity to feel pain and therefore deserve moral protection (13). He reasoned that even though there are important differences between humans and nonhuman animals, the most relevant similarity was the capacity for **sentience**, that is, the capacity to experience pleasure, pain, and suffering. Bentham argued that the capacity to experience pain was, itself, significant enough to confer at least some significant moral standing. This reasoning underlies a famous, and often cited, quote made by Bentham: "The question is not, can they reason? Nor, can they talk? But, can they suffer?" The implications of such a quote have endured, for it is pain, suffering, and overall welfare, not rationality or self-awareness, that provide the reason many critics object to the use of nonhuman animals in research and food production.

Contemporary utilitarians, such as Peter Singer, acknowledge that many nonhuman animals have desires and preferences about their future and that they experience pain and suffering. Singer maintains that we must justify our involvement of nonhuman animals using a basis that takes into account their interests per the impartiality requirement of utilitarian theory (14). He further argues that one must point to morally relevant differences between species to justify differences in their treatment (3). However, commonly used citations of morally relevant differences including autonomy and self-consciousness do not apply to all human beings. Thus, a newborn baby or comatose patient may not meet the morally relevant difference standards. Therefore, according to Singer, such marginalized humans could not receive differential treatment over nonhuman species. Any attempt to justify animal-based research on the basis of morally relevant differences would therefore have to include certain populations of marginalized humans, who also don't meet the morally relevant difference standard. Armed with these convictions, Singer concludes that it is much more difficult to justify animal experimentation (15). Singer does not completely discount the possibility of animal-based research: "Those that do not involve any, or very much, suffering for the nonhuman animals, and promise major benefits for humans or animals, may be defensible on utilitarian grounds" (15).

Another contemporary utilitarian is Raymond Frey. His practical implications of utilitarianism cause him to reach different conclusions than Singer. Frey argues that the value of any life, human or nonhuman, is contingent upon its quality and that goods in life, such as those defined under utilitarian theory, measure quality (16). Although nonhuman animal life is typically not as rich in goods as human life, some animals have lives that are more valuable than other animals, including humans. Frey believes that the lives of dogs, cats, and chimpanzees, for example, are more valuable than the lives of mice, rats, and worms. Like Singer, Frey believes that the life of a human infant is less rich than the life of an adult chimpanzee and therefore the human infant would have less moral standing than the chimpanzee. According to Frey, life is valuable to human and nonhuman alike only under certain conditions. As life becomes less valuable, it has progressively less moral standing. As the degree of moral standing in nonhuman animals decreases, it becomes increasingly more justifiable to use them in research.

For both Singer and Frey, species membership is not a factor in making moral judgements. It is not one's species, but the quality of one's life, or its utility, that matters most in determining degree of moral standing. Many ethicists reject utilitarianism because it requires too much unfound speculation about consequences, lacks the backbone of any firm principle and requires a balancing of goods and harms that seem, on occasion, to violate human rights or leave minorities vulnerable to abuse.

B. KANTIAN OR DEONTOLOGICAL THEORIES

Deontology is the study of moral obligation and responsibility and has its origin in Immanual Kant (1724–1804). For Kantians, the rightness or wrongness of some actions can be determined no matter what the consequences. In contrast to utilitarianism, there is no requirement for balancing of consequences. Each action can be viewed independently as having intrinsic moral consequences.

Kant's primary principle is the requirement never to treat a person as a means towards one's own end (17). His theories are intended to apply only to rational humans and he explicitly excludes animals from his scope. Kant demands that we must treat persons as "ends in themselves," as having their own autonomously established goals. According to Kant, humans could be used as research subjects but only with proper consent, which must be obtained in a non-manipulative manner. Kant believed that nonhuman animals "must be regarded as man's instruments ... as means to an end. That end is man." Using this philosophy, nonhuman animals have a reduced value because of their status as subhuman animals. This reduced value permits humans to use them in terms of their value to humans.

Kant felt that humans have no direct obligations to nonhumans, however, humans do have *indirect* obligations, from the perspective that actions directed toward nonhumans reflect potential actions toward fellow humans. Using this argument, cruelty toward nonhuman animals does not violate any obligation toward the animals but it does represent an inhumane act by a human, which suggests a proclivity toward cruelty, which may later be directed towards other humans.

Another form of deontologic theory, which uses similar principles but reaches different conclusions, is referred to as "**inherentism**." This is best represented by the writings of Tom Regan. Regan uses the arguments from marginalized humans and concludes that nonhuman animals must also be included in the scope of his theories. Regan argues that both human and nonhuman animals have inherent value because they are "subjects of life." Regan further argues that once this "subject of life" criterion has been met, all other classification traits are arbitrary and of less significance. Therefore, unlike Kant, Regan suggests that all animals that experience life have a moral standing that directly protects them from being treated in certain ways that reduce their lives to the status of mere resources for others. Regan views all other traits used to characterize humans, such as beliefs, desires, and reasoning, as insignificant in the determination of standing. The capacity to experience life is unsurpassed and singular in its conference of standing.

Upon further dissection of Regan's theories, however, one finds definitions of nonhuman animals that contain, among other requirements, a belief system, desires, and intentional acts. This suggests that inherentism does, in fact, embrace a broader definition of standing and leaves his theories open to attack by critics who claim this proves the level of trait is precisely important in determining standing. Reagan's theories also make it exceedingly difficult to draw lines to differentiate which nonhuman animals are subjects of life and which are not. Are insects, cephalopods, and arthropods to be included? In contrast to utilitarian theory, inherentism does not provide the latitude to weigh traits in a utilitarian manner in which the value of life is related to the quality of the primary goods of the subject that possesses them.

Inherentism is an abolitionist philosophy and is used by many animal rights groups to oppose recreational hunting, sports that exploit animals, scientific research involving animals, and the use of animals for food. Inherentism is controversial for a number of reasons. It does not adequately define a set of criteria that attributes inherent values to animals; it rules out all balancing of costs and benefits characteristic of utilitarian theories and it confers too many rights upon animals, while depriving humans of some of their rights.

C. RIGHTS THEORIES

Modern ethical theory revolves around the language of animal rights. Historically, the concept of rights developed as a means by which underrepresented groups of people checked the authoritarian power assumed by the governing authority. Rights are designed to protect individuals from such actions as oppression, unequal treatment, intolerance, and invasion of privacy. To have a right is to be in a position to control what others are required to do (19). Rights give parties a claim, based on a system of rules, which authorizes those parties to affirm, demand, or insist upon what is due to them. Thus, it follows that rights confirm obligations by others (20). If someone holds a right, then others have an obligation (21). Some, but not all, people would further adopt the corollary that any obligation confers a right. If, for example, one assumes an obligation to a nonhuman animal to alleviate pain and distress, then, according to this logic, one acknowledges that nonhuman animals have a right to live without pain and distress. This concept is fundamental to understanding the ethics of nonhuman animal use in research. If one assumes that humans have certain obligations to nonhumans, then by correlation to some, one confers corresponding rights to those obligations upon the nonhumans. Given this logic, it is not surprising that many advocates for animal protection choose to frame their argument on the basis of rights. During the last quarter century, the movement to protect the interests of animals has been co-opted into the movement known as animal rights. It is not difficult to imagine taking this another step and conferring equal rights to nonhuman animals.

The concept that animals have rights and that these rights provide the basis for ethical and political theory has been resisted by many. Utilitarians, for example, see the idea of animal rights as undermining the risk-benefit analysis that provides the basis for utilitarian reasoning. Carl Cohen argues that the ability to claim a right exists only within a community of individuals who can make claims against one another and are authorized to do so (22). He argues that rights are necessarily human because the possessors of rights are persons with the ability for moral judgement and the ability to exercise moral claims. Because animals lack these abilities, Cohen claims they cannot have rights.

This brief historical overview summarizes the major concepts and theories in the field of bioethics. There are other bioethical philosophies and models including contractualism, Humean ethics, and coherence models, but these extend beyond the scope of this overview. It is also important to consider the limitations of each theory and to understand that ethical problems are often complex and must be viewed using multiple perspectives and considerations. It is noteworthy that the values espoused in these theories can, and have been, utilized in different capacities to reach very different conclusions. The remainder of this chapter will focus on laws, regulations, and public perceptions surrounding the use of animals. Specific ethical issues relevant to a laboratory animal facility and the unique role of the manager in this complex environment will be highlighted.

V. LAWS AND REGULATIONS GOVERNING THE CARE AND USE OF RESEARCH ANIMALS

It is important to be well versed in the laws, regulations, and guidelines that comprise the basic framework for providing humane care of research animals before considering the management of specific ethical concerns that may arise in the animal facility setting. Prior to 1963 there were few laws specifically regulating the humane care and use of laboratory animals. Between 1963 and 1985, due to the involvement of numerous groups including the National Institutes of Health (NIH), the Institute for Laboratory Animal Resources (ILAR), and the Public Health Service (PHS), laws, regulations, and guidelines were put into place to assure that animals used in a research setting were used humanely, including the Animal Welfare Act (PL89-544, PL91-579, PL94-279, PL99-198), the United States Department of Agriculture (USDA) regulations (23), PHS Policy (24), and the *Guide for the Care and Use of Laboratory Animals* (the *Guide*) (25). The formation, content, and revision of these regulatory laws and guidelines are discussed in detail in Chapter 6 of this text and in two excellent articles found in the May 1999 issue of the *ILAR Journal* (26, 27).

Two noted animal welfare cases, involving alleged mistreatment of non-human primates in the early 1980s, caused a major public outcry and set many regulatory changes in motion: the monkeys in Edward Taub's laboratory in Silver Spring, Maryland and the baboon studies performed at the Head Injury Clinic at the University of Pennsylvania. The People for the Ethical Treatment of Animals (PETA) and the Animal Liberation Front (ALF) were involved in bringing these cases into the public light. The overwhelming public response to these incidents was instrumental in eliciting increased Congressional pressure to tighten regulations involving the use of research animals. Since the late 1980s, there has been an increasingly cooperative effort between the agencies who regulate and provide oversight of animal research facilities including the USDA (which enforces the Animal Welfare Act), the Office of Laboratory Animal Welfare (OLAW, previously known as the Office for the Protection from Research Risks, which is responsible for the administration of the PHS Policy), and the Association for the Assessment and Accreditation of Laboratory

Animal Care International (AAALAC), a voluntary accrediting organization that utilizes the *Guide,* as well as the aforementioned standards during their accrediting process.

This cooperative process, or "harmonization of standards," is a collaborative effort to institute performance-based standards that evaluate the success of an animal care and use program by observing the direct effects of the program on the animals' health and behavior. This effort has met with approval by the research community who have seen positive results, such as improved daily care, healthier animals, a decrease in the number of painful procedures, and modification of procedures that may cause pain or distress, due to the implementation of performance-based standards.

The animal rights community, however, believes that performance-based standards give institutions too much leeway because they rely on the use of professional judgement in the creation and implementation of animal care programs. They believe that the use of professional judgement leads to inconsistent and inappropriate review of animal care and use programs and a lack of documentation and accountability regarding compliance with animal welfare regulations. Animal rights groups, therefore, argue for the use of engineering-based standards, which measure technical compliance with specifically stated requirements. The controversy over which specific standard will provide the greatest level of protection for laboratory animals remains heated and includes a recent suit by the animal rights groups against the USDA (26).

While the regulatory framework governing the humane care and use of laboratory animals is in place, there is no nationally accepted ethical code pertaining to how, or if, animals should be used in research. Instead, IACUCs, through USDA regulation, PHS Policy, and the *Guide*, have been given the authority to identify and adjudicate animal-related ethical issues at their respective institutions. Committees are charged with the responsibility to assure that pain and distress experienced during proposed procedures is minimized, the number and species of animals used is scientifically justified, alternatives to animal use and procedures are properly explored, and that the proposed research has value to the advancement of scientific knowledge and/ or the benefit of human or animal health. Therefore, each committee independently addresses and institutes animal welfare related policies at its own institution without the benefit of national ethical standards for guidance. Once these policies are enacted, an institutional ethical standard is established, and personnel interacting with the animals are responsible for adherence to these standards.

The philosophical debate over whether or not animals should be used in research has been discussed for centuries, and, due to the complexity and volatility of the issue, may never be completely resolved. The scope of this chapter prevents further discussion of this debate, however, since animals are currently housed and used in biomedical research throughout the world, and detailed laws and regulations are in place to govern their physical care and well-being. The rest of this chapter will address: (1) public perceptions about the use of animals and how these perceptions affect personnel working within the research environment; (2) the role of the animal resource manager in handling ethical concerns; (3) common ethical concerns encountered in the research facility; and (4) communication skills and basic managerial techniques for resolution of animal welfare concerns.

VI. PUBLIC PERCEPTION ABOUT THE USE OF ANIMALS

Public opinion about the ethics of animal use as pets, sources of food and clothing, for entertainment, sport, or as research subjects differs widely and generates a great deal of emotional response. An Associated Press poll, conducted in November 1995, showed that 67% of Americans believed that animals have as much right to live without suffering as humans; 59% felt it was wrong to use animals for their fur; 67% opposed the use of animals in cosmetic testing, but 70% believed it was right to use animals to test medical treatments; and 98% of the people polled ate meat (28). While the majority of the American public support the use of animals in research, this support is not without qualification (29–32). The use of animals may be necessary to pursue medical advancements but animals must be humanely treated, not subjected to painful procedures without the use of analgesics, and the study must be essential for obtaining usable information. Animal rights groups counter that animals should not be used in biomedical research because alternatives such as cell culture, epidemiological studies, and computer simulation can produce similar or better results. This philosophy has not met with wide public acceptance. The majority of the public endorse the view that alternatives such as cell culture and computer simulation play an important role in research, but these alternatives are not always a viable option because they cannot predict how a substance or treatment will react within a complex biological system. It is the issue of humane care and potential pain and distress for research animals that causes the greatest concern with the public. Animal rights groups have specifically targeted these issues in their media campaigns and, as a result, have made a significant impact on public perception. Unfortunately, the biomedical research community has historically been silent on these important issues. Researchers and research advocates need to reach out to the community to educate the public about how animals are actually maintained and cared for in research institutions. National and state biomedical advocacy groups can be a valuable information source for the research community. These groups can provide historical and current information and a balanced perspective between the issues of ethics, animal welfare and the value of research. So, while Americans in general support animal research, it remains an uneasy acceptance and the topic continues to be both controversial and potentially volatile.

The public's uneasy perceptions about what happens to animals in research facilities can cause personnel involved in all facets of animal research to be defensive about the work they do. The reluctance of technicians, managers, veterinarians, investigators, and administrative support staff to discuss specific work duties and responsibilities occurs not only in a public setting but also when socializing with family and friends (33, 34). The reticence to speak is often due to personnel encountering negative perceptions and misconceptions about research facilities. Common misconceptions include beliefs such as: horrible conditions are the norm within animal facilities; most animals experience unrelieved pain and distress during experiments; stolen pets are often used as research subjects; investigators do not like animals and are free to act without recourse; and that research involving animals is unregulated, unnecessary, and repetitive. There is a reluctance to discuss these issues in public for fear of drawing the attention of animal rights activists, leading to reprisals and/ or harassment, either personally or against family members. Laboratory animal personnel should confront these misplaced perceptions and tell the truth so that they can pro-actively redress the animal rightists' mis-information campaign and solicit public support for the appropriate use of animals in research. Personnel need to become familiar with the range of ethical theories that has historically shaped, and continues to shape, current ethical perspectives. Understanding basic ethical tenets allows them to formulate and become comfortable with their own ethos. Once a personal ethos is in place, the individual is better equipped to effectively deal with animal welfare related issues, whether they occur within the research facility or in a public setting.

VII. THE ANIMAL RESOURCE MANAGER AND ETHICAL CONCERNS

Ethical concerns routinely occur in the laboratory animal setting and the animal resource manager is often called upon to appropriately identify, investigate, and resolve these issues. The selection of specific ethical concerns to discuss is relatively easy but the role of an animal resource manager in handling these issues, due to their unique position in the administrative hierarchy, is inherently difficult. Managers are often caught "in the middle" of ethical concerns. They receive information from front line staff members and then function as the conduit of that information to clinical veterinarians, facility directors, principal investigators, research technicians, and/or IACUC members. Managers may then collect the facts surrounding an issue, and find themselves again "in the middle" between front line staff members who are hoping, expecting, or demanding immediate action and resolution of the issue; veterinarians and directors searching for an acceptable "middle ground" and ways to identify mutually acceptable compromises that meet everyone's needs; and principal investigators who demand, expect, or hope for a final resolution of the issue that will ultimately support the ongoing research effort.

Managers are often responsible for assuring that problems involving ethical issues are properly reported. They may be directly responsible for the proper training of animal care staff members or for assuring, through front line supervisors, that staff members are properly trained and are following standard operating procedures. Managers may be held administratively responsible if animal health issues are not reported by animal caretakers, if animals are mishandled by untrained or poorly trained caretakers or supervisory staff, or if investigative staff members do not adhere to IACUC protocols within the facility. The institution may expect the animal resource manager to promptly handle these difficult issues and the manager may, or may not, have the expertise to deal with these problems. To gain expertise and proficiency in managing these issues, the manager should attend continuing education programs, be in a position to provide practical input when animal welfare policies are being formulated, and, if an animal welfare incident occurs, receive consistent administrative support and guidance while the problem is reviewed and resolved.

VIII. COMMON ETHICAL ISSUES ENCOUNTERED IN THE RESEARCH ANIMAL FACILITY

There is no standard biomedical research facility. Facilities vary markedly in their physical size and location; numbers and types of species of animals housed; housing systems used; types of experiments performed; number, type, and educational level of personnel; and administrative structure and function. Notwithstanding these major differences, there are still ethical issues that appear to be universal among facilities. Six ethical concerns, separated into procedural and facility-related concerns, are outlined in an attempt to illustrate the complexity of these types of issues (pros and cons) and to highlight pertinent ethical/policy questions that IACUC members, facility directors, veterinarians, and animal resource managers must consider or address when formulating institutional ethical policies or during problem resolution.

A. ETHICAL CONCERNS INVOLVING COMMON PROCEDURES

1. Tail Clipping for Tissue Collection in Unanesthetized Rodents (35, 36)

Pros
- Tail clipping has a wide margin of safety when performed without anesthesia.
- Sufficient tissue for Southern blot testing can be collected using this method. This test requires the collection of greater amounts of tissue but gives more genetic information than other tests.
- The procedure is quick and easy to perform.
- Minimal personnel training is required to perform the procedure.
- Neonatal rodents experience little or no pain due to immature neural circuitry.

Cons
- Alternative tissue is available for collection (saliva, ear punch tissue, hair) and the methods are less invasive and potentially less painful.
- It is difficult to determine the specific age when anesthesia should be required for the tail clipping procedure.

- Post-procedural complications can occur (bleeding, infection, self-induced trauma).
- Tail clipping without anesthesia causes pain and distress for the animal.
- The use of general anesthesia would increase the time to perform the procedure and the risk of animal death.
- Performing the procedure on unanesthetized animals is stressful for staff personnel.

Ethical/Policy Considerations
- Is, or should, tail clipping be allowed?
- Is tail clipping, without anesthesia, a painful procedure? If the procedure is painful, at what age?
- If tail clipping is allowed, is anesthesia required or just recommended?
- How old should the animal be before administration of anesthesia is required, if at all?
- If the animal is genetically altered and/or "valuable," will anesthesia then be recommended, but not required?
- What is the maximum number of tail clips allowed per animal?
- What is the maximum amount of tail that can be initially clipped and what is the amount of tail that can be clipped in subsequent procedures?
- Are alternative tissue collection methods possible to perform and still obtain the genetic information needed (e.g., ear punch, saliva, hair)?
- Is special training required to perform this procedure?
- Is performing this procedure without anesthesia stressful for technical staff?
- Should post-procedural care of the animals be routinely provided? If so, what level of care will be recommended or required?
- Are there any identifiable early endpoints for animals undergoing this procedure?
- Who is responsible for monitoring adherence to institutional standards?

2. Hypothermia as a Sole Anesthetic Agent in Neonatal Rodents (37–41)

Pros
- Neonates are easily anesthetized with hypothermia.
- Good post-procedural survival rates are seen when hypothermia is used.
- Recovery from hypothermia anesthesia is rapid.
- Animals can be protected during the cooling process.
- Neonatal rodents experience little or no pain due to immature neural circuitry.

Cons
- There is a concern that hypothermia just immobilizes the animals and does not provide anesthesia.
- There are better anesthetic agents available for use in neonatal rodents.
- Hypothermia is not acceptable in other animals as a sole anesthetic agent.
- It is difficult to monitor the degree of cooling in neonatal rodents.
- Animals experience pain and distress caused by the cooling process during induction and by the re-warming process during recovery.

Ethical/Policy Considerations
- Is, or should, hypothermia be used as a sole anesthetic agent in neonatal rodents?

- Will hypothermia provide an adequate plane of anesthesia for the proposed procedures?
- What degree of hypothermia is required (i.e. cooling to what core body temperature) to provide an adequate anesthetic level?
- What is the best cooling method and how will the animal's depth of anesthesia and degree of cooling be monitored during the anesthetic procedure?
- What is the maximum age of the animal that can be anesthetized using this method?
- Are alternative anesthetic agents available and what are their margins of safety in neonatal rodents?
- At what age do rodents experience pain and distress? What steps should be taken to alleviate pain and distress?
- How are pain and distress monitored in neonatal rodents?
- Are the induction and recovery phases of this anesthetic procedure painful?
- Are there any identifiable early endpoints for animals undergoing this procedure?

3. Creation and Use of Animal Models of Chronic Disease (42–45)

Pros
- The technology for creating chronic models of disease by genetic manipulation of animals is now available. Until these techniques became available, there were no good models for most disease conditions.
- Animal models for severe and devastating chronic diseases may closely mimic the human or animal condition.
- Use of chronic animal models allows for rapid discovery of new drugs and treatment regimens.
- Chronic animal models are needed to address conditions in the aging human population and new, emerging transmissible diseases.

Cons
- Animal model development sometimes creates chronic, severe disease conditions in animals.
- It can be difficult to predict (i.e., during the planning phase of the experiment) what adverse clinical effects will be seen in the animal model.
- It can be difficult to predict early experimental endpoints due to lack of information on the nature of the disease that will be induced.
- There is a potential for unrelieved, chronic pain and distress for the animals.
- Working with chronically ill animals can increase stress for technical and animal care staff members.
- Specialized husbandry and veterinary care may be required for chronically ill animals.

Ethical/ Policy Considerations
- Is the creation of this model of chronic disease justified, in relation to the potential amount of pain and distress that may be induced?
- Will the disease created cause unrelieved pain and distress in the animal?
- Have the adverse effects caused by the genetic alteration/ or disease induction been described in the species of animal to be used? If so, what are the adverse effects and how will they be monitored?

- If the adverse effects are not known, how will animals be monitored to assess if adverse effects do occur?
- What is the anticipated duration of the study or life span of the animal?
- How will the presence of pain and distress be assessed?
- Can analgesics be administered without affecting the experimental results? Can other types of supportive care be provided?
- Are animal resources available (housing, space, personnel) to properly care for and clinically manage these animals?
- What specific criteria will be used to determine study endpoints and early endpoints?
- Do personnel working with the animals understand the endpoints?
- Are detailed standard operating procedures in place to care for these animals on weekends and holidays and to euthanize them, in a timely manner, once the early endpoints are met?
- Can early endpoints be met and still maintain the value of the experimental data?

B. ETHICAL CONCERNS INVOLVING FACILITY-RELATED ISSUES

1. Are Animal Care and Research Personnel Adequately Trained?

Pros
- USDA regulations require, and the *Guide* recommends, training of personnel working with animals.
- Professional staff is available at most institutions to provide personnel training.
- Certification and licensing programs in laboratory animal medicine and science are readily available.
- Scientific literature and the Internet are available as information resources for training purposes.

Cons
- The level of training or skill required to enable personnel to perform procedures properly is not specified in the regulations or recommendations.
- An individual's demonstrated knowledge or skill level may not match the training or experience stated in the IACUC protocol.
- High staff turnover requires institutional mechanisms to provide ongoing training and tracking.
- Cultural and language barriers can affect training efforts.
- Institutional training programs and documentation can be costly.
- Resources may not be available at the institution if highly advanced training is required.

Ethical/Policy Considerations
- How is the level of training of personnel working with animals obtained, assessed, and documented?
- Does the information requested adequately address the degree of proficiency required in USDA regulations?

- Is the training information provided by personnel accepted "as is" by the IACUC or is the information checked further?
- If personnel have received animal-related training or experience at another institution, do personnel have to be re-trained?
- Who is responsible for training "untrained" individuals?
- Is training mandatory for any (or all) levels of personnel working with animals (i.e. animal caretakers, supervisors, students, fellows, residents, research technicians, investigators) or is training voluntary?
- If training is provided, should the training be didactic, hands-on, or both?
- Does training need to be provided for all species used and all procedures performed in the facility? Is re-training of current personnel required, and if so, how often?
- If an animal welfare incident occurs, and it is determined that an individual involved in the incident lacks the necessary skills or training to perform the approved procedures, are there institutional procedures in place to recommend or require additional training?
- If training is to be provided by the institution, who provides the training, pays for the training program, and maintains documentation of the training?

2.　Are Animal Welfare Concerns Properly Addressed by the Institution?

Pros
- The IACUC has the responsibility to formulate, review, and enforce institutional policies.
- Community animal welfare interests are represented on the IACUC by the non-affiliated (lay) member.
- External agencies are available to review animal welfare complaints.
- "Whistleblowers" are protected because it is illegal to retaliate against them for raising animal welfare concerns.

Cons
- There are no formal national ethical standards for institutions to use as guidelines in setting or adjudicating animal welfare issues.
- Institutional politics may interfere with the review and resolution of an animal welfare concern.
- IACUC members may not take "Whistleblower" concerns seriously.
- The potential "Whistleblower" may not report concerns, fearing retaliation.
- "Whistleblowers" may experience informal retaliation for raising concerns despite institutional prohibition against retaliation.
- Animal care or research staff members may not know how to report an animal welfare concern.

Ethical/Policy Considerations
- Does the institution have a policy in place to properly identify, review, and resolve animal welfare concerns?
- If an animal welfare incident has occurred, were the procedures outlined in the policy followed and did they work?
- Is the "Whistleblower" policy readily understood and available to all personnel working with animals (i.e., posted in animal facilities, on an institutional Web

page, handed out with other IACUC policy and procedural material, discussed during training sessions)?

- Is the policy reviewed on a regular basis to ensure that all the information is accurate and the procedural steps are still viable?
- Are there major animal welfare concerns in the institution that have been overlooked or that are unresolved due to internal politics? If so, how can these concerns be properly addressed?
- Do lay members on the committee have the authority, knowledge and/or ability to represent the full range of community animal welfare interests?
- Are policies in place to ensure anonymity of the complainant?
- Have staff members either expressed concern about or experienced retaliation for raising animal welfare concerns? If retaliation is suspected, what steps will be taken to protect staff members?
- Is there administrative support from the institutional official for the IACUC and the animal welfare policy decisions that are made?

3. Are Standard Operating Procedures (SOPs) Being Followed and Is Documentation Accurate?

Pros

- SOPs for most procedures are scientifically or medically based and are written to protect animals and/or humans.
- Written procedures are specific and easy to use. These SOPs can be utilized as a reference.
- SOP-oriented training is an effective management tool and provides consistent information for all staff members.
- Staff and supervisors can document completion of SOPs.
- Written SOP documentation can be reviewed by site inspectors and site visitors to determine if procedures are performed properly.

Cons

- Personnel may not follow the SOPs, as written.
- SOP violations can invalidate research data and can endanger animal and/or human health.
- SOP documentation may differ from the procedures that were actually performed.
- Inaccurate documentation can lead to disease outbreaks in animals and humans, regulatory citations, or loss of accreditation status.

Ethical/Policy Considerations

- How does your institution monitor SOP compliance?
- Who performs this type of monitoring (animal facility supervisory staff, veterinary staff, safety officer, occupational health officer, principal investigator)?
- Are there conflicts of interest between monitoring groups, and if so, how are these conflicts resolved?
- If SOP violations occur, is there a policy in place to review the violation and determine the severity of the violation (in terms of animal health, human health, and/or alteration of scientific data interpretation). Are there adequate procedures to handle the incident and monitor for compliance after the incident?

- If the violation involves endangerment of animal health or research integrity (e.g., breaking a barrier facility protocol, mixing up animals between investigators, not checking automatic watering devices leading to an animal's death from dehydration) or human health (e.g., not wearing proper protective clothing required in a biohazard room, not following a Herpes B prevention protocol after exposure to a macaque), who within the institution is notified?
- Who within the institution determines the consequences for SOP violations?
- If personnel become aware of an issue that involves potential scientific fraud involving animals, are they responsible for reporting this and, if so, to whom?

There are currently no nationally recognized standards in place for institutions to use as guidelines when dealing with ethical concerns involving routine procedures, creation of animal models of chronic disease, or any of the facility-related concerns outlined above. IACUCs function independently. The committee, using performance-based standards, has the latitude to determine specific institutional policies or guidelines for each type of concern. The effectiveness of these policies should be evaluated by the IACUC during its semi-annual review of the animal care and use program. The institution's adherence to its own internal policies and guidelines is externally monitored. If the institution is AAALAC accredited, the AAALAC site visitors will review the animal welfare-related policies during their tri-annual program review. The USDA also will review these policies and guidelines during its routine facility inspections.

IX. EFFECTIVE MANAGEMENT OF ETHICAL CONCERNS

Animal resource managers can equip themselves with the knowledge and skills necessary to effectively manage ethical concerns in the laboratory animal facility through education, institutional involvement, and by utilizing basic managerial techniques. Tools that are useful in this regard are listed below.

A. CONTINUING EDUCATION AND TRAINING

The major laboratory animal organizations including AAALAC International, the American Association for Laboratory Animal Science (AALAS), and the American College of Laboratory Animal Medicine (ACLAM) provide didactic or hands-on training opportunities that address animal welfare issues, training methodology, animal rights theories, and regulatory issues. Additionally, the Animal Welfare Information Center, the Scientists Center for Animal Welfare, and local state associations for biomedical research are excellent resources for a wide variety of topics related to the care and welfare of animals. Managers can also find current information available in the laboratory animal scientific literature (*Contemporary Topics*, *Laboratory Animals*, and *Comparative Medicine*). Working knowledge of all laws, regulations, and guidelines pertaining to the proper care and use of laboratory animals and an understanding of ethical theory is essential for the manager to formulate innovative methods to resolve ethical issues. Training personnel about the importance of humane care and use of research animals will also expand the animal resource manager's knowledge base and improve his/her interactive skills. Opportunities for teaching include preparing and presenting lectures, posters, and/or workshop instruction as a part of the institution's in-house training program or at local, regional, or national AALAS meetings. Managers should also become involved in educational programs or events sponsored by schools or civic organizations within the local community.

B.   IACUC MEMBERSHIP

The animal resource manager can serve a unique role as an IACUC member. The institutional official is responsible for appointing IACUC members and often selects members who, among other qualities, have demonstrated a high standard of ethical behavior, have previous experience working with animals, and exhibit a willingness to address difficult issues. IACUC rosters are typically filled with facility directors, clinical veterinarians, scientists, and laypersons but often may lack the additional breadth of technical /administrative personnel. Managers can utilize their administrative, managerial, supervisory, and technical skills to provide a "global" perspective during protocol review, semi-annual program review, and during the investigation of animal welfare incidences. Often, the manager has a historical perspective of previously approved protocols, familiarity with the progress of currently approved studies, and practical insight about potential animal welfare concerns involving new studies or protocols undergoing annual renewal. Managers also can inform the committee if the type of animal resource support being requested in the proposed project is currently available, including appropriate vendors, caging, space within the facility, and special environmental needs. The IACUC has the responsibility to institute policies regarding how certain experimental procedures will be performed (e.g., monoclonal antibody production, tumor production, tail clipping, animal models), procedures for the investigation of animal welfare complaints (i.e., "Whistleblowing" policies), and all other animal welfare related policies. As an active IACUC member, the animal resource manager can become an integral part of the research community by participating in the formulation and review of animal welfare policies that become the working institutional ethical standards.

C.   COMMUNICATION SKILLS AND BASIC MANAGERIAL TECHNIQUES FOR RESOLUTION OF ANIMAL WELFARE CONCERNS

The animal resource manager should strive to create and maintain an open, supportive work environment so that potential or existing ethical concerns are readily identified, discussed, and resolved. The working environment within an animal research facility is inherently difficult. A wide variety of personnel interact with the animals on a daily basis, and these personnel differ greatly with regard to level of education and training, the types and degree of direct experimental involvement they have with animals, and their individual cultural and societal beliefs regarding animal use. These differences create conflicting and overlapping ethical perceptions of each person's role as an animal caretaker, supervisor, manager, veterinary technician, research technician, veterinarian, or research investigator and how that person should or could or does interact with the animals. For example, an individual may perceive his or her specific role to be that of a protector, advocate, data collector, scientific investigator, or care provider. The individual may likewise view the animal as a research subject, clinical patient, data-point, animal model, production unit, or friend.

An additional, overlying nuance in this human-animal interactive environment, which generates strong differences of opinion, is the varying levels of importance that may be assigned to different species of animals. For example, some staff members may consider rodents less important than larger animals, such as dogs, cats, or nonhuman primates. Animals that are considered to be more important are sometimes treated differently. To further complicate the picture, ethical perceptions of the various roles and importance of the animals may overlap or change over time. This change may be seen if the research study starts using a different species of animal (e.g., moves from small animals to larger animals), or if procedures change (e.g., moving from non-survival studies to survival studies), or if specific animals start being housed for a longer period of time (e.g., leading to more interaction which can create a stronger human-animal bond). All of these perceptions and circumstances work together to create a challenging work environment.

Conflicts and disputes surrounding what constitutes proper care and use of animals and issues of pain and distress can rapidly escalate to critical levels if there is not strong leadership within the facility. The animal resource manager is situated in a pivotal administrative position and can utilize this position to be an integral member of the leadership team. When an incident involving animal welfare occurs, the manager can investigate the allegation through a fact-finding mission. After obtaining and documenting the pertinent information submitted from all parties involved, the manager can piece together what most likely occurred and recommend a course of action. Finally, the manager can implement steps or procedures necessary to resolve the incident and coordinate ongoing monitoring to assure that such incidents do not recur. The following managerial techniques can assist managers working through complex situations:

1. Be Responsive

Take on the difficult issues when they arise; don't put them off because they will not go away. As a manager, strive to be an effective resource. If you are willing to address situations openly, fairly, and in a timely manner, personnel will feel comfortable bringing up difficult ethical issues and concerns. While the final outcome of any specific incident may not meet everyone's needs, the manager who is willing to address and is adept at handling these situations will gain the respect of his employees, co-workers, and colleagues.

2.   Be Consistent

Although creative management of animal welfare concerns involves adjudicating a wide range of perceptions, interests and needs, consistency is essential for maintaining credibility and effectiveness as a manager.

3.   Have Standard Operating Procedures in Place

To appropriately identify, address, and resolve ethical issues, it is essential to pro-actively formulate and institute standard policies and procedures and use them as a framework for working through specific issues. If all personnel responsible for the humane care and use of research animals, including IACUC members and animal facility personnel, can agree upon a working philosophy that is tailored to their institutional needs, this will provide a uniform approach to resolving animal welfare issues.

4.   Do Not Blame

Assigning blame creates a negative, hostile environment that is rarely conducive to effective resolution of any problem. If staff feel blamed they are often reluctant to bring up problems or supply accurate information about an ongoing issue.

5.   Encourage Dialogue and Develop Communication Skills

Do not judge. Feelings are being expressed and these feelings should be validated. Be available to talk with personnel when issues arise and listen, with an open mind, to all sides of the issue.

Using these managerial techniques will help the animal resource manager set a positive tone within the facility that will foster a good working relationship between animal care, research, and facility support staff and encourage the timely resolution of ethical concerns.

Identification and management of ethical concerns in the laboratory animal research setting is a complex and difficult task, but one that can be extremely rewarding. The animal resource manager can effectively manage these issues by studying the historical ethical theories of animal protection, developing a personal ethical standard, understanding the progression and current state of animal use laws and regulations, providing input during policymaking decisions, and fine-tuning personal communication skills by utilizing basic managerial techniques. This multifaceted managerial approach will give the animal resource manager the information, skills, and confidence needed to identify and resolve ethical concerns within the institution.

REFERENCES

1. **British Cruelty to Animals Act of 1876.**
2. **Orlans, F.B., Beauchamp, T.L., Dresser, R., Morton, D.B., and Gluck, J.P.,** Moral issues about animals, in *The Human Use of Animals*, Oxford University Press, New York, 1998.
3. **Russow, L.M.,** Bioethics, animal research, and ethical theory, *ILAR J.,* 40,15, 1999.
4. **Descartes, R.,** Animals are machines, in *Animal Rights and Human Obligations*, 2nd ed., Regan, T. and Singer, P., Eds., Prentice-Hall, Englewood Cliffs, NJ, 1989.
5. **Hume, D.,** A treatise of human nature, in *Hume's Enquiries*, Selby-Bigge, L.A. and Nidditch, P., Eds., Oxford University Press, Oxford, 1978.
6. **Darwin, C.,** The descent of man (1871), in *Philosophy and the Human Condition*, 2nd ed., Beauchamp, T.L., Feinberg, J., and Smith, J.M., Eds., Prentice-Hall, Englewood Cliffs, NJ, 1989.
7. **Francione, G.L.,** *Animals, Property, and the Law*, Temple University Press, Philadelphia, 1995.
8. **Lamborn, C.,** Court upholds ALDF suit, *Lab Anim.*, 27, 10, 1998.
9. **Cavalieri, P. and Singer, P.,** *The Great Ape Project*, St. Martin's Press, New York, 1993.
10. **DeGrazia, D.,** *Taking Animals Seriously – Mental Life and Moral Issues*, Cambridge University Press, New York, 1996.
11. **Singer, P.,** *Animal Liberation*, 2nd ed., New York Review/Random House, New York, 1990.
12. **Rowan, A.N.,** Formulation of ethical standards for use of animals in medical research, *Toxicol. Lett.* 67, 1, 1993.
13. **Benthem, J.,** *Introduction to the Principles of Morals and Legislation* (1789), Hafner, New York, 1948.
14. **Singer, P.,** *Practical Ethics*, 2nd ed., Cambridge University Press, New York, 1993.
15. **Singer, P.,** Animal experimentation: philosophical perspectives, in *The Encyclopedia of Bioethics,* Reich, W., Ed., Free Press, New York, 1978.
16. **Frey, R.G.,** Moral standing, the value of lives, and speciesism, in *Between the Species* 4, no. 3, Clarendon Press, Oxford, 1988.
17. **Kant, I.,** *Foundations of the Metaphysics of Morals* (1785), Beck, L.W., Trans., Bobbs Merrill Company, Indianapolis, IN, 1959.
18. **Regan, T.,** *The Case for Animal Rights,* University of California Press, Berkeley, 1983.
19. **Hart, H.L.A.,** Bentham on legal rights, in *Oxford Essays in Jurisprudence*, 2nd ser., Simpson, A.W.B., Ed., Oxford University Press, Oxford, 1973.
20. **Feinberg, J.,** *Social Philosophy*, Prentice-Hall, Englewood Cliffs, NJ, 1973.
21. **Braybrooke, D.,** The firm but untidy correlatively of rights and obligations, *Can. J. Phil.*, 1, 351, 1972.
22. **Cohen, C.,** The case for the use of animals in research, *New England J. Med.,* 315, 865, 1986.
23. **CFR (Code of Federal Regulations), Title 9; parts 1, 2, and 3 (Docket No. 89-130),** Federal Register, Vol. 544, No. 168, August 31, 1989, and **9 CFR Part 3 (Docket No. 90-218)**, Federal Register, Vol. 56, No. 32, February 15, 1991.
24. **Public Health Service Policy on Humane Care and Use of Laboratory Animals**, U.S. Department of Health and Human Services, National Institutes of Health, Bethesda, MD, 1996.

25. Committee to Revise the *Guide for the Care and Use of Laboratory Animals*, *Guide for the Care and Use of Laboratory Animals*, National Research Council, National Academy Press, Washington, D.C., 1996.

26. **Sideris, L., McCarthy, C., and Smith, D.H.**, Roots of concern with nonhuman animals in biomedical ethics, *ILAR J.*, 40, 3, 1999.

27. **Vandeberg, J.L., Blangero-Williams, S., and Wolfle, T.L.**, U.S. laws and norms related to laboratory animals, *ILAR J.*, 40, 34, 1999.

28. **Masci, D.**, Fighting over animal rights, *The CQ Researcher*, 6, 673, 1996.

29. **Tannenbaum, J.**, Animal research, in *Veterinary Ethics – Animal Welfare, Client Relations, Competition and Collegiality,* 2nd ed., Duncan, L.L., Ed., Mosby Year Book, Inc., St. Louis, 1995, chap. 24.

30. **Orlans, F.B.**, Current attitudes and ethical arguments, in *In the Name of Science – Issues in Responsible Animal Experimentation,* 1st ed., Oxford University Press, Inc., New York, 1993, chap. 2.

31. **Trull, F.L.**, The research movement, *Lab Anim.*, 23, Apr. 1994.

32. **Macrina, F.L. et al.**, Use of animals in biomedical experimentation, in *Scientific Integrity*, Macrina, F.L., Ed., ASM Press, Washington, D.C., 1995, chap. 5.

33. **Szymczyk, J.**, Animals, vegetables and minerals: I love animals, and can still work with them in a research laboratory, *Newsweek*, 10, Aug. 1995.

34. **Goodwin, F.K.**, Animal rights: medical research and product testing: is this a "hang together or together we hang" issue? *Contemp. Top.*, 31, 6–11, Jan. 1992.

35. **Irwin, M.H., Moffatt, R.J., and Pinkert, C.A.**, Identification of transgenic mice by PCR analysis of saliva, *Nature Biotech.*, 14, 1146, 1996.

36. **Hogan, B., Bedington, R., Costarini, F., and Lacy, E.**, in *Manipulating the Mouse Embryo: A Laboratory Manual*, Cold Spring Harbor Laboratory Press, Cold Spring Harbor, NY, 1994.

37. **Phifer, C.B. and Terry, L.M.**, Use of hypothermia for general anesthesia in preweanling rodents, *Phys. and Behavior*, 38, 887, 1986.

38. **Davis, P.J.**, Pain in the neonate: the effects of anesthesia, *ILAR News*, 33 (1–2), 1991.

39. **Danneman, P.J. and Mandrell, T.D.**, Evaluation of six anesthesia regimens in neonatal rats, *Contemp. Top.*, 35(4), 60, 1996.

40. **Park, C.M.**, Improved techniques for successful neonatal rat surgery, *Lab. Anim. Sci.*, 42(5), 508, 1992.

41. **Preparation and Maintenance of Higher Mammals during Neuroscience Experiments**, U.S. Department of Human Health and Human Services, NIH Publication #91-3207, 23, 1991.

42. **Rollin, B.**, An ethical dilemma for animal research: the creation of transgenic animal "models" for human genetic disease, in *Genetic Engineering and Animal Welfare: Preparing for the 21st Century*, Gonder, J.C., Prentice, E.D., and Russow, L., Eds., Scientists Center for Animal Welfare, Greenbelt, MD, 1999, 96–108.

43. **Gordon, J.**, Transgenic technology and its impact on laboratory animal science. *Scand. J. Lab. Anim. Sci.*, 23, 235, 1996.

44. **Gordon, J.**, Transgenic animals and laboratory animal science, *ILAR J.*, 38, 32, 1997.

45. **Gordon, J.**, Transgenic animal models of disease, in *Biological Aspects of Disease: Contributions of Animal Models*, Iannacone, P.M. and Scarpelli, D.G., Eds., Gordon and Breach, Abingdon, U.K., 1997, 15–37.

5 Animal Health and Medicine

Mark A. Suckow, D.V.M., Dipl. ACLAM
and Brent J. Martin, D.V.M., Dipl. ACLAM

I. BACKGROUND

A critical aspect of proper management of the animal resource program involves provision of adequate veterinary care. Such efforts optimize animal health and facilitate humane conditions for animals and eliminate the costs associated with disease outbreaks, while assuring investigators that healthy and acceptable research subjects are being provided.

This chapter will describe a number of facets related to management of animal health and medicine. A key to effective management of the laboratory animal care resource is to understand the role and responsibilities of veterinary care. Methods to approach management challenges associated with the role of the veterinarian, medical facilities and equipment, and medical care programs are discussed. Descriptions of approaches are not exhaustive, but are offered as examples of strategies the authors have found to be effective.

Because the veterinarian is the individual most often recognized by regulatory agencies as the person responsible for veterinary care, this chapter will focus on the role of the attending veterinarian. It should be recognized, however, that several other individuals play an important role in delivery of veterinary care, including those listed below.

A. Veterinary Technician

Individuals with specific training in the care, health, and basic biology of animals are valuable members of the veterinary team. Often, such individuals have a 2- or 4-year degree in veterinary technology and are designated as a "Registered," "Certified," or "Licensed" Veterinary Technician (RVT, CVT, or LVT), depending upon state licensure. Through experience and training, veterinary technicians typically are skilled at animal handling, record keeping, and technical procedures such as injections and blood sampling; familiar with procedures for aseptic surgery; and adept at assessing the needs of animals and providing appropriate care. Many institutions rely heavily on veterinary technicians to provide the "hands-on" care to the animals, under the direction of a veterinarian. Small institutions often choose to employ a veterinary technician and use a veterinarian on a part-time consulting basis. Veterinary technicians provide a valuable interface between the animal care unit and investigators. Not only are they in a position to help ensure adequate animal health, but their technical skills are also of great value to investigators who need to perform surgery, sampling, compound administration, or other procedures involving animals.

B. Animal Technician

Individuals with background in laboratory animal science can become certified by the American Association for Laboratory Animal Science (AALAS) as an Assistant Laboratory Animal Technician (ALAT), a Laboratory Animal Technician (LAT), or a Laboratory Animal Technologist (LATG). The training typically required to pass the certification examination includes information relevant to animal health. Such individuals are usually well prepared to recognize and record signs of disease and understand procedures for reporting sick animals. They are generally familiar with basic requirements for animal health, such as proper nutrition, environmental conditions, environmental enhancement, sanitation, and the need for proper care of animals following procedures such as survival surgery.

C. Institutional Official

Although not directly involved in hands-on animal health, the Institutional Official (IO) plays a critical role. The IO is designated as the individual who is authorized to legally commit on behalf of the research facility that regulatory requirements will be met. In this regard, the IO wields considerable leverage to promote proper animal care and health. Along with the Chief Executive Officer (CEO) of the institution, the IO is in a position to coordinate resources to support efforts directed at animal health.

II. ROLE OF THE VETERINARIAN

A. ROLE OF THE VETERINARIAN AS DEFINED BY REGULATIONS

Veterinarians play a variety of roles in the research environment. While these roles are generally based on practical job development, the expectations and descriptions of the veterinarian's role as defined by regulatory guidelines cannot be ignored. The words "veterinary" and "veterinarian" appear more than 150 times in the the Animal Welfare Act Regulations (AWAR), thus demonstrating the importance that this key legal document lends to the role of the veterinarian in humane animal care and use. The AWAR define the "attending veterinarian" as follows:

"***Attending veterinarian*** *means a person who has graduated from a veterinary school accredited by the American Veterinary Medical Association's*

Council on Education, or has earned a certificate issued by the American Veterinary Medical Association's Education Commission for Foreign Veterinary Graduates, or has received equivalent formal education as determined by the Administrator; has received training and/or experience in the care and management of the species being attended; and who has direct or delegated authority for activities involving animals at a facility subject to the jurisdiction of the Secretary."

The USDA has not specifically defined the quality or quantity of the required training or experience. A common interpretation of this requirement is that the graduate veterinarian has completed several years of post-doctoral training under the tutelage of experienced veterinarians. Board certification by the American College of Laboratory Animal Medicine (ACLAM) is generally considered to be evidence of sufficient knowledge and experience for the veterinarian. Many facilities successfully utilize veterinarians who are not ACLAM board certified; however, caution must be exercised, as the basic veterinary education usually includes little information about laboratory animals and even less with respect to veterinary care issues in the research environment.

As a practical matter, it is worthwhile for the attending veterinarian, or another veterinarian at the facility, to be licensed in the state in which the institution is located. For example, the AWAR (§2.38.h) state that the health certificate accompanying an animal to be shipped must be issued by a licensed veterinarian. Acquisition of controlled substances requires a valid veterinary license. Beyond the practical aspects, many research facilities require a state veterinary license even though the institutional veterinary care activities may not fall within the individual state veterinary practice regulations. In this regard, veterinarians and institutions should review the requirements for licensure within their states.

B.   ROLE OF THE VETERINARIAN AS DEFINED BY VETERINARY CARE RESPONSIBILITIES

The most readily understood role of the veterinarian is the administration of veterinary medical care. This encompasses the standard concepts of disease diagnosis, treatment, control, and prevention (§2.31.d.1.vii and §2.33.b.2). A prudent approach to the delivery of veterinary care will accommodate reasonable and necessary limitations dictated by the nature of the research project. In some cases, proper medical care may be inconsistent with the research goals. However, the veterinarian still retains ultimate and complete authority and responsibility for veterinary medical care. In some cases, euthanasia or removal of the animal from the study may be the only reasonable alternatives when research goals cannot be met if proper veterinary care is delivered. It is reasonable to presume that serious medical problems that cannot be properly treated within the confines of the research project may represent significant variables that could invalidate the research. Time and effort in such cases is often best spent in planning future procedures in light of the lessons learned from the failed case.

An attempt at definition of "adequate veterinary care" is provided in the AWAR (§2.33.a). However, because veterinary care is administered through a filter of professional judgement with respect to a great variety of factors, it is an inexact science not well suited to precise definition (1–5). In any event, the care provided should be comparable to that currently accepted in veterinary practice (AWAR §2.33.b.5). This encompasses pre- and post-operative care, maintenance of medical records, aseptic technique, availability and use of appropriate methods to diagnose and treat illness and injury, daily observation of animals, and facilities, equipment and personnel sufficient to perform these functions. The USDA has further clarified several features of adequate veterinary care in its Policy Manual. These policies address issues such as the use of expired pharmaceuticals and other medical materials, euthanasia, medical records, and the availability of necropsy capabilities (6, 7). Adequate veterinary care should be available at all institutions, regardless of the research mission.

A key feature of adequate veterinary care is that it should be available at all times. This can present logistical problems when the veterinary staff consists of a single individual, and the situation is further compounded when veterinary care is exclusively provided through a part-time consulting arrangement. The need for medical care can develop at any time, in effect putting the veterinarian on call 24 hours a day. Medical care needs can be controlled to some extent by effective preventive medicine programs. In addition, veterinary medical care can often be administered by trained technical staff such as veterinary technicians functioning under the purview of the veterinarian. In this regard, it is important that sufficient personnel are on staff for adequate delivery of veterinary care.

With respect to part-time and consultant veterinary care, there is no diminution in the veterinarian's responsibilities related to veterinary care. In the case of facilities using only part-time veterinary services, regularly scheduled visits are required although the frequency of these visits is not dictated by regulations. However, the AWAR require that the schedule be included in a written program of veterinary care (§2.33.a.1). An outline for the program of veterinary care is available from the USDA and is usually included with the application for registration sent to new facilities. This program is a document that is likely to be reviewed during visits by the USDA inspector.

By default, the veterinarian usually carries the responsibility for legal use of pharmaceuticals in the animal care and use program. A number of state and federal regulations control the use and dispensing of pharmaceuticals in animals (8). Few pharmaceuticals are approved for use in laboratory animals. Use of drugs that are not approved for a particular species constitutes "extra label" use and carries additional responsibilities. The prevailing, and perhaps the only viable, view is that such extra label use is being done either as part of an approved animal use protocol or under veterinary supervision as an authentic veterinarian-client relationship (9). In this regard, the veterinarian needs to develop systems and policies that eliminate or minimize drug use which does not incorporate either direct or indirect supervision. This is particularly critical regarding drug use in animals, such as cattle, that could end up in the human food chain. Reputable pharmaceutical suppliers who require veterinary license information for purchases provide some assistance with this issue.

Part of an adequate program of veterinary care includes assurance that pharmaceuticals work as intended. In this regard, the USDA has stipulated that **expired pharmaceuticals cannot be used in survival procedures and expired drugs used to control pain cannot be used under any circumstance (6). Expired drugs also should not be used for treatment of clinically ill animals.** Sometimes, pharmaceuticals are formulated at the facility from chemical grade compound if the needed material is not otherwise available. Because such formulations can be of dubious efficacy and sterility and may be contaminated with pyrogens, use of such material is not permitted if a pharmaceutical grade product is available (6).

The use of controlled substances presents special challenges for the veterinarian. Controlled substances are those pharmaceuticals that have the potential for human abuse and therefore require registration with the U.S. Drug Enforcement Administration (DEA) for purchase. For example, many anesthetics and analgesics are controlled substances. Considerable variation exists among facilities with respect to mechanisms for procurement and use of controlled substances. Possible methods of management range from requiring that all such drugs be purchased by the veterinarian, to individual investigators obtaining DEA "research use" registrations (which do not require a medical degree) for acquisition and use of such compounds. In any case, when drugs are purchased under the veterinarian's registration, that veterinarian is responsible for secure storage and accurate records of use.

C. ROLE OF THE VETERINARIAN ON THE INSTITUTIONAL ANIMAL CARE AND USE COMMITTEE

Both the AWAR (§2.31.b.i) and the Public Health Service (PHS) Policy (IV.A.3.b.1) require that the Institutional Animal Care and Use Committee (IACUC) include as a full voting member a veterinarian with training or experience in laboratory animal science and medicine and who has direct or delegated responsibility for activities involving animals at the institution. The general interpretation is that this individual is the attending veterinarian for the institution, but neither document offers further guidance on the expected role of the veterinarian. It has been argued that the veterinarian has special authority in matters of humane treatment of animals, but there appears to be no statutory basis for that belief (10). There exists a tacit expectation by both USDA and Office for Laboratory Animal Welfare (OLAW) officials that the veterinarian's contributions should carry particular weight in deliberations concerning animal health and welfare, although no official documents exist in this regard. Generally, most IACUC members seem to acknowledge the training and expertise of the veterinarian with respect to animal care, behavior, biology, and medicine and rely upon that knowledge. Typically, the veterinary member of the IACUC advises the committee with respect to aseptic technique and peri-operative care, recognition of pain, appropriate use of anesthetics and analgesics, overall medical care and preventive care for the animals, and any other issue that might affect animal health and welfare. The veterinarian should also be qualified to provide the IACUC with insight into animal behavior and means of environmental enrichment, alternative methods to minimize the likelihood of pain and distress to animals, and acceptable standards for husbandry of animals.

A veterinarian trained and certified (by ACLAM) in laboratory animal medicine is often the most knowledgeable individual at the facility in matters related to regulatory requirements, and thus helps define the role of the IACUC. It should be noted that as a recognized expert, the veterinarian may also have some liability for advising the institution on animal regulatory matters (11, 12).

Aside from the general role as an IACUC member, the veterinarian has some special responsibilities as described in the AWAR. Critical reading of the AWAR shows that the veterinarian is required to be involved with the planning stages of projects that include potentially painful or distressful procedures (§2.31.d.1.iv.B). In many cases, a well-trained veterinarian can provide advice with respect to animal care and handling, and in this way help to lessen animal pain and distress. In addition, programs for environmental enhancement for nonhuman primates and canine exercise must be approved by the attending veterinarian (§3.8 and 3.81). The veterinarian is to determine specifics of these programs, including frequency, duration and methods. Investigator training and exceptions to regulations are also veterinary responsibilities according to the AWAR.

D. ROLE OF THE VETERINARIAN IN TRAINING

According to the AWAR and the PHS Policy (IV.C.1.f), the institution has a responsibility to assure that personnel conducting animal research are adequately trained to perform their duties, and that this training is reviewed by the IACUC. According to the AWAR, training must be provided in the following areas:

1. The basic needs of each species being used
2. Proper handling and care for the species being used
3. Proper pre- and post-procedural care of animals
4. Aseptic surgical methods
5. Methods to limit the use of animals or minimize animal distress
6. Proper use of anesthetics, analgesics, and tranquilizers for the species used
7. Procedures to report deficiencies in animal care and treatment
8. Use of services such as the National Agricultural Library and National Library of Medicine to find information related to proper methods for

animal care and use, alternatives to the use of live animals in research, the intent and requirements of the Animal Welfare Act, and to prevent unnecessary duplication of research involving animals

In addition, the AWAR indicate that adequate veterinary care includes guidance on handling, immobilization, anesthesia, analgesia, tranquilization, and euthanasia (§2.33.b.4). The *Guide* repeats this guideline and specifically indicates that it is the veterinarian's responsibility.

The veterinarian is often assigned the task of providing the training to research personnel. This is appropriate, since the typical veterinary education includes many of the relevant topics, including aseptic technique, surgical methods, anesthesia, analgesia, and euthanasia. Methods of handling, care, and species-specific needs and biology are usual components of specialized training in laboratory animal medicine. Often, the overall training program records are overseen by another individual who coordinates training and recruits the veterinarian to actively participate with instruction. The veterinarian and ancillary personnel, such as veterinary technicians, are often experienced and effective at "wet lab" instruction involving hands-on training in procedures and methods.

Guidance from the veterinarian with respect to the use of pharmaceuticals to control pain can generally be accomplished through two methods. First, the veterinarian often develops a formulary of useful drugs, dosages, routes, and frequencies of administration for individual species. The formulary can be distributed to investigators as either a paper booklet or as an electronic document. Second, the veterinarian can provide guidance prior to and during the IACUC protocol review process.

E.   ROLE OF THE VETERINARIAN IN HUSBANDRY AND PROGRAM OVERSIGHT

Of the roles expected of the veterinarian as described in the regulations, the one addressed in the most obscure way is that of "program responsibility." In several places, the AWAR indicate a role that is clearly broader than that traditionally viewed as veterinary practice. For example, in defining the veterinarian who is assigned to the IACUC, the regulations indicate that the veterinarian must have "direct or delegated program responsibility for activities involving animals" (§2.31.b.i and §2.33.a.3). The PHS Policy contains a similar definition (IV.A.3.b.1). While these statements could be interpreted to suggest "activities" of a veterinary medical nature, the AWAR go on to indicate that facilities:

"....shall assure that the attending veterinarian has appropriate authority to ensure the provision of adequate veterinary care *and to oversee the adequacy of other aspects of animal care and use*;" (emphasis added) (§2.33.a.2 and §2.40.a.2).

Presumably, this requirement is in recognition of the veterinarian's "generalist" training in animal care, biology, behavior, herd health, and factors that affect physiological stability and animal welfare and that should be incorporated into overall facility programs. The *Guide* offers some additional guidance with respect to what may constitute "other aspects" by listing animal husbandry and nutrition, sanitation practices, zoonosis control, and hazard containment. Because program decisions such as which bedding and food are used can have unintended effects on research, the veterinarian should be included in such decisions (13, 14).

In practice, the attending veterinarian is often appointed as the director of the laboratory animal resource and subsequently has extensive program responsibility inherent in that position. In any event, the attending veterinarian is often a key contributor to management decisions related to regulatory compliance.

F.   ROLE OF THE VETERINARIAN IN ALLOWING EXCEPTIONS TO STANDARDS

Regulatory documents indicate specific requirements for a number of parameters related to the care and use of animals. In general, these requirements must be adhered to without exception. Still, in some unusual circumstances, the veterinarian may determine that the needs of the animal are met by conditions other than those specifically described by regulations. For example, the AWAR indicate temperature ranges for dogs and cats (§3.2.a and §3.3.a) and nonhuman primates (§3.77.a). Temperatures outside of the specified ranges can be allowed following approval by the attending veterinarian. In some situations, the veterinarian may be able to approve housing situations that are not generally acceptable under the AWAR. This might occur in a situation such as a bitch or queen with a litter size that is larger than is typically anticipated. If the cages were not able to legally accommodate the group, the veterinarian could assess whether this crowding situation actually impacted animal welfare (§3.6.c.ii). Similarly, canine exercise requirements described in the AWAR (§3.8) require that the attending veterinarian approve the plan for provision of exercise.

The regulations are somewhat flexible to allow for adjustments based upon the professional judgement of the attending veterinarian (§3.8.b.2 and §3.8.d.1). For example, the AWAR require feeding of rabbits at least once daily, unless otherwise required to provide adequate veterinary care (§3.54.a). With respect to nonhuman primates, the AWAR require environmental enhancement (§3.81). Certain nonhuman primates must be provided special attention regarding enhancement of their environment, based on the needs of the individual species and in accordance with the instructions of the attending veterinarian. The attending veterinarian is also allowed the flexibility to exempt specific animals from the program of environmental enhancement or specific program components, such as group housing.

It should be clearly understood that all exemptions and exceptions to regulatory standards are allowed only under circumstances in which the exception would still allow delivery of proper veterinary care. Although some exemptions to standards can be granted to accommodate specific research needs, the IACUC, rather than the attending veterinarian, must approve such exceptions.

G. ROLE OF THE VETERINARIAN BASED UPON PROFESSIONAL KNOWLEDGE

1. Aseptic Technique

Introduction of foreign material into surgically exposed tissues imposes the risk of infection to an animal. Even an amount of material too small to visually discern may carry potentially harmful bacteria. Although many, if not most, surgical wounds are exposed to bacteria, the use of aseptic procedures minimizes the likelihood that such exposure will develop into an actual infection.

The AWAR (§2.31.d.ix) and the *Guide* both state the need for the use of aseptic technique and procedures during survival surgery. In this regard, it is the role of the attending veterinarian to develop, implement, and ensure compliance with policies and procedures consistent with the goal of reducing microbial contamination during survival surgery.

First, the attending veterinarian should assure that the **location** of the surgery is amenable to asepsis. Ideally, surgical facilities will be located in an area that has an air pressure which is positive to the outside room or corridor. Some surgical facilities utilize a HEPA-filtered air supply, either by use of a biological safety cabinet or by use of a clean room, as a means of controlling airborne contaminants. It is preferable to have the surgery location apart from areas used for other, unrelated purposes but near surgical support areas.

Second, the attending veterinarian should ensure that proper **procedures** are used. In general, proper aseptic technique includes use of sterile instruments and equipment, use of sterile apparel by the surgeon(s), and appropriate preparation of the animal.

Sterile instruments and equipment must be used for all survival surgeries. The most common method of sterilization is by steam autoclave. Some facilities choose to soak equipment in sterilant chemicals; however, sterilization times are generally long and this method may therefore be impractical (15). It should be noted that ethyl alcohol is neither a sterilant nor a high level disinfectant. Equipment made of material that cannot withstand the autoclaving process can be sterilized by exposure to ethylene oxide or other chemical sterilants.

In some circumstances, multiple animals undergo surgery in sequence and the same instruments are used between animals. Glass bead sterilizers have been shown to be an effective means of quickly sterilizing the working tips of instruments in such situations (15).

A critical aspect of proper procedure is that the surgeon(s) prepare him/herself for aseptic surgery. This generally involves performing a surgical scrub on the hands and forearms with an antiseptic solution and wearing of appropriate apparel including sterile gloves, gown, face mask, and hair bonnet. The exact apparel worn depends upon the species and the procedure to be performed, but at a minimum sterile gloves and a face mask should be worn. In addition, it is advisable for the surgeon to wear a sterile gown. For procedures involving nonhuman primates or other animals that might potentially harbor infectious zoonotic agents, it is also important that personnel wear eye protection such as goggles.

The animal should be properly prepared for aseptic surgery. This usually involves clipping the hair at the designated incision site, scrubbing the incision site with an antiseptic such as 10% povidone-iodine, and isolating the incision site with sterile drapes.

Third, the attending veterinarian should ensure that proper **training** in aseptic and surgical technique has been provided to personnel. This may be accomplished through classroom lecture in basic surgical methods, although hands-on practice is usually very effective. The attending veterinarian should also help ensure that personnel can competently practice the methods they have learned. It is important that a member of the veterinary staff observe and document acceptable competency and ability of personnel in aseptic technique and other practices related to invasive procedures. The attending veterinarian should ensure that records of training and documentation of competency are maintained for all personnel involved in surgical procedures on animals.

2.   Surgical Technique and Method

As described above for training in aseptic procedures, it is the responsibility of the attending veterinarian to ensure that individuals performing invasive procedures on animals are adequately qualified and competent. This is frequently accomplished with initial classroom instruction and subsequent hands-on practice. The basic handling of surgical instruments and suturing of incisions can be practiced on inanimate objects such as foam rubber or even an orange. Personnel should be familiar with different types of instruments and how to properly handle them. Some institutions may even allow practice on anesthetized animals being used in nonsurvival procedures. Those undergoing training should observe and even assist with actual surgeries to obtain experience with aseptic procedure, anesthesia, hemostasis, and postoperative care.

In some instances it is more practical for a trained member of the veterinary staff to conduct invasive procedures. In this way, the facility can be more certain that proper basic procedures will be followed for the overall care of the animal. Indeed, many facilities choose to create and staff surgical support services that provide a location, staff, and all basic equipment needed to conduct studies involving surgery. Some even choose to provide individuals skilled in veterinary surgery, while others allow investigators to conduct the procedure. In either case, it is common for use of such facilities to be accessed on a recharge system to the investigator.

3.   Occupational Health and Zoonotic Disease

A variety of occupational health risks exist within the typical research animal facility, including physical, chemical, radiologic, and infectious hazards. The attending veterinarian should play a key role in developing and implementing procedures to minimize these risks, and work to identify risks within the facility and animal research programs.

An important component of the occupational health program is education of personnel. The veterinarian should coordinate training with the extant risk management group for the facility. In some cases, this will include the veterinarian developing written materials summarizing the risk and steps that should be taken to minimize the risk; in other cases this material may be communicated through actual discussions between the veterinarian and personnel.

The veterinary staff should help establish standard operating procedures (SOPs) for handling of hazardous materials such as animals infected with zoonotic pathogens and related waste materials, radioisotopes, and chemicals (experimental or chemicals used in facility sanitation). SOPs should describe the type of hazard and likely routes of exposure and then specifically detail protective equipment to be worn and procedures to be followed.

Some hazards, particularly those involving infectious pathogens, require special housing and ventilation systems to contain the hazard. Quarantine/isolation areas should be located distant from common use areas. Special caging systems such as cubicles, microisolators, and ventilated racks can be used to contain animals posing a zoonotic risk. In all cases, the veterinarian should play a key role in planning for the facilities and equipment needed for risk management.

The veterinarian can also play a role by advising investigators about the specific animal to be used. For example, the veterinarian might advise the investigator to acquire specific pathogen-free (SPF) animals rather than conventional animals. Although most commercially available rodents are SPF, the veterinarian should regularly scrutinize vendor health reports to assure that testing has proven the source to be free of infectious zoonotic pathogens such as lymphocytic choriomeningitis virus. For other species, the veterinarian should also assist in identifying sources of low-risk animals. For example, the veterinarian might locate a source of SPF sheep that would pose a lower risk for zoonotic diseases such as contagious ecthyema. The veterinarian might further advise the investigator about animal behavior. For example, if a less aggressive species might serve as an adequate research or teaching model, the veterinarian should suggest that species to the investigator, thereby lowering the risk of traumatic injury to handlers and researchers.

4.   Sanitation

Recommendations for appropriate sanitation of equipment, caging, and facilities should be developed with input from veterinary staff members, who are uniquely qualified to understand the nature of infectious disease and the risk it poses to animals, particularly research animals. The veterinarian should provide advice about infectious pathogens likely to be encountered with particular groups of animals and what steps should be taken toward disinfection. For example, if rhesus monkeys are to be housed in a certain area, the veterinarian might consider that many quaternary ammonium compounds are tuberculocidal and would be useful in this situation. In addition, the veterinarian should advise personnel about safe use of disinfectant chemicals.

It is critical that the efficacy of products and procedures used in sanitation be evaluated on a periodic basis. The veterinarian should work with the facility manager to develop methods to evaluate sanitation adequacy. For example, the veterinarian might help outline a plan to sample equipment and locations within the facility on a periodic basis using rodac plates or sterile swabs plated onto microbiologic media.

5. Acquisition of Food and Bedding

The attending veterinarian typically has the training and experience to understand needs of the animals, particularly those with unique or unusual needs. For this reason, the veterinarian should work with the facility manager to ensure that feed and bedding that meets the requirements of the animals is acquired. The veterinarian should be familiar with various vendors of supplies and have some sense of relative quality. Quality assurance statements from vendors should be requested and closely evaluated on an ongoing basis. For example, quality assurance statements for feed should be routinely reviewed to determine that the feed contains adequate levels of nutrients and is free of specified contaminants. In some cases, feed for livestock obtained from vendors unfamiliar with the requirements for research animals may contain added antibiotics.

III. MEDICAL FACILITIES AND EQUIPMENT

A. SURGICAL FACILITIES

In general, facilities for survival surgery (surgery in which the animal recovers from anesthesia) should be designed to facilitate conduct of aseptic procedures. Nonsurvival surgery does not require the same conditions, although the location should be isolated from other concurrent activities and is constructed in such a way that clean-up and sanitation are easily performed.

Surgical equipment for research use is typical of that used for veterinary surgery (16–18). Anesthesia machines, recovery cages, and surgery tables may need to be set up for animals smaller than those for which they were designed. Many facilities conducting surgery on non-rodent mammals have equipment such as EKG machines and equipment to monitor oxygen saturation and blood pressure. Specialized equipment not typical to veterinary practice is sometimes required in the surgical research facility. Microsurgical apparatus and physiological recording equipment are examples (19–21).

Facilities for survival surgery can be divided into those relevant for rodents and those relevant for non-rodent mammals.

1. Rodents

The facilities needed to conduct survival surgery on rodents are substantially less complicated than those needed for non-rodent mammals. According to the *Guide*, surgery for rodents may be performed in a small area, even a "dedicated space in a laboratory appropriately managed to minimize contamination from other activities in the room during surgery." Often, a clean benchtop in a secluded area of the laboratory is acceptable if other aseptic surgical procedures are practiced.

As with all surgical areas, surfaces should be nonporous to facilitate sanitation. In this regard, commercially available rodent surgery boards constructed out of durable plastics are particularly useful. Such boards not only facilitate sanitation, but also are an efficient means for animal positioning during surgery. Body temperature of the animal subject is easier to maintain, because most plastics do not conduct heat very well.

In facilities where a high volume of surgical procedures is performed, a dedicated, shared surgical facility may be advantageous. By having a centralized resource of this type, expensive equipment such as instruments, autoclaves, and anesthesia machines can be shared in a cost-effective manner (22). High volume rodent surgical facilities often have several surgery "stations" fed by a single gas anesthesia machine connected to a manifold distribution system. HEPA-filtered "clean benches" or even Class II biological safety cabinets are sometimes used to augment other aseptic techniques during surgery.

2. Non-Rodent Mammals

When survival surgery is performed on non-rodent mammals, full, dedicated surgical facilities are needed. In many cases, the required surgical facilities are extensive and may rival state-of-the-art suites found in human hospitals. The basic facility requirements have been extensively reviewed elsewhere (17, 20, 23–25).

The entire facility must be designed and operated for contamination control in support of aseptic surgery. Basic features include fresh air changes to minimize airborne contaminants and air balance to bias airflow from least contaminated to more contaminated areas. The room layout should facilitate movement of personnel and animals from less clean to more clean areas while isolating clean areas from nonessential traffic. To minimize contamination of the facility, surfaces must be smooth, substantially seamless, impervious to water, and contain a minimum of horizontal surfaces that are prone to collect dust.

Facilities for survival surgery of non-rodent mammals typically include areas to address the following specific functions.

a. *Surgical Support*

An area should be included that provides for storage of materials related to the care of animals involved in surgical procedures. This is typically the area where surgical instruments are cleaned, sterilized, and repackaged for use. Storage cabinets should be located in this area, including a double-locked cabinet or box for storage of controlled substances. A sink with running water for cleansing of surgical instruments should be within this area, and some facilities further utilize ultrasonic cleaners for this function. Many facilities sterilize surgical equipment by means of a small autoclave, often located in this area of the surgical facility.

b.   *Animal Preparation*

The animal preparation area is the location where animals often are administered pre-medications and where anesthesia is sometimes initially induced. In addition, the surgical site on the animal is prepared by clipping and cleaning. If inhalant anesthetics are used in this location, an appropriate system to scavenge waste gases should be included either in the infrastructure or within the anesthesia machine. Because of the potential for sudden, untoward effects of anesthesia, this area should be equipped with medications appropriate for emergencies. Running water, ground fault interrupting circuitry (GFI), and a preparation table with a fenestrated top are standard. Some type of vacuum device is advisable for disposal of clipped hair.

c.   *Surgeon's Scrub*

An area is needed where surgical personnel can decontaminate themselves prior to surgery by donning surgical apparel and disinfecting their hands and arms. A typical arrangement is for a locker room to be available for personnel to don nonsterile items such as surgical scrubs. Separate locker rooms for men and women are generally provided.

Usually, an area adjacent to the locker rooms and the operating room is designated the "surgeon's scrub." Here the surgical personnel don surgical masks and hair covers. The surgeon's scrub area must have a sink with running water that permits a thorough scrub of the surgeon's hands and forearms without recontamination by operating valves. Elbow, foot, or knee controls and even automatic sensors are used to operate the water supply. An antiseptic such as betadine scrub is typically part of this preparation.

Finally, sterile gloves are donned following entry into the operating room. Nonsterile, "floating" personnel assist surgical personnel with fastening gowns and making adjustments to nonsterile apparel for the comfort of the surgical personnel.

d.   *Operating Room (OR)*

The OR is the location where the invasive procedure is performed on the animal. Disinfection of surfaces within the OR is critical to minimize the likelihood of postoperative infection of surgical wounds. Stainless steel is the preferred material for surfaces within the OR due to simplicity of disinfection of such a nonporous, durable surface.

Some facilities choose to place multiple surgery tables within a single OR. Such an arrangement allows a team of personnel to conduct surgery on several animals simultaneously, although this set-up should be used only if the procedures are related and are being conducted on the same species at the same time.

As with the animal preparation area, the OR should have provisions for scavenging of waste anesthetic gases. This may involve the use of scavenging substances through which gases flow prior to exhaust or may involve attachment of the anesthetic machine to lines that exhaust to a chemical fume hood or to outside of the building.

Other equipment within the OR will depend upon the nature of the procedures being conducted. For example, imaging equipment (e.g., x-ray, sonography, magnetic resonance imaging) may be required in some circumstances. Equipment to evaluate and maintain homeostasis of the animal might include an ECG monitor, heating pads (circulating water type is preferable) for the animal to lay upon, an esophageal stethoscope, and IV infusion pump, emergency pharmaceuticals, and any specialized equipment that might be needed for individual procedures.

e. *Postoperative Recovery*

An area where animals recover from anesthesia is required for surgery on nonrodent mammals. This area should be quiet and allow variable intensity illumination, since animals will sometimes experience a less distressful recovery in a quiet, darkened room. This area should include or be near a supply of emergency medical supplies in the event of an unexpected complication during recovery. Typically, animals are recovered in cages, often lying upon or wrapped in a blanket. Circulating water heating pads are useful to help the animal maintain normothermia.

3. Nonsurvival Surgery

Ideally, nonsurvival surgery should be performed in facilities designed for survival surgery. By doing so, the animal will be close to needed equipment and pharmaceuticals if an emergency develops that threatens to cause the animal distress or to interfere with the successful use of the animal through completion of the study. Nonsurvival surgery can be performed within laboratories if a location amenable to cleanup and disinfection of surfaces is used. Surfaces should be impervious to moisture, and a sink with running water is useful. In addition, if inhalant anesthetics are used, provisions for scavenging of waste gases must be made. If a site other than a central surgical resource is used, provisions for safe and discreet transportation of carcasses to the carcass storage site should be made.

B. Treatment Facilities

An area for treatment of sick animals should be included in the facility, although the specifications for such an area will vary substantially based upon the number and species of animals, and the scope of the research being conducted. Facilities maintaining species such as rabbits and other larger animals may need separate space for medical examination and treatment. In some cases, this may be a separate, dedicated room. In other cases, examination and treatment of animals can be performed in the regular animal housing room.

If an animal is being treated for a contagious condition or if frequent handling or monitoring is needed, a separate treatment area is warranted. Even when the routine housing area will suffice, space may be needed for convenient organization of materials, supplies, and equipment. A comfortable, easily sanitizable worktable with adjustable lighting is useful for examination of animals. In this regard, a stainless steel table with running water and a fenestrated top near GFI circuitry is standard in veterinary hospitals and is valuable for research facilities. A small refrigerator with freezer for storage of some pharmaceuticals and vaccines should be included as basic room equipment. The freezer is needed for storage of serum samples prior to shipping for analysis. Maintaining "blue ice" packs for shipping along with such samples is advisable.

Generally, the equipment used for treatment of ill laboratory animals is the same as that used in standard veterinary practice (16). Because of the small size of rodents, a source of magnification is a useful adjunct for physical examination and intravenous injection. A 20-30 diopter hand lens is recommended for ophthalmological examination of rats (16). For oral medication of rodents, if the drug is not reliably consumed voluntarily, ball-tip gavage needles of varying sizes are useful.

Equipment for diagnostic evaluation of samples is useful, again depending upon the type and number of animals present in the facility. Often, no specialized facilities are needed, but a few simple pieces of equipment to spin microhematocrit tubes, separate serum, measure total protein, do fecal flotation, and examine slides are sufficient. This equipment would include a centrifuge and a light microscope. In more complex situations, such as facilities with extensive surgical programs, full clinical pathology and microbiology support may be needed.

C.   ISOLATION FACILITIES

"Isolation" refers to separation of animals to prevent one group or individual from influencing or affecting another. Isolation is typically implemented through utilization of techniques, personnel, equipment, and physical space. A common goal of isolation is to prevent spread of infectious agents between animals. Because infectious agents are often transmitted by surface contamination of shared supplies or equipment or by carriage upon personnel moving through the facility, it is critical that personnel understand the concepts of contamination and disinfection. Sometimes the term **"barrier"** is used to refer to isolation within research facilities.

A number of circumstances may require the need for isolation of animals. For example, immunodeficient animals, such as nude mice, which must be protected from infectious agents are typically placed within isolation. Animals harboring infectious agents, acquired either naturally or through purposeful experimental infection, are usually isolated to prevent spread of infection to other groups of animals. In this regard, animals exhibiting signs of illness are often isolated from other animals, so that the disease may not be spread if it is of an infectious origin. In addition, this allows sick animals to receive greater individual attention. An overview of biocontainment management has been published elsewhere (26).

For practical reasons, research animals are often housed in dense colonies with no practical barrier to cross-infection within individual rooms and often across several rooms. Once an animal has been identified as ill, it has likely already shed the infectious agent and movement to an isolated location is unlikely to be productive in protecting that group. Under such conditions, isolation procedures should focus on assessing the extent of disease within the exposed group and implementing isolation for that entire group.

Isolation is used in a general way to stop cross-contamination between groups of animals that are different. A common use of isolation procedures is for the quarantine of newly arrived animals from those already in the facility. During a typical quarantine, animals are closely observed and evaluated for evidence of disease and infectious agents not currently present in the existing colonies. Rodents are often tested for parasites such as pinworms and for evidence of surreptitious agents by serological analysis. Larger animals may be vaccinated and even treated for common bacterial and parasitic infections while in quarantine. Nonhuman primates are generally tested for tuberculosis.

Since isolation is utilized for a variety of situations and reasons, the facilities used for isolation can vary. In some cases, an area within the treatment facility or an empty animal room may suffice. Ideally, though, a number of features are desirable. The physical plant should be designed for ease of sanitation, with floor drains and moisture-impervious surfaces. In addition, access to the isolation should be strictly controlled to allow entry of only essential personnel (27).

It is sometimes difficult to maintain effective isolation when the facilities are also used for other activities. Well-defined transition zones where personnel can decontaminate and don protective gear during entry and/or exit to/from the isolation area are desirable. Small anterooms that are traversed before entering the isolation area are effective. Locker room/shower facilities serve as an effective transition zone for more extensive isolation areas. When retrofitting an isolation area into limited existing space, it may be adequate to define a "virtual" transition zone surrounding the doorway into the isolated room/area.

When isolation is utilized to control infectious agents, an autoclave of appropriate size, and in close proximity to the isolation area, is desirable. Particularly useful are double-door, "pass-through" autoclaves that are situated in a wall between the isolated area and the "outside." Such an arrangement allows materials to be sterilized either upon entry into, or exit from, the isolation area.

Air that is balanced to augment the other isolation procedures is standard practice. Specifically, air pressure differentials should be such that air is directed from the area least likely to the area most likely to be contaminated. In many cases, air undergoes HEPA filtration prior to entry into the cage (e.g., in the case of immunosuppressed mice). A number of specialized caging systems have been developed for isolation. A great variety of such cages exist, ranging from the standard sealed bubble (Trexler) isolator, to microisolator cages that operate on a petri dish concept, to racks that ventilate each cage

individually. A more thorough review of ventilated racks can be found elsewhere (28). The use of cubicles has also been advocated in isolation programs
(29). Each type of caging system can be a cornerstone to procedures and
policies that form an effective isolation program when rodents are involved.

D.   NECROPSY FACILITIES

Necropsy is the study of dead animals in order to understand the processes that
lead to death. The capability to necropsy animals that are euthanized or found
dead is an important diagnostic aspect of proper veterinary care, since it may
provide information that will benefit future management of the operation with
the goal of eliminating the problem. In the case of animals included in the
AWAR, provisions for necropsy of animals that die without readily apparent
cause are required (7).

Necropsy involves direct observation and study of the whole carcass, as
well as subsequent tests of selected samples. Interpretation of the findings must
be done within the context of historical information encompassing: (1) the life
history of the individual; (2) previous knowledge of colony health/disease
status; (3) husbandry and care procedures; and (4) experimental procedures in
which the animal has been involved.

Although a few specialized techniques exist with respect to animal necropsy,
facility and equipment needs are fairly standard (30). The initial phase of necropsy,
called **gross necropsy** as it is a general examination of the carcass, requires space
appropriate for opening and observing the carcass. Facilities appropriate for gross
necropsy are basically the same as for other veterinary facilities (31). Key facility
and equipment features are influenced by the species being used, but a stainless
steel table with integral water supply and drainage, and good lighting are usually
needed. Typically, a set of surgery-type instruments, including such items as
scalpel handle and blades, forceps, and operating and iris scissors, are used (32).
Syringes, neutral buffered formalin, and microbiological supplies should be available. Since the most meaningful information will come from the examination of
a fresh carcass, a refrigerator dedicated to exclusive storage of animal carcasses
should be available. For safety reasons, this refrigerator should not be used for
storage of other items such as food or pharmaceuticals.

Because infectious agents may be responsible for the animal's death, it is
important that the space be isolated from cross-contaminating traffic patterns
and from other animals. Ideally, the necropsy area is under negative air
pressure relative to adjacent areas. Some facilities pass exhaust air from
necropsy areas through HEPA filtration. Downdraft necropsy tables are particularly useful, as they direct the flow of air away from personnel, and through
a filter. The area should be easily sanitized, with surfaces being smooth and
impervious to water, and having as few seams and ledges as possible. The use
of hands-free audiorecording equipment for dictation of necropsy findings may
be useful in facilities with high use (33).

E.   GENERAL FACILITIES ISSUES

The preceding sections have briefly described facility and equipment issues that directly impact veterinary care. Veterinary care in the research facility should be focused on preventive medicine aimed toward excluding health problems that can adversely affect animal health and research. As such, the programs and facilities of the entire animal care program have an impact on the veterinary care program and need to work in conjunction with it. For example, the use of disinfectant chemicals must be coordinated in such a way that exposure of animals to harmful agents is limited. Improper use and exposure of animals to such materials can result in harm to the animal and thus impact veterinary care.

Lack of space is a consistent problem in most animal research facilities and is a concern that frequently causes conflict between husbandry (and research) needs and veterinary care. Proper handling of veterinary medical problems often involves isolation of different groups of animals from one another. Unfortunately, such separation is usually synonymous with less efficient use of space, since only a few animals might be housed in a relatively large isolation area. Isolation also often involves specialized entry and handling procedures for isolation equipment, thereby imposing personnel, space, and equipment utilization restrictions on the rest of the animal care program. Violating these restrictions can sometimes create veterinary medical problems.

Noise is another basic characteristic of facilities that may impact the veterinary care program. Many animals and activities related to animal husbandry can generate noise that may adversely affect some animals. For example, excessive noise can result in poor reproductive performance in rodents. While all sources of noise cannot be eliminated from animal care, design and utilization of the facility to minimize its impact on animals is an important adjunct to veterinary care. Similarly, illumination of animal rooms can impact both animal health and research results. It should be sufficient to permit husbandry and examination of animals, but should not be of excessive intensity or duration. Light cycles should be regularly timed.

IV.   MEDICAL PROGRAMS

An effective program of veterinary care has several components, including preventive medicine, routine veterinary care, perioperative care, behavioral management, and euthanasia. A key concept is that a veterinarian with experience and training should provide direction and oversight for the program of veterinary care. Often, trained veterinary technicians or other personnel are delegated the responsibility for observation and "hands-on" care of the animals; however, the ultimate responsibility for ensuring proper clinical care remains with the attending veterinarian. The veterinarian should establish a mechanism for receiving animal health information that will ensure fulfillment of this responsibility.

For all veterinary care procedures it is important to maintain documentation, either written or electronic. All records should be detailed enough to adequately explain what occurred to a person knowledgeable in the field.

A.   PREVENTIVE MEDICINE

Preventive medicine and health monitoring programs are undertaken to ensure that healthy animals are acquired initially and that these animals remain healthy. These efforts should be active and ongoing. The following are aspects of a sound program of preventive medicine.

1.   Vendor Surveillance

Vendor surveillance is the initial step in a sound program of preventive medicine. A high quality commercial animal vendor typically supplies the customer with a written report of animal health. Such information tends to be most comprehensive for rodents; however, it is often available for other species as well. Reports usually provide a description of methods used to evaluate the health of the animals followed by results of the most recent evaluation. It is advisable to maintain a file of these reports so that one can evaluate changes in the monitoring programs or results of individual vendors over time. Common methods used to evaluated colony health include serologic testing for bacterial and viral pathogens, fecal flotation for endoparasites, pelt examination for ectoparasites, and necropsy and histopathology of representative individuals. The precise testing methods will vary with the vendor and the species, but preferably should be conducted by an independent laboratory. Testing should be frequent enough to detect significant changes in colony health, usually quarterly or semi-annually at a minimum. When practical, it is also useful to conduct on-site visits of vendors, perhaps annually, to evaluate the overall system for maintenance of animal health, including housing, sanitation, feed storage, and veterinary care. If problems are identified either on the vendor reports or during an on-site visit, the veterinary staff should coordinate arrangements to identify alternate vendors or implement other means to ensure that healthy animals are being used.

2.   Evaluation of Transportation

Specific regulations govern several aspects of animal transport. These regulations are included in the AWAR (§2.38.f) and the *Live Animal Regulations* of the International Air Transport Association (IATA) (34). Beyond meeting the regulatory requirements, focus should also be placed on provisions to ensure the well-being of the animal(s). The following issues should be evaluated with respect to transport:

a.   Shipping Container

The device in which the animals are housed during transport should be sturdy enough to withstand the rigors of transportation. It should allow for adequate ventilation and be large enough to comfortably house the animals. The shipping container should be constructed such that the animals inside are protected from microbial or traumatic insults and so that personnel are protected from aggressive animals or possible zoonotic agents harbored by the animals. Animals arriving at the research facility in damaged containers should be closely inspected for signs of injury or disease, or the animals should be rejected.

b.   Time of Shipping

Attention should be paid to the time of shipping so that animals are not transported during severe weather conditions or just prior to weekends or holidays when personnel are not available at the research facility to accept and process the shipment. The International Air Transport Association (IATA) has specifications for the allowable time animals may spend within shipping containers.

c.   Food and Water

Provisions should be made so that animals being transported do not endure excessive periods of time without food and water.

d.   Conveyance

The condition of the transport vehicle should be reviewed when possible. Ideally, such vehicles will have a controlled environment for shipments so that animals will not be exposed to environmental extremes. Animals should not be shipped together with potentially hazardous materials, such as toxic chemicals. The vehicle should be clean and ideally is sanitized prior to animal shipments.

e.   Personnel

It is preferable for individuals transporting animals to have understanding and knowledge of issues related to animal health and welfare as they relate to transportation. Furthermore, personnel should be educated with respect to possible zoonotic diseases, and they should be instructed to wear personal protective equipment when needed. Damaged shipping containers may indicate that procedures or equipment used in transportation are inadequate.

3.   Examination of Animals

Examination of animals upon arrival at the facility is an additional component of an effective program of preventive medicine. Newly received animals should be examined by either a veterinarian or a trained technician. Attention should be directed toward any signs suggestive of disease, such as lethargy, poor hair coat, diarrhea, any obvious abnormal masses or wounds, lameness, or abnormal discharge from an orifice. For some larger species such as dogs, cats, and nonhuman primates, body temperature of individuals may be taken and blood samples submitted for determination of hematocrit, hemoglobin content, and white blood cell count. Testing for tuberculosis is initiated during this time for nonhuman primates. For random source dogs, it is common to also evaluate a blood sample for heartworm (*Dirofilaria immitis*). During the initial examination, the behavior of animals should also be evaluated. Overly aggressive animals may present a danger to personnel and are therefore undesirable as research subjects. Vaccinations or routine deworming medication can be administered during this initial examination. Animals that are found to have medical problems should be treated, euthanized, or returned to the vendor.

Once newly received animals have been examined they should undergo a period of quarantine and acclimation. During this time, they are separated from animals that have been at the facility for longer periods of time and are being used in research or teaching projects. Quarantine/acclimation allows continued evaluation of the health and behavior of the animal over a short period of time so that problems which may have not been clinically apparent during the initial examination have an additional opportunity for detection. In addition, quarantine/acclimation allows a period for physiologic stabilization of the animal after shipping, since the process of transport can produce significant alterations in physiologic processes of animals (35–37). During this time, animals can become accustomed to their new environment, cage, food, water, and other aspects of their surroundings. Typical periods for quarantine vary, but often range from 7 to 10 days (38). Quarantine of rodents often includes evaluation for specific pathogens (39). For nonhuman primates, a quarantine period of 90 days is recommended for completion of tuberculosis testing (40).

4.   Ongoing Preventive Medicine

Ongoing preventive medicine should be provided for animals that remain on a long-term basis at the facility after release from quarantine. Typical aspects of this effort include the following.

a.   Scheduled Physical Exams

All animals should be examined every day, including weekends and holidays by trained personnel, usually an ALAT, LAT, or LATG. A closer evaluation of the animals can be done during transfer to a clean cage. Again, this is usually the responsibility of an ALAT, LAT, or LATG. It is further useful to perform a hands-on physical examination of animals on a routine basis, either annually, semi-annually, or more frequently if necessitated by the study. Species typically included are rabbits, dogs, cats, and nonhuman primates. In some cases, livestock are included, although physical examination is not usually practical when large herds are housed outdoors. At a minimum, the animal should be weighed, the body temperature should be taken, the teeth and external features examined, and feces sampled for endoparasite examination. More detailed examinations might include sampling of blood for routine hematologic evaluation.

b.   Tuberculosis Testing

It is important that nonhuman primates, particularly Old World species, be tested on a regular basis for tuberculosis (TB). Semi-annual intradermal testing with tuberculin is recommended for Old World species (41). Animals that test positive for TB should be removed from the colony and either isolated and treated with an appropriate medication recommended by the attending veterinarian, or euthanized.

c.   Rodent Colony Health Monitoring

It is important that a program be maintained to periodically evaluate the microbial status of resident rodent populations. Even though many rodent infectious agents cause little or no disease, infection may cause perturbations in experimental data.

It is common for groups of mice, rats, hamsters, gerbils, and guinea pigs to be included in a monitoring program. A list of agents commonly screened for is provided in Table 1. Some basic principles and methods associated with monitoring of rodent colonies follow.

Animals evaluated should have had exposure to the colony for approximately four weeks. In this regard, animals to be evaluated may be culled from the colony or may be **sentinel animals** purchased specifically for the purpose of exposure to and evaluation of the colony. Sentinel animals may be exposed to the colony by a variety of means, including housing within the same room, housing within the same cage, housing in a cage to which soiled bedding from the colony has been added, or a combination of these methods. In any case, the sentinels used should be initially free of infectious pathogens.

Monitoring of colonies often includes immunoassay of serum specimens; bacterial culture of respiratory and gastrointestinal tracts; gross pathologic examination; and histopathologic evaluation.

Evaluation is usually by a variety of methods, including serologic testing, pelt examination, fecal testing, and necropsy/histopathology. In this regard, blood is sampled and the serum evaluated for the presence of antibody to specific infectious agents. Fecal samples can be evaluated for some pathogens, such as *Helicobacter hepaticus*, by means of polymerase chain reaction (PCR) (42). In addition, feces can be examined by means of fecal floatation for some oxyurids such as *Aspicularis tetraptera*. In general, because these procedures can be performed on samples obtained without the need to euthanize the animal, it is possible to monitor the colony without the use of sentinel or cull

TABLE 1. Infectious Agents Commonly Included in Rodent Health Monitoring

Infectious Agent	Species
Mycoplasma pulmonis	Mouse, rat
Sendai virus	Mouse, rat, gerbil, guinea pig
Sialodacryoadenitis virus/rat coronavirus	Rat
Kilham's rat virus (KRV)	Rat
Toolan's H-1 virus	Rat
Rat parvovirus	Rat
Mouse parvovirus	Mouse
Pneumonia virus of mice (PVM)	Rat, mouse, hamster, gerbil, guinea pig
Reovirus-3	Rat, mouse, hamster, gerbil, guinea pig
Hantaan virus	Rat, mouse
Theiler's mouse encephalomyelitis virus	Rat, mouse
Mouse adenovirus	Mouse
Lymphocytic choriomeningitis virus	Rat, mouse, hamster, gerbil, guinea pig
Mouse hepatitis virus (MHV)	Mouse, gerbil
Minute virus of mice (MVM)	Mouse
Rotavirus	Mouse
Ectromelia (mousepox virus)	Mouse
Mouse adenovirus	Rat, mouse
Polyoma virus	Mouse
Mouse thymic virus	Mouse
Cytomegalovirus	Mouse, guinea pig
K virus	Mouse
Lactate dehydrogenas-elevating virus (LDV)	Mouse
SV-5	Guinea pig
Encephalitozoon cuniculi	Mouse, guinea pig
Helicobacter spp.	Rat, mouse, hamster, gerbil
Clostridium piliforme	Hamster, gerbil
Endoparasites	Rat, mouse, hamster, gerbil, guinea pig
Ectoparasites	Rat, mouse, hamster, gerbil, guinea pig

Monitoring of colonies often includes immunoassay of serum specimens; bacterial culture of respiratory and gastrointestinal tracts; gross pathologic examination; and histopathologic evaluation.

animals. It is worthwhile, however, to euthanize some animals and perform a necropsy followed by histopathologic examination of representative tissues such as liver, kidney, spleen, intestinal tract, and lungs.

Examination for ectoparasites is often done by examination of the pelt or carcass of a euthanized specimen beneath a dissecting microscope. As the pelt (or carcass) cools, the ectoparasites locomote toward the surface of the hair coat and are readily visible. If an animal is not to be euthanized, a piece of cellophane tape is applied to the dorsal surface of the animal, between the shoulders, gently applied and removed, and then examined under a microscope while attached to a glass slide. This same technique can be used to examine for Oxyurids such as *Syphacia obvelata* in the mouse, by applying the tape to the perineal region.

d.   *Monitoring of Injectable Biological Materials*

Biologic materials such as cell lines and biologic fluids such as serum may be contaminated with infectious agents. Because such materials are often administered to rodents, attention must be paid to ensure that pathogens are not present. The **mouse antibody production (MAP) test** is a common method for making this determination. Similar methods are used in other rodent species.

Briefly, MAP testing involves injection of a small volume (0.1 to 0.25 ml) of the material being evaluated into a mouse. It is common to administer the material intraperitoneally; however, subcutaneous injection also may be used. During this time, the test animal should be considered as potentially infectious for other mice and should be isolated. After 4 weeks, the mouse is euthanized; samples are taken for serologic evaluation and tissues examined by necropsy and histopathology as for routine monitoring as described above. If the results are positive and suggest contamination of the biological material, it should be discarded. In contrast, results suggesting lack of contamination indicate that the material can be used in live rodents.

Specific recommendations for policies and procedures related to monitoring of rodent colonies have been described in detail elsewhere (43).

B.   ROUTINE VETERINARY CARE

Routine veterinary care involves the diagnosis and treatment of clinical illness that occurs either spontaneously or as a result of experimental manipulation. It is important that veterinary care be available at all times, including weekends and holidays, in the event of an emergency. Toward this end, veterinary staff must remain accessible at all times. Many facilities utilize cellular phones and pagers to establish this line of emergency communication. Routine aspects of the veterinary care program include the following.

1.   Diagnosis and Treatment of Ill Animals

A proper program must be in place to evaluate and treat those animals which experience clinical illness. The basis of diagnostic medicine is the physical examination, which should be performed by a veterinarian or a trained designate, such as a trained veterinary technician. Findings should be recorded and additional diagnostic procedures or recommendations for treatment made based upon the findings. Other common diagnostic procedures are summarized in Table 2.

There are numerous other diagnostic procedures that can be performed in support of the veterinary care program. Those listed above are a sample of some of the more commonly used techniques. Because of the cost of equipment needed to perform many of these procedures, laboratories outside of the institution are frequently used. Such labs may be commercial, for-profit enterprises, while others may be associated with academic institutions. One of the most versatile pieces of equipment is a binocular light microscope capable of a range of magnifications, and facilities should consider purchase of such an item.

TABLE 2. Common Veterinary Diagnostic Procedures

Diagnostic Procedure	Usual Purpose
Measurement of body temperature	To detect hyperthermia or hypothermia
Measurement of body weight	To assess body condition, adequacy of nutrition, detect changes in body weight as an indication of underlying disease
Determination of hematocrit	To assess adequacy of red blood cell number
Determination of blood hemoglobin	To assess oxygen transport capacity of the blood and to characterize the nature of anemia if present
White blood cell count	To provide information relevant to infectious processes
Blood cytology	To provide morphologic information on red and white blood cells relevant to various disease processes including anemia, infection, and neoplasia
Plasma total protein	To assess multiple scenarios including possible hemmorhage, enteric protein loss, hepatic disease, and gammopathies
Serum enzyme levels (e.g., ALT, AST, SDH, SAP)	To assess dysfunction in tissues such as the liver and muscle
Cytology	To characterize abnormal fluids
Urinalysis	To assess cellular and chemical composition of urine for evidence of disease
Radiography	To evaluate internal structures for evidence of disease

Once diagnosis has been made, a specific treatment plan should be prepared under the authority of the attending veterinarian. The specific medications and equipment needed will vary with the species being housed and the scope of activity at the institution; however, basic equipment useful to most facilities would include:

- An assortment of sterile syringes (1.0 to 20 ml)
- An assortment of sterile hypodermic needles (18 to 26 ga; 5/8" to 1")
- An ophthalmoscope
- A thermometer
- A scale of appropriate size to weigh animals
- A stethoscope; an esophageal stethoscope is valuable for monitoring during anesthesia
- Stainless steel ball-tipped feeding needles for rodents

- Blood collection tubes (red top for serum; lavender for whole blood)
- Assortment of bandaging materials
- Sterile gauze pads
- Circulating water heating pad
- Rodent and rabbit restrainers
- Sterile fluids such as lactated Ringer's and 0.9% saline
- Assortment of intravenous catheters and intravenous fluid sets
- Nail clippers
- Assortment of surgical scissors, forceps, clamps, scalpel blades, suture material (exact equipment will depend upon individual needs of the facility)

An assortment of medication should be available for use. The specific needs of the facility will determine the type and quantities needed. Many pharmaceuticals used for anesthesia and analgesia are controlled by the DEA. A safe or locked cabinet should be used for storage of these drugs. Provision of adequate veterinary care necessitates that a stock supply of a variety of pharmaceuticals is maintained unless they can be acquired from nearby sources quickly enough to responsibly treat an ill animal. In any event, a small variety of antibiotics and emergency drugs should be kept on hand (16). Although very few pharmaceuticals are approved for use in laboratory animals, thus making such use "extra-label," the prevailing view is that such extra-label use is being done under veterinary supervision and is described in the experimental protocol or is done under an authentic veterinarian-client relationship (9). Pharmaceuticals should be routinely monitored to ensure that they have not exceeded the expiration date indicated on the package.

2. Perianesthetic/Operative Care

Many experimental procedures involve anesthesia and surgery. Proper care before, during, and after surgery is critical to success, and many of these same principles apply to procedures that involve anesthesia without a subsequent surgery. It is important, then, that adequate perianesthetic/operative care be provided to animals undergoing surgery. Typical components of perianesthetic/operative care include the following.

a. Pre-Anesthetic/Operative Care

It is critical that the animal be appropriately prepared for anesthesia and surgery. Useful practices are summarized in Table 3.

b. Care during Anesthesia/Surgery

Anesthesia and surgery represent major challenges to the animal's homeostasis. To minimize complications a number of common practices are summarized in Table 4.

c. Post-Anesthetic/Operative Care

Because animals remain vulnerable to complications following anesthesia and surgery, proper post-anesthetic/operative care is crucial. Typical practices are summarized in Table 5.

C. ANESTHESIA AND ANALGESIA

A key aspect of the experimental use of animals is that pain and distress be minimized. Indeed, reduction of pain is a regulatory requirement. The *Guide*, the AWAR (§2.31.d.1.iv.A), and the Public Health Service Policy on Humane Care and Use of Laboratory Animals (IV.C.1.b) all specify this principle. Toward this end, it is the duty of the attending veterinarian to ensure that methods used are appropriate to the species and to the procedure being conducted. General principles of anesthesia apply to research use as well (44). Equipment and compounds are available. A variety of special techniques and uses of equipment have been described to augment general veterinary methods (45–47). The choice of a particular method will largely be determined by the species, expected length of anesthesia, and the procedure to be performed.

Compounds used in anesthesia, sedation, and analgesia can produce states that may be defined as follows:

TABLE 3. Summary of Pre-Anesthetic/Operative Care Practices

Practice	Purpose
Clinical evaluation	To confirm that the animal is healthy and likely to withstand the challenge of anesthesia and surgery
Fasting for 8 to 12 hours	To decrease the possibility of vomiting and aspiration during anesthesia (note: some species such as the rabbit, mouse and rat do not vomit and therefore fasting is not necessary)
Removal of drinking water 60 minutes prior to surgery	To ensure adequate fluid balance while decreasing the possibility of vomiting water during anesthesia (as above, the rabbit, mouse and rat do not vomit and water does not need to be withheld)
Placement of intravenous catheter	To provide access for pharmaceuticals and fluids
Administration of atropine	To decrease respiratory tract secretions during anesthesia
Administration of tranquilizers/sedatives	To decrease apprehension of the animal and lower the amount of anesthetic required
Administration of analgesics	To decrease the dose of anesthetic required and to initiate analgesia for the post-operative period
Pre-anesthetic antibiotic administration	To provide the animal an advantage against post-operative infection; generally used during potentially contaminating procedures such as when the gastrointestinal tract is penetrated

---

TABLE 4. Summary of Common Practices during Anesthesia/Surgery

Practice	Purpose
Place animal on circulating water heating pad	To minimize development of hypothermia
Administration of intravenous fluids	To maintain fluid balance during procedures that are long or involve loss of body fluids
Assessment of anesthetic depth	To ensure that the level of anesthesia is neither too light nor too deep
Frequent evaluation of body temperature, mucous membrane color, respiratory rate and character, and heart rate and character	To determine adequacy of perfusion and maintenance of body temperature, and to identify perturbations in respiration or cardiac function

Analgesia — Loss of sensitivity to pain.

Anesthesia — Total loss of sensation in either a specific area (regional) or site (local) or in the whole body (general). General anesthesia also usually involves the loss of consciousness and ideally includes analgesia.

Hypnosis — An induced state of sleep or a trance mimicking sleep in which the patient can be aroused by stimuli.

Neuroleptanalgesia — A state of hypnosis and analgesia resulting from a combination of a neuroleptic drug and an analgesic drug.

Sedation — A state in which the patient remains conscious but has decreased awareness of its surroundings. Generally, the patient can be aroused by sufficient stimuli.

Tranquilization — A state in which the patient is calm and conscious, but unconcerned or indifferent.

A number of pharmaceutical compounds can be used to produce anesthesia, analgesia, sedation and tranquilization in animals (48). Often, they are used in combination so that the dosage of one compound with undesirable side effects can be reduced. Specific dosages should be based upon the recommendation of the attending veterinarian. Compounds used to induce anesthesia or to provide analgesia in animals include the following.

1.   Inhalant Anesthetics

Inhalant anesthetics are best administered through a vaporizer, thereby allowing precise control of the amount of anesthetic administered. Usually, the anesthetic is poured in liquid form into the vaporizer and the concentration to be administered is selected on a dial. The vaporizer allows mixture of air with anesthetic gas to reach a specific concentration. The gas is then administered to the animal by a tube placed into the trachea (intubation), a face mask that fits over the nose and mouth, or an induction chamber into which the animal is placed. Intubation allows for the most accurate delivery of inhalant anesthetic doses. In addition, supplemental oxygen can be readily supplied if

TABLE 5. Common Post-Anesthetic/Operative Practices

Practice	Purpose
Placement of animal on heating pad or beneath warming lamp or inside incubator	To minimize development of hypothermia
Administration of fluids	To correct or avoid dehydration
Frequent monitoring of body temperature, mucous membrane color, respiratory rate and character, and heart rate and character	To determine adequacy of perfusion and maintenance of body temperature, and to identify perturbations in respiration or cardiac function
Frequent monitoring of activity	To assess return to normal behavior; alterations in appetite, grooming, or locomotion could suggest complications such as post-operative pain
Monitoring of incision site	To evaluate for evidence of infection, dehisence, or self-trauma to the sutures or tissues
Administration of analgesics	To minimize post-operative pain
Administration of antibiotics	To minimize the likelihood of post-operative infection; generally used during procedures with high likelihood of contamination such as those involving penetration of the gastrointestinal tract

needed by the animal. Commonly used inhalant anesthetics include halothane, isoflurane, and nitrous oxide. Ether was commonly used in the past due to ease of vaporization and ready availability; however, it is highly flammable and explosive and thus represents a significant hazard. Because other, safer agents are available, the use of ether as an anesthetic should be avoided.

Alternatively, some individuals administer inhalant anesthetics to small animals, usually rodents, by placing a cotton ball soaked with the anesthetic liquid into a jar. This method does not allow for accurate administration of anesthetic and carries a high risk of overdose. If this method is used, it is important that a grid separate the animal from the liquid anesthetic, since contact may be irritating to the animal.

An important concern with administration of any inhalant anesthetic is the occupational risk posed by waste gases. There is some concern that individuals exposed to waste anesthetic gases over time may develop a variety of ailments, including hepatic and renal disease, neurological abnormalities, and hematopoietic perturbations (49). In particular, pregnant women should minimize their exposure, since waste anesthetic gases may result in spontaneous abortion and birth defects. Recommended acceptable levels of waste anesthetic gases are < 2 ppm when used alone, < 0.5 ppm when used in combination with nitrous oxide, and < 25 ppm of nitrous oxide. Some method to scavenge waste gases must be provided. Common methods for scavenging of waste gases utilize either an **active** system in which gas is drawn by a vacuum, fan, or pump to an evacuation site (usually to the outside) or a **passive** system in which the flow of waste gas is controlled by ventilation into a non-recirculating ventilation system, to the outside, or to a canister containing an absorptive compound. In general, passive systems tend to be easier to install and less expensive, but are typically less efficient.

2. Injectable Anesthetics

A large number of compounds have been used as injectable anesthetics. Here, we describe only a few representative examples of those commonly used in animal research. A more complete review of injectable anesthetics used for anesthesia of laboratory animal can be found elsewhere (48, 50).

A number of routes of injection are routinely used for administration of anesthetics, analgesics, and other pharmaceuticals. These routes include intravenous (i.v.), subcutaneous (s.c.), and intraperitoneal (i.p.).

Commonly used injectable agents for anesthesia include the following.

a. Ketamine Hydrochloride

Ketamine is classified by the DEA as a Schedule III controlled substance, thereby necessitating special storage and record keeping procedures.

b. Lidocaine

Lidocaine is usually infused into a specific anatomic area to provide regional or local anesthesia. Infusion of lidocaine rarely causes any tissue irritation.

c. Bupivicaine

Bupivicaine is a local anesthetic used similarly to lidocaine, but it has a much longer duration of action. It is the agent of choice for local anesthesia for many surgical procedures (52).

d. Sodium Pentobarbital

Sodium pentobarbital is a short-acting barbiturate used to produce general anesthesia. It depresses the respiratory and cardiovascular systems and may cause hypothermia. Sodium pentobarbital is classified by the DEA as a Schedule II controlled substance.

e. Tribromoethanol

Used principally for anesthesia of rodents, tribromoethanol produces surgical anesthesia when administered intraperitoneally. Use of this compound is disadvantaged by its irritancy, which may result in peritoneal adhesions and death of the animal.

3. Analgesics

Analgesics are compounds used to relieve pain associated with experimental procedures or spontaneous disease and injuries. Analgesics should be used even if the potential for pain exists. Although exceptions to the use of analgesics can be made if justified for scientific reasons, such exceptions must be approved by the IACUC on a case-by-case basis. The following are analgesics commonly used in laboratory animals.

a. Aspirin

Aspirin is a non-steroidal antiinflammatory drug that provides sufficient analgesia for mild to moderate pain.

b. Buprenorphine

A long-lasting potent analgesic, buprenorphine is classified by the DEA as a Schedule V controlled substance.

c. Butorphanol

Butorphanol is a potent analgesic with less duration than buprenorphine. It is classified by the DEA as a Schedule IV controlled substance.

d. Fentanyl

Fentanyl is relatively short acting, with an analgesic duration of 30 minutes or less in most species. It is often used for post-operative pain relief as a continuous infusion. In addition, a slow-release skin fentanyl patch has been used successfully for post-operative analgesia. The DEA classifies fentanyl as a Schedule II controlled substance.

e. Morphine

Morphine is a potent opioid agonist that has a relatively short analgesic duration (2–4 hours), although some longer-lasting preparations are available. Morphine is classified as a Schedule II controlled substance by the DEA.

D. MEDICAL RECORDS AND OVERSIGHT

Documentation of observations, treatments, and outcomes are an important part of the veterinary care program. Properly maintained records assist in facility management and document an adequate veterinary care program to regulatory officials. The veterinary staff often uses medical records retrospectively to "fine tune" procedures and treatments.

The specific contents of the records depend somewhat on the species being maintained and the types of procedures being performed. It is advantageous for records to be maintained after the animal has been euthanized, so that retrospective evaluation of procedures can be made if necessary. However, the logistical difficulties with archiving a large number of records, usually results in a more practical approach to retain records for a minimum of 3 years following completion of the study and euthanasia of the animal. Of course, studies being conducted under Good Laboratory Practices need to archive records indefinitely. Such GLP records should be stored under conditions that prevent tampering and damage due to extreme environmental conditions.

The following types of records have been suggested as important to veterinary care (53).

1. Standard Procedures and Animal Health

Many aspects of veterinary care are checked frequently, even daily, and observations should be recorded. Examples include evaluation of environmental parameters, behavioral/environmental enrichment efforts, provision of feed and water, and observation of animals. An effective method to accomplish this is to develop a standard operating procedure detailing what is to be included in routine animal husbandry. A daily check-off form can then be used to document that a procedure has occurred or that an observation has been made. It is practical to also employ a monthly room care check-off sheet to document activities occurring less frequently such as cage changing or disinfection. Perhaps the most efficient method of monitoring environmental conditions employs an online monitoring system that feeds information into a central computer that documents conditions and initiates an emergency response when upper or lower limits are exceeded. Several systems that provide this oversight are commercially available.

2. Medical Care Records

The veterinary staff should be alerted to any animal that is exhibiting abnormal behavior or signs suggestive of illness. Written documentation should describe the veterinary staff's findings, diagnostic procedures performed and results, treatments prescribed and provided, and follow-up care and progress of the animal. All procedures and information related to preventive medicine should also be recorded. Individual record files are often maintained for larger, less numerous species such as dogs, cats, nonhuman primates, exotic species and occasionally farm animals. For other, smaller animals such as rodents, which are members of a much larger group, colony/room/group records are generally sufficient. The exact format for these records is flexible but should allow easy retrieval of information.

An alternative to written medical care records is to store the information in an electronic format. A number of commercially available programs are available to accommodate this method. In addition, many facilities have chosen to develop their own electronic record-keeping systems through collaboration with their institutional information technology resources.

3.   **Breeding Colony Records**

It is important that accurate and accessible records be maintained for breeding colonies so that offspring of the desired lineage can be produced in an efficient manner. As the desirability of genetically pure animals for many types of research has increased, so too has the complexity of maintaining adequate records. An excellent review of colony record keeping and computerized colony management is described in detail elsewhere (54–56). Some basic principles follow.

a.   *Identification Number*

Each animal should have a unique identification number. A universal numbering system does not exist and many facilities have developed their own. Typically, an identification number will include characters that reference back to items such as the year (or even month and day) of birth, the source or lineage, the parity of the dam (e.g., 1st litter, 2nd litter, etc.), and the number of the mouse within its lineage (e.g., 4th offspring born to a specific dam). Of course, other information can be referenced in the code, but it is important to keep the numbering system as simple as possible while facilitating easy retrieval of key information.

b.   *Basic Background Information*

In addition to the information reflected in the identification number, additional basic information on each mouse should be maintained in the database. For example, the following information is useful:

- Parents
- Location within the facility
- Breeding history
- Sex
- Identification numbers of siblings
- Genotype
- Medical history (key components; may refer back to medical care records if detailed information is required)

Often, some, if not most, of this information is also reflected on the cage card.

4.   **Anesthetic and Peri-Procedural Care**

Records should detail pre-anesthetic and pre-procedural preparation of the animal, use of anesthetics, analgesics and other medications, monitoring of the animal during the procedure and during recovery, and supportive care. Records should be sufficiently detailed and organized so that it is clear that care consistent with accepted veterinary standards is being provided. In addition, it should be apparent that the veterinary staff has responded expeditiously to any significant problems. The records should begin with the initial pre-procedural evaluation of the animal and conclude following successful recovery of the animal after the procedure. For animals that have only undergone anesthesia for minor or noninvasive procedures, the records for each episode might conclude once the animal has resumed normal behavior and feed and water consumption, usually within 24 hours after anesthesia. For more invasive procedures, the records might extend over several days or even weeks.

The veterinary staff, in particular the attending veterinarian, should ensure that proper care is being provided to animals when procedures involving anesthesia or invasive methods are being performed. Ultimately, the IACUC is charged with making the determination that the veterinary staff is responsive. For this reason, the records should be clearly formulated and accessible to the IACUC. Standard forms are valuable for recording such information in a useable format.

Documentation should be made for any procedure and relevant outcome described in Tables 3, 4, and 5. This includes all pre-operative evaluation and preparation, administration of anesthetics, tranquilizers, sedatives, and analgesics, results of monitoring, and any supportive measures provided. All records of procedures should be accompanied by the date and time when the procedure was conducted and the initials of the individual performing the procedure. The dosage and route of administration should be recorded for any pharmaceutical provided. If catheters, sutures, endotracheal tubes or other devices have been placed, removal of such equipment should be recorded in the records.

E. BEHAVIORAL MANAGEMENT

The term "behavioral management" refers to potential enhancements and enrichments to the animal's cage environment, social environment, and activity level. Enrichment of the animal's environment should strive to present the animal with complex stimuli that alleviate the occurrence of abnormal behaviors (57). Examples of abnormal behaviors include self-injury, repetitive bar chewing in rodents (58), repetitive flipping in rodents, and repetitive pacing or circling (59).

A provision was made to the Animal Welfare Act, in 1985, which mandates conditions "adequate to promote the psychological well-being of nonhuman primates." Indeed, much focus has been given to methods for environmental enrichment of nonhuman primates; however, the possibility that other species can also benefit from steps taken to promote species-typical behavior has led to enrichment strategies for most species. It should be noted that many methods of enrichment are based on extrapolation of the species' behavior in the wild and subsequent observational analysis of the method in captivity.

The general goals of enrichment should be to stimulate the expression of species-typical behaviors and to allow the animal to exert some control over its environment. Specific methods for enrichment will vary with the species, and even the individual animal. A thorough knowledge of the typical behavior of the species is advantageous. Under no circumstances should forced activity, such as treadmill running, be used as an enrichment strategy. All efforts at environmental enrichment should be undertaken only after the potential for interference with the objectives of the research have been considered. Some examples of enrichment strategies are described below.

1. Group Housing

Group housing of compatible conspecifics is a valuable means to provide enrichment to social species. The positive interaction afforded by a cagemate is perhaps the richest form of environmental enhancement. Of course, it is important to determine that animals housed together are not aggressive toward one another (60, 61). Optimally, animals should be housed so that they are able to have physical contact with one another; however, when this is not possible animals may also benefit from visual, auditory, or olfactory contact. When housing animals in groups, one must also ensure that the cage size provides adequate space for each individual and is consistent with regulatory guidelines.

2. Encouragement of Foraging Behavior

The search for food occupies a significant portion of an animal's time in the natural environment. Many species seem to retain an interest in practicing this behavior in captivity; therefore, methods to encourage foraging behavior are considered useful as a means of environmental enrichment.

A number of approaches to provide opportunities to forage have been attempted. For example, specially designed puzzle feeders and other devices that allow the animal to retrieve a food reward by successfully guiding it out of the device have been used for nonhuman primates. Consumption of rawhide bones is a form of foraging for dogs. Seeds or other food treats can be mixed into bedding to allow rodents to forage for small treats. Foods that require additional processing by the animal for consumption can be used, such as provision of non-shucked corn-on-the-cob to nonhuman primates. For large animals such as ruminants and horses, grazing areas free from toxic plants can provide an opportunity to forage.

It is important that any food item provided for enrichment be palatable and free of contaminants. Food items should be provided in moderation so that the animals consume a normal portion of their regular, nutritionally balanced diet and do not become obese.

3. Provision of Inanimate Objects

A number of inanimate objects have been used to enhance the environment of captive animals. Objects should encourage exploration, be sanitizable or replaced when soiled, and be reasonably resistant to chewing and subsequent ingestion if not intended as a foodstuff. Examples include provision of nesting material, cardboard rolls, wooden blocks, marbles, and sections of PVC pipe to mice (62, 63); hard nylon bones or balls for chewing to rats (64); perches and harborage made of PVC pipe to bullfrogs (65); suspended chains and ropes, large balls, and straw rooting areas for swine (66); large wood climbing spools and other perches for goats (66); empty soft drink cans, balls, and wood blocks to rabbits (67); and swings, perches, balls, ropes, pads of synthetic fleece, and Kong toys to nonhuman primates (68–70). Many more examples exist beyond those indicated above. It is useful to rotate specific objects in and out of the animal's environment to maintain the novelty of the object.

4. Visual and Auditory Stimulation

Some research facilities have employed means to provide visual and auditory stimulation to animals, usually nonhuman primates. For example, when group housing with conspecifics is not possible, cages can be organized in such a way that animals have visual, auditory, or even minor tactile contact. When this is not possible, some facilities have used mirrors, televisions, and video systems. Others have utilized systems that provide the animal with a food treat for successful completion of a visual task through manipulation of a video game joy stick (71–74). Some auditory stimuli such as that provided by calm, soothing music or recordings of jungle sounds have been anecdotally noted to have a calming behavioral effect on rhesus monkeys (authors' personal observation).

F. EUTHANASIA

Euthanasia has been defined as a "good death," one that occurs without pain and distress (35). A commonly referenced document for discussions related to euthanasia is the 2000 Report of the AVMA Panel on Euthanasia (75). This document provides guidelines and recommendations for euthanasia of animals, including research animals. Revision of this document occurs periodically and the most current version should be reviewed.

The Report of the AVMA Panel describes a number of key considerations that should be used in evaluating methods of euthanasia, including:

- The ability to induce loss of consciousness and death without causing pain, distress, anxiety, or apprehension
- The time required to induced unconsciousness; ideally, this time will be short
- Reliability
- Safety to personnel
- Irreversibility
- Compatibility with the purpose (including the scientific objectives for research animals)
- Emotional effect on observers
- Compatibility with subsequent evaluation or use of tissue
- Availability and human abuse potential of drugs, if pharmaceuticals are to be used

- Age and species limitations
- Ability to maintain equipment in proper working order

In addition, it is important that those individuals performing euthanasia be properly trained so that distress and pain to the animal and potential for human injury are minimized.

It is important that death of the animal be ensured following the euthanasia procedure, since animals can sometimes recover following some methods, such as carbon dioxide overdose. Cessation of the heartbeat should be ensured. For smaller animals, a quick incision to lacerate the thorax and induce bilateral pneumothorax is useful. Alternatively, cervical dislocation can be used for animals that have been overdosed with carbon dioxide or anesthetics.

1.   Equipment Used for Euthanasia

A number of specialized pieces of equipment have been designed for euthanasia of animals. Table 6 lists some of the more common equipment within research animal facilities.

a.   *Carbon Dioxide Inhalation Chamber*

Chambers with a tubing connection to a compressed carbon dioxide gas cylinder are useful for euthanasia of many rodent species. Optimally, such chambers should be pre-charged to a carbon dioxide concentration of approximately 70% prior to introduction of the animal. The chamber should be large enough that animals are not crowded.

b.   *Guillotine*

Guillotines are available for euthanasia of small animals, including rodents and amphibians. Guillotines should be used only by trained individuals so that risk of injury to the operator and distress to the animal are minimized. Special plastic sleeves (Decapicones®) that fit around the animal as a restraint aid are available to facilitate use of the guillotine.

c.   *Cervical Dislocator*

Similar in appearance and use to the guillotine, the mechanical cervical dislocator does not result in decapitation, but instead results in euthanasia by dislocation of cervical vertebrae and subsequent disruption of critical brainstem function.

2.   Disposal of Carcasses

Carcasses are usually stored under refrigeration or in a freezer prior to disposal. Refrigeration is advisable if carcasses are being saved for later necropsy. In contrast, freezing is advisable to decrease putrefaction during longer-term storage. Carcasses contaminated with hazardous materials often require special disposal procedures. Disposal of medical waste, including carcasses, is regulated under the Medical Waste Tracking Act, which was written as an amendment to the Resource Conservation and Recovery Act (76, 77). In addition, many facilities are covered by state and local regulations for waste disposal.

Although several methods for disposal exist, animal carcasses are commonly disposed in one of three fashions.

a. Incineration

Extremely high burn temperatures are typically required for safe disposal of medical waste by incineration. Typical minimum temperatures range from

TABLE 6. Common Methods for Euthanasia of Laboratory Animals

Method	Species Commonly Used for	Comments
Carbon dioxide overdose	Rodents	Chamber should be precharged with CO_2 to approximately 70% concentration
Decapitation	Rodents, reptiles, amphibians, fish	Method should be used following anesthesia, if possible; mechanical guillotine should be used; use without anesthetics should be scientifically justified; sometimes used following stunning or pithing of amphibians and reptiles
Overdose with injectable anesthetics or euthanasia agents	Rodents, rabbits, cats, dogs, nonhuman primates	Agents should be administered intravenously (intraperitoneally is acceptable in rodents)
Cervical dislocation	Mice and rats less than 200 grams in body weight, chickens	Use of mechanical cervical dislocators is encouraged; use without anesthetics should be scientifically justified
Exsanguination	Rodents, rabbits	Animal must first be anesthetized; usually used when terminal blood or serum samples are needed
Immersion in tricaine methanesulfonate (MS-222)	Fish, amphibians	Typically, MS-222 solutions or 1-3 grams/liter of water are used
Overdose of inhalant anesthetics	Mammals, reptiles	Precautions should be taken so that animals do not experience distress during induction; note that some animals can hold their breath and euthanasia may require a very long exposure to the gas

1,400 to 1,800°F, depending upon the regulations of the state (78). Some facilities maintain their own incinerators, while others contract with a commercial disposal enterprise. Incineration of animal carcasses has been associated with ash barium levels in excess of standards (79).

b.   Rendering

Disposal of carcasses by rendering to animal by-products for other uses is utilized by some facilities. Typically, this is carried out by a commercial rendering service that transports the carcasses from the facility to the rendering plant. This method should not be used for disposal of carcasses contaminated with chemical, radiologic, or infectious hazards.

c.   Landfill

Carcasses are sometimes disposed with other waste to landfill sites. Commercial firms are usually contracted to transport carcasses to their landfill site. Routine landfill disposal should not be used for disposal of carcasses contaminated with hazardous materials.

3.   Distress of Personnel Associated with Euthanasia

Loss of a pet animal is a well-recognized emotional event that, for some people, rivals the loss of a family member (80). Similarly, a bond between humans and research animals often develops, which can create anxiety, even grief, when the animal is euthanized for either experimental or health reasons (81). It is important for those charged with management of laboratory animal resources to recognize this possibility and to address the needs of affected individuals. For example, individuals other than those having regular contact with the animal could be trained and instructed to perform the euthanasia. The manager should ensure that proper training in euthanasia procedures has been provided so that pain and distress to the animal is minimized. Likewise, animals should be accorded respect in the process of euthanasia. Some facilities use rituals, such as a moment of silence following euthanasia, to allow individuals an opportunity to process their emotions. Finally, it is important that the manager be sympathetic and provide consolation to personnel who are deeply affected by euthanasia of animals. Referral to counseling services can be beneficial for such individuals.

V.   FINANCIAL ASPECTS OF VETERINARY CARE

Funding of the program of veterinary care must be considered, so that adequate resources are available. A number of approaches exist, including recharge of costs to investigators or departments, subsidization of the veterinary care program by the institution, or incorporation of costs into per diem charges to create a "health maintenance organization" for the animals within the facility.

The approach adopted may depend upon the type of institution, whether it is an academic, commercial, or government institution. For academic institutions, the NIH *Cost Analysis and Rate Setting Manual for Animal Research Facilities* (82) is a useful document to follow. That publication indicates that costs associated with animal health care should be allocated to direct cost centers and included in billing rates. More information on rate setting can be found in Chapter 10.

REFERENCES

1. **Pakes, S.P.**, Adequate veterinary care as viewed by the American Association for Accreditation of Laboratory Animal Care, *J. Am. Vet. Med. Assoc.*, 168, 519, 1976.
2. **Anchel, M.**, Beyond "adequate veterinary care," *J. Am. Vet. Med. Assoc.*, 168, 513, 1976.
3. **Schwindaman, D.F.**, An evaluation of adequate veterinary care by the U.S. Department of Agriculture, *J. Am. Vet. Med. Assoc.*, 168, 517, 1976.
4. **Melby, E.C., Jr.**, What does "adequate veterinary care" mean to the American College of Laboratory Animal Medicine? *J. Am. Vet. Med. Assoc.*, 168, 508, 1976.
5. **Weisbroth, S.**, Guest editorial: Defining adequate veterinary care, *J. Med. Primatol.*, 5, 1, 1976.
6. **USDA Policy Manual, Policy #3, Veterinary Care**, April 14, 1997.
7. **USDA Policy Manual, Policy #22, Necropsy Requirements**, October 13, 1998.
8. **Jenkins, W.L.**, Educating veterinarians to prescribe and use drugs in a responsible manner, *J. Am. Vet. Med. Assoc.*, 202, 1708, 1993.
9. **Sojka, N.J.**, Extra-label drug use — veterinary practitioner views: Laboratory animals, *J. Am. Vet. Med. Assoc.*, 202, 1648, 1993.
10. **Banks, R.**, The unwritten duties of the LAM veterinarian: The IACUC experience, *Lab Anim.*, 21, 37, 1992.
11. **Hannah, H.W.**, The liability potential for laboratory animal and public veterinarians, *J. Am. Vet. Med. Assoc.*, 197, 1140, 1990.
12. **Hannah, H.W.**, Liability protection for laboratory animal and public veterinarians, *J. Am. Vet. Med. Assoc.*, 197, 1456, 1990.
13. **Chwalibog, A.**, Nutrition and the importance of nutrients to animal experiments, in *Handbook of Laboratory Animal Science, Vol. I, Selection and Handling of Animals in Biomedical Research*, Svendsen, P. and Hau, J., Eds., CRC Press, Boca Raton, 1994, chap. 13.
14. **Svendsen, P.**, Environmental impact on animal experiments, in *Handbook of Laboratory Animal Science, Vol. I, Selection and Handling of Animals in Biomedical Research*, Svendsen, P. and Hau, J., Eds., CRC Press, Boca Raton, 1994, chap. 14.
15. **Callahan, B.M., Hutchinson, K.A., Armstrong, A.L., and Keller, L.S.F.**, A comparison of four methods for sterilizing surgical instruments for rodent surgery, *Contemp. Top.*, 34, 57, 1995.
16. **Harkness, J.E. and Wagner J.E.**, *The Biology and Medicine of Rabbits and Rodents*, Williams & Wilkins, Baltimore, 1995.
17. **Waynforth, H.B. and Flecknell, P.A.**, *Experimental and Surgical Technique in the Rat*, 2nd ed., Academic Press, New York, 1992.
18. **Lang, C.M. and Mancuso, C.A.**, Instruments and sutures, in *Animal Physiologic Surgery*, 2nd ed., Lang, C.M., Ed., Springer-Verlag, New York, 1976, chap. 2.

19. **Steinbruchel, D.**, Microsurgical procedures in experimental research, in *Handbook of Laboratory Animal Science, Vol. I, Selection and Handling of Animals in Biomedical Research*, Svendsen, P. and Hau, J., Eds., CRC Press, Boca Raton, 1994, chap. 22.

20. **Lang, C.M. and Mancuso, C.A.**, Operating room procedures, in *Animal Physiologic Surgery*, 2nd ed., Lang, C.M., Ed., Springer-Verlag, New York, 1976, chap. 1.

21. **Nolan, T.E. and Conti, P.A.**, Centralized surgical service: the nuts and bolts, *Lab Anim.*, 8, 18, 1979.

22. **Conti, P.A.**, Why should you consider a centralized surgery service, *Lab Anim.*, 8, 30, 1979.

23. **White, W.J. and Blum, J.**, Design of surgical suites and postsurgical care units, in *Anesthesia and Analgesia in Laboratory Animals*, Kohn, D.F., Wixson, S.K., White, W.J., and Benson, G.J., Ed., Academic Press, New York, 1997, chap. 8.

24. **Olesen, H.P.**, Surgical procedures, in *Handbook of Laboratory Animal Science, Vol. I, Selection and Handling of Animals in Biomedical Research*, Svendsen, P. and Hau, J., Eds., CRC Press, Boca Raton, 1994, chap. 21.

25. **Brown, M.J. et al.**, Guidelines for animal surgery in research and teaching. *Am. J. Vet. Res.*, 54, 1544, 1993.

26. **King, C.S., Hessler, J.R., and Broderson, J.R.**, Management of a biocontainment research facility, *Lab Anim.*, 28, 26, 1999.

27. **Sorensen, D.**, Laboratory animal facilities, in *Handbook of Laboratory Animal Science, Vol. I, Selection and Handling of Animals in Biomedical Research*, Svendsen, P. and Hau, J., Eds., CRC Press, Boca Raton, 1994, chap. 9.

28. **Lamborn, C.**, The new ventilated rack systems: a look at emerging technology, *Lab Anim.*, 28, 42, 1999.

29. **Hessler, J., Broderson, R., and King, C.**, Rodent quarantine: facility design and equipment for small animal containment facilities, *Lab Anim.*, 28, 34, 1999.

30. **Feldman, D.B. and Seely, J.C.**, *Necropsy Guide: Rodents and the Rabbit*, CRC Press, Boca Raton, 1988.

31. **Andrews, E.J. and Lang, C.M.**, Necropsy of the dog, in *Animal Physiologic Surgery*, Lang, C.M., Ed., Springer-Verlag, New York, 1976, chap. 20.

32. **Feinstein, R.**, Necropsy procedures, in *Handbook of Laboratory Animal Science, Vol. I, Selection and Handling of Animals in Biomedical Research*, Svendsen, P. and Hau, J., Eds., CRC Press, Boca Raton, 1994, chap. 23.

33. **Berndt, T.L. and Burns, J.M.**, Voice recognition technology in the necropsy lab, *Lab Anim.*, 21, 37, 1992.

34. **International Air Transport Association**, *Live Animal Regulations*, 26th ed., IATA, Montreal, 1999.

35. **Wallace, M.E.**, Effects of stress due to deprivation and transport in different genotypes of house mouse, *Lab. Anim.*, 10, 335, 1976.

36. **Landi, M.S.**, Effects of shipping on the immune function in mice, *Am. J. Vet. Res.*, 43, 1654, 1982.

37. **Tuli, J.S., Smith, J.A., and Morton, D.B.**, Stress measurements after transportation, *Lab. Anim.*, 29, 132, 1995.

38. **Smith, M.W.**, Safety and hygiene, in *The UFAW Handbook on The Care and Managment of Laboratory Animals*, Vol. 1, 7th ed., Poole, T., Ed., Blackwell Science, Ltd., Oxford, 1999, chap. 10.

39. **Rehg, J.E. and Toth, L.A.**, Rodent quarantine programs: purpose, principles, and practice, *Lab. Anim. Sci.*, 48, 438, 1998.

40. **Butler, T.M., Brown, B.G., Dysko, R.C., Ford, E.W., Hoskins, D.E., Klein, H.J., Levin, J.L., Murray, K.A., Rosenberg, D.P., Southers, J.L., and Swenson, R.B.**, Medical Management, in *Nonhuman Primates in Biomedical Research: Biology and Management*, Bennett, B.T., Abee, C.R., and Henrickson, R., Eds., Academic Press, San Diego, 1995, chap. 13.

41. **Baskerville, M.**, Old world monkeys, in *The UFAW Handbook on The Care and Management of Laboratory Animals*, Vol. 1, 7th ed., Poole, T., Ed., Blackwell Science, Ltd., Oxford, 1999, chap. 39.

42. **Beckwith, C.S., Franklin, C.L., Hook, R.R., Besch-Williford, C.L., and Riley, L.K.**, Fecal PCR assay for diagnosis of *Helicobacter* infection in laboratory rodents, *J. Clin. Micro.*, 35, 1620, 1997.

43. **Committee on Infectious Diseases of Mice and Rats**, National Research Council, Health surveillance programs, in *Infectious Diseases of Mice and Rats*, National Academy Press, Washington, D.C., 1991, chap. 4.

44. **Muir, W.W. and Hubbell, J.A.E.**, *Handbook of Veterinary Anesthesia*, 2nd ed., Mosby, St. Louis, 1995.

45. **Vogler, G.**, Anesthesia equipment: types and uses, in *Anesthesia and Analgesia in Laboratory Animals*, Kohn, D.F., Wixson, S.K., White, W.J., and Benson, G.J., Eds., Academic Press, New York, 1997, chap. 7.

46. **Horne, D., Ogden, B., Houts, J., and Hall, A.**, A nonbreathing anesthetic delivery system for mice, *Lab Anim.*, 27, 32, 1998.

47. **Dubin, S.**, Use of biocompatible adhesive paste to improve the performance of rodent anesthesia face masks, *Lab Anim.*, 28, 50, 1999.

48. *Anesthesia and Analgesia in Laboratory Animals*, Kohn, D.F., Wixson, S., White, W.J., and Benson, G.J., Eds., Academic Press, New York, 1997.

49. **Skarda, R.T., Bednarski, R.M., Muir, W.W., and Hubbell, J.A.E.**, Anesthetic toxicity, oxygen toxicity, and drug interactions, in *Handbook of Veterinary Anesthesia*, Mosby Year Book, Inc., St. Louis, 1995, chap. 12.

50. **Flecknell, P.A.**, Anaesthesia, in *Laboratory Animal Anesthesia: A Practical Introduction for Research Workers and Technicians*, 2nd ed., Academic Press, San Diego, 1996.

51. **Branson, K.R. and Booth, N.H.**, Injectable anesthetics, in *Veterinary Pharmacology and Therapeutics*, Adams, H.R., Ed., Iowa State University Press, Ames, 1995.

52. **Steffey, E.P. and Booth, N.H.**, Local anesthetics, in *Veterinary Pharmacology and Therapeutics*, Adams, H.R., Ed., Iowa State University Press, Ames, 1995.

53. **Suckow, M.A. and Doerning, B.J.**, Assessment of veterinary care, in *The IACUC Handbook*, Silverman, J., Suckow, M.A., and Murthy, S., Eds., CRC Press, Boca Raton, 2000.

54. **Larkins, D.N.**, Computerized colony management, in *Systematic Approach to Evaluation of Mouse Mutations*, Sundberg, J.P. and Boggess, D., Eds., CRC Press, Boca Raton, 1999.

55. **Sundberg, B.A. and Sundberg, J.P.**, Necropsy methods for laboratory mice: biological characterization of a new mutation, in *Systematic Approach to Evaluation of Mouse Mutations*, Sundberg, J.P. and Boggess, D., Eds., CRC Press, Boca Raton, 1999.

56. **Festing, M.F.W. and Peters, A.G.**, Animal production and breeding methods, in *The UFAW Handbook on The Care and Management of Laboratory Animals*, Vol. 1, 7th ed., Poole, T., Ed., Blackwell Science, Ltd., Oxford, 1999, chap. 5.

57. **Bayne, K., Dexter, S., Mainzer, H., McCully, C., Campbell, G., and Yamada, F.,** The use of artificial turf as a foraging substrate for individually housed rhesus monkeys (*Macaca mulatta*), *Anim. Welfare,* 1, 39, 1992.

58. **Ödberg, F.O.,** The influence of cage size and environmental enrichment on the development of stereotypies in bank voles (*Clethrionomys glareolus*), *Behav. Processes,* 14, 155, 1987.

59. **Hubrecht, R.C., Serpell, J.A., and Poole, T.B.,** Correlates of pen size and housing conditions on the behaviour of kennelled dogs, *Appl. Anim. Behav. Sci.,* 34, 365, 1992.

60. **Bayne, K., Haines, M., Dexter, S., Woodman, D., and Evans, C.,** Nonhuman primate wounding prevalence: a retrospective analysis, *Lab Anim.,* 24, 40, 1995.

61. **Reinhardt, V.,** Social enrichment for laboratory primates: a critical review, *Lab. Primate Newsl.,* 29, 7, 1990.

62. **Hobbs, B.A., Kozubal, W., and Nebiar, F.F.,** Evaluation of objects for environmental enrichment of mice, *Contemp. Top.,* 36, 69, 1997.

63. **Coviello-McLaughlin, G.M. and Starr, S.J.,** Rodent enrichment devices — evaluation of preference and efficacy, *Contemp. Top.,* 36, 66, 1997.

64. **Watson, D.S.B.,** Evaluation of inanimate objects on commonly monitored variables in preclinical safety studies for mice and rats, *Lab. Anim. Sci.,* 43, 378, 1993.

65. **Bang, D. and Mack, V.,** Enriching the environment of the laboratory bullfrog (*Rana catesbiana*), *Lab Anim.,* 27, 41, 1998.

66. **Hays, J.T., Suckow, M.A., Jackson, G.E., and Douglas, F.A.,** Considerations in the design and construction of facilities for farm animal species, *Lab Anim.,* 27, 22, 1998.

67. **Huls, W.L., Brooks, D.L., and Bean-Knudsen, D.,** Response of adult New Zealand White rabbits to enrichment objects and paired housing, *Lab. Anim. Sci.,* 41, 609, 1991.

68. **Bryant, C.E., Rupniak, N.M.J., and Iversen, S.D.,** Effects of different environmental enrichment devices on cage stereotypies and autoaggression in captive cynomolgus monkeys, *J. Med. Primatol.,* 17, 257, 1988.

69. **Lam, K., Rupniak, N.M.J., and Iversen, S.D.,** The use of a grooming and foraging substrate to reduce stereotypies in macaques, *J. Med. Primatol.,* 20, 104, 1991.

70. **Kessel, A.L. and Brent, L.,** An activity cage for baboons, part I, *Contemp. Top.,* 34, 74, 1995.

71. **Hopkins, W.D., Washburn, D.A., and Rumbaugh, D.M.,** Note on hand use in the manipulation of joy-sticks by rhesus monkeys (*Macaca mulatta*) and chimpanzees (*Pan troglodytes*), *J. Comp. Psychol.,* 103, 91, 1989.

72. **Washburn, D.A., Hopkins, W.D., and Rumbaugh, D.M.,** Automation of learning-set testing: the video-task paradigm, *Behav. Res. Meth. Instrum. Comput.,* 21, 281, 1989.

73. **Richardson, W.K., Washburn, D.A., Hopkins, W.D. Savage-Rumbaugh, E.S., and Rumbaugh, D.M.,** The NASA/LRC computerized test system, *Behav. Res. Meth. Instrum. Comput.,* 22, 127, 1990.

74. **Andrews, M.W. and Rosenblum, L.A.,** Relative efficacy of video versus food-pellet reward of joystick tasks, *Percept. Mot. Skills,* 78, 545, 1994.

75. **AVMA Panel on Euthanasia,** 2000 Report of the AVMA panel on euthanasia, *J. Am. Vet. Med. Assoc.,* 218, 669, 2001.

76. **Code of Federal Regulations 40, §259.30.**

77. **U.S. Environmental Protection Agency,** Medical waste management in the United States: first interim report to Congress, p. 4-11, Office of Solid Waste, EPA, Washington, D.C., 1990.

78. **Brunner, C.R. and Brown, C.H.**, Hospital waste disposal by incineration, *J. Air Pollut. Contr. Assoc.*, 38, 1297, 1988.
79. **Gordon, B.E., Skoula, C.M., and Pulliam, C.L.**, Pyrolytic incineration of medical waste containing animal carcasses may result in excessive barium ash levels, *Contemp. Top.*, 34, 68, 1995.
80. **Beck, A. and Katcher, A.**, Breaking the bond, in *Between Pets and People: The Importance of Animal Companionship*, Purdue University Press, West Lafayette, IN, chap. 10.
81. **Walshaw, S.O.**, Animal death and human emotion in the laboratory, *Lab Anim.*, 23, 24, 1994.
82. **Cost Manual Revision Committee**, *Cost Analysis and Rate Setting Manual*, National Institutes of Health, National Center for Research Resources, Bethesda, MD, 2000.

6 Regulatory Compliance

Janet C. Gonder, D.V.M, Ph.D.

Management of a laboratory animal resource facility requires knowledge and understanding of federal, state, and local laws and regulations pertaining to the operation of the facility. The nature and extent of the regulations that apply to laboratory animal facilities may at first appear daunting. However, by breaking the requirements into smaller segments and enlisting the help of appropriate individuals, the task is less onerous. The importance of involving many different individuals in this process will become clear. At most institutions the animal care and use committee becomes the focus of many regulations that apply to the animal facility. There are, however, other institutional functions that participate in development of programs to comply with the many applicable regulations. Examples include departments of occupational health and safety and environmental safety.

A brief discussion of the regulatory process will help the reader understand how regulations and standards are developed and how institutions can contribute to the rule-making process. The process typically begins with a **Public Law** or **Act** passed by the United States Congress. The Law generally requires that an agency (e.g., United States Department of Agriculture) develop regulations and standards to ensure that the wishes of Congress stated in the Law are carried out. The regulations and standards basically define to whom the regulations apply and the requirements for compliance with the regulations. The agency generally publishes the proposed regulations in the **Federal Register** for a period of written public comment. The process can also involve public hearings where the agency gathers additional oral and written input from interested parties. Both of these mechanisms offer ways in which institutions can influence the regulations that affect them. Following the public comment period, the agency reviews all comments, and issues the **final rule**, which specifies the effective date of the regulation.

The extent and applicability of the regulations for animal facilities varies somewhat based on the species housed and type of research, teaching, and testing procedures performed. There are, however, fairly general regulations that apply to most facilities, as well as professionally accepted standards of practice that apply. It is these more general, or commonly encountered, regulations and practices that will be the focus of this chapter. State and local requirements, which may also have an impact on animal facility management (such as zoning and fire ordinances), must also be considered but are beyond the scope of this publication.

In this chapter, the main features of common regulations and standards are presented as they apply to typical animal research facilities, and examples are given to provide guidance concerning the implementation or application of these requirements.

I. ANIMAL WELFARE ACT AND REGULATIONS

The **Animal Welfare Act** (AWA), passed by the United States Congress in 1966, addressed a variety of activities involving animals in interstate and foreign commerce. The specific intent was to ensure that animals used in research, for exhibition, or in production for the pet trade were provided humane care and treatment, appropriate transportation, and to protect owners of animals from theft.

Subsequent amendments to the AWA, the latest in 1985 (1), have focused increased attention on the use of animals in research, testing, and teaching. The regulations and standards published by the U.S. Department of Agriculture (USDA) pursuant to the AWA include very specific requirements for research facilities (2). The AWA itself is quite specific regarding some of the requirements that were to be addressed by the USDA when writing the regulations. In addition to the development of minimum standards for housing, feeding, watering, sanitation, and other standards for most species, the AWA specifies that minimum standards be developed for the exercise of dogs, and for a physical environment adequate to promote the psychological well-being of nonhuman primates. It also specifies that research facilities must:

- Consider procedures to minimize pain and distress
- Consider the use of alternatives to animals
- Require veterinary consultation for use of anesthetics and for pre- and postsurgical care
- Prohibit the use of paralytics without anesthesia
- Restrict the use of animals in more than one major operative procedure
- Provide training
- Establish an **Institutional Animal Care and Use Committee (IACUC)** with specific responsibilities to oversee its animal-related activities

The detail included by Congress in the 1985 Amendments to the AWA was considered unusual at the time and provided the Secretary of Agriculture and the USDA little flexibility in developing the regulations and standards in some areas. However, in many areas, the standards have taken the approach of performance expectations, rather than more specific "engineering-based" standards.

The following discussion focuses on a few of the requirements of the **Animal Welfare Act Regulations (AWAR)** (2) that have an impact on management of animal facility programs today.

A. THE INSTITUTIONAL ANIMAL CARE AND USE COMMITTEE (IACUC)

Although the Animal Welfare Act itself is very specific with respect to the establishment and function of the IACUC, it is Subpart C — Research Facilities of the AWAR (Part 2) that defines detailed requirements of the IACUC. Management should refer to the regulations for information on committee appointment and membership, program review and inspection responsibilities, protocol review and approval, and authority for the animal care and use program.

A key responsibility of the IACUC is the semi-annual inspection of the animal facility and review of the animal care and use program. The requirement to inspect the animal care facility and animal use areas is generally well understood. The IACUC, or a designated inspection sub-committee, typically tours the facility and evaluates the physical plant and associated animal care procedures such as husbandry in accordance with the AWAR. The requirement to review the entire program of animal care and use is sometimes neglected. Program review entails review of all aspects of the program from function of the IACUC to the adequacy of training programs. Some IACUCs include in the review standard operating procedures and facility policies related to the animal care and use program. The semi-annual program review process is also an opportunity to follow up on adherence to protocols and procedures that the committee has previously approved, although this is not a specific requirement.

The regulations do specify certain record-keeping requirements related to the function of the IACUC. The IACUC is required to maintain minutes of its meetings that include attendance, activities of the committee, and results of deliberations. Records of proposed activities, commonly referred to as **"protocols,"** must be kept as well as a record of the IACUC decision to grant or withhold protocol approval. The semi-annual inspection and program review must be documented, and the report must contain results of the review, any deficiencies (designated as either minor or significant), timelines for deficiency correction, and any minority reports. The semi-annual report is to be signed by a majority of committee members and forwarded to the designated Institutional Official. The regulations also require that each registered facility submit to the USDA an annual report that includes a number of assurances as well as information on the numbers of animals used and the categorization of animal use. The report must be signed and certified by the Institutional Official. The AWAR require that records be retained for a minimum of three years after the completion of the activity. A thorough review of the IACUC requirements is presented elsewhere (3). Subpart C of Part 2 of the AWAR addresses the programmatic requirements for qualifications and training of personnel, and provision of veterinary care, covered in depth in Chapters 2 and 5 of this book.

B. EXERCISE FOR DOGS

The requirement for exercise of dogs has been the subject of considerable discussion since the AWA was passed. In the case of dog exercise, the AWA provided little guidance other than that the exercise program be determined by the attending veterinarian and be in accordance with the standards to be developed. The subsequent AWAR (Part 3 – Subpart A) establishes several requirements worthy of comment.

The facility is required to develop, document, and follow a plan (approved by the attending veterinarian) to provide dogs with the opportunity for exercise. In practice, and in certain parts of the standard, this has been interpreted to require involvement of the IACUC in the process. The plan must be a written program with specific procedures for implementation. The expected approach is to define program-specific ways of achieving the goal of exercise. The "opportunity for exercise" need only be addressed if certain minimum requirements for housing space are not met. For dogs housed individually, additional opportunity for exercise need not be provided if the floor space provided in the enclosure is at least twice the minimum space required by the AWAR for individually housed dogs. When housed in groups, no additional exercise is required if the total floor space is at least 100% of the AWAR required space for each dog if maintained separately. This standard has generated significant controversy. The standards provide little guidance for the provision of exercise if the above space requirements are not met, other than that dogs be provided access to a run or open area. The frequency and duration of exercise is not specified, but is to be determined by the attending veterinarian.

Most institutions have been able to comply with the regulations by first developing a written plan that simply outlines or specifies how dogs will be housed in their facilities (i.e., space requirements) and how they will be exercised, if required. The plan is typically approved by the IACUC and reviewed on a schedule consistent with the review of protocols (annually) or in conjunction with the IACUC's semi-annual program review. Because of the lack of specific requirements in the AWAR, many facilities have selected a frequency and duration of exercise opportunity consistent with the available exercise space, the average daily canine population, and personnel resources. With that as a starting point, periodic observation (with documentation) of the behavior of the animals serves as a means of evaluating the success of the program. A conscientious effort to plan, implement, evaluate, and improve the exercise program for dogs, if appropriately documented, is generally sufficient to demonstrate compliance to the standard. Additional guidance can be found in the National Research Council publication, *Laboratory Animal Management: Dogs* (4).

C.   PSYCHOLOGICAL WELL-BEING OF NONHUMAN PRIMATES

While the AWA states that facilities housing non-human primates must provide a "physical environment" adequate to promote the psychological well-being of primates, the AWAR (Part 3 – Subpart B) specifies that "environmental enhancement" be provided. An environmental enhancement plan must be developed that is consistent with appropriate professional standards as cited in appropriate professional journals or reference guides. Initial plans developed by institutions utilized numerous and varied strategies. While it was clear that a certain degree of flexibility was essential to developing and implementing effective programs, the need for guidelines was recognized. The National Research Council, Institute for Laboratory Animal Research (ILAR) subsequently published guidelines specifically addressing this requirement. That report, *The Psychological Well-Being of Nonhuman Primates* (5), provides considerable information on environmental enhancement strategies for different species and for different situations. The report supports the performance-based standard approach as distinct from engineering-based standards, but emphasizes the need for scientific approaches to meeting the standards so that results can be measured and evaluated. When using this document as a guideline, it is important that professional judgement is used in interpreting and applying the recommendations. As in the case with the care of any animal species, the specific knowledge, experience, and skills of the facility personnel involved in the implementation of the program is critical.

The AWAR for environmental enhancement do specify areas that must be addressed, including social grouping, environmental enrichment, special considerations, and restraint devices. The facility plan must address the social needs of any nonhuman primate species known to exist in social groups in the wild. Exceptions to the requirement for social interaction may include animals that exhibit overly aggressive behavior or those that are debilitated as a result of age or other conditions. It is recognized that animals suspected of having contagious disease, would need to be isolated from other animals, as would animals undergoing diagnosis and treatment of a disease condition. Compatibility of animals housed in groups is stressed. If housed individually, the animals must be able to see and hear others of their species unless this is contraindicated for medical or scientific reasons and so documented.

The AWAR suggest several approaches to environmental enrichment designed to provide a means for the animals to express species-typical activities. Examples include:

- Perches, swings, mirrors, and various cage complexities
- Objects to manipulate
- Varied food items and foraging opportunities
- Interaction with caretakers where appropriate
- Housing with compatible conspecifics

It is recognized that special circumstances may exist that will influence the approach to housing and environmental enrichment. These include provisions for infants and juveniles, research-based protocol restrictions, and the housing of large great apes.

The AWAR prohibit the use of restraint devices unless required for health reasons (determined by the attending veterinarian) or as part of a research protocol approved by the IACUC. The restraint should be for the shortest time possible. If restraint exceeds 12 hours, the animal should periodically be provided with the opportunity for unrestrained exercise if the research protocol or situation permits.

The institution's approach to meeting the requirement for environmental enhancement can be very similar to that for exercise for dogs. A written plan is developed taking into consideration the species, existing facility and equipment, and personnel resources. The plan is typically approved by the IACUC and reviewed on a regular basis. The plan should include methods of data collection that allow for evaluation of the success of the program. The ILAR report, *The Psychological Well-Being of Nonhuman Primates* (5), provides guidance not only on strategies for implementation, but also on measures that can be used to evaluate success. By using the ILAR report and other available information, compliance with the standard can be achieved with diligent planning, implementation, evaluation, and improvement that is well documented.

D.   OTHER AWA REQUIREMENTS

The AWAR (Part 3 – Subparts A–F) contain the majority of the requirements specific to the care of various species including, requirements for facilities, operations, animal health and husbandry, and transportation. Detailed standards are provided for areas such as indoor and outdoor housing, primary enclosures (cages and pens), feeding, watering, cleaning and sanitation, and pest control. In some cases the standards are quite specific (engineering-based standards). However, the concept of performance-based standards and use of professional judgment is evident throughout the section.

In 1998 the USDA amended the regulations under the Animal Welfare Act to address issues of comfort and foot injury associated with housing of dogs and cats on suspended mesh or slatted flooring (6). Following a phase-in period for new purchases, the requirements of this amendment became effective for all primary enclosures in January 2000.

The standards for primary enclosures for dogs and cats (Part 3, Subpart A, Section 3.6) state that the enclosures must have "floors that are constructed in a manner that protects the dogs' and cats' feet and legs from injury, and that, if of mesh or slatted construction, do not allow the dogs' or cats' feet to pass through any openings in the floor." The standards require that suspended flooring for dogs and cats either be constructed of metal strands greater than 1/8" (9 gauge) in diameter or coated with a material such as plastic or fiberglass. Primary enclosures with such flooring must also be constructed so that the floor does not bend or sag between the structural supports.

The intent of this amendment was to address concerns that certain types and designs of suspended flooring contributed to foot injuries, and that appropriate modification would decrease the incidence of such problems. In addition, sagging, unstable floors were thought to cause psychological trauma for dogs trying to balance on the floors. The modifications to the standards were intended to improve comfort for dogs and cats housed in primary enclosures with suspended floors. With the exception of the most recent changes, requirements included in the AWAR were incorporated into the 1996 Revision of the

National Research Council *Guide for the Care and Use of Laboratory Animals (Guide)* (7), covered later in this chapter.

II. PUBLIC HEALTH SERVICE POLICY

In 1985 Congress passed the **Health Research Extension Act of 1985**, "Animals in Research" (8), which directed the National Institutes of Health (NIH) to establish guidelines for the proper care, treatment, and monitoring of animals used in biomedical and behavioral research. Like the AWA that was enacted in the same year, this funding agency act mandated the organization and operation of IACUCs at all institutions that received funds from the PHS.

In 1986 the *Public Health Service Policy on Humane Care and Use of Laboratory Animals* (**PHS Policy**) (9) was developed in order to implement the Health Research Extension Act of 1985. PHS Policy applies to all PHS-conducted or supported activities involving animals. Many activities at U.S. institutions, particularly academic centers, are directly or indirectly supported by funds from the PHS.

The PHS Policy emphasizes adherence to the **U.S. Government Principles for the Utilization and Care of Vertebrate Animals Used in Testing, Research and Training** (9). Briefly, the principles address:

- The care and use of animals
- Consideration of alternatives to animal use
- Anesthesia and analgesia
- Minimization of discomfort, distress, and pain
- The provision of adequate veterinary care
- Qualifications and experience of personnel

The PHS requires institutions to use the *Guide* as the basis for the operation of their animal care and use programs. Several specific requirements are delineated as part of PHS Policy, while others are incorporated in the *Guide*. PHS Policy requires that institutions engaged in activities involving animals that are supported by the PHS submit a written **Animal Welfare Assurance** to the NIH **Office of Laboratory Animal Welfare (OLAW)**. The submitted Assurance is reviewed by OLAW staff members to assess the institution's compliance with PHS Policy.

The PHS Policy specifically requires the involvement of the IACUC and specifies the membership and functions of the committee as well as the recordkeeping and reporting requirements for the institution. One primary IACUC function is the review of proposed animal studies and ongoing (every 6 months) review of the animal care and use program. The program is expected to comply with the *Guide* and AWAR.

The institution's Assurance is generally prepared with input from the management of the animal care and use program and the IACUC and forwarded by the Institutional Official to OLAW for approval. Each application for project funding from an institution must include the institution's Animal Welfare Assurance number. The institution must also submit annual reports to OLAW. In addition to requiring that an Assurance be on file, the PHS stipulates that the institution provide verification of IACUC approval for all animal activities included in the grant application. Helpful information on compliance with PHS Policy can be found on the OLAW Web site (http://grants.nih.gov/grants/olaw/olaw.htm).

A. GUIDE FOR THE CARE AND USE OF LABORATORY ANIMALS

The National Research Council's *Guide for the Care and Use of Laboratory Animals (Guide)* (7) has for many years been the primary guidance document for the operation of animal research facilities. This document has become the recognized standard of animal care and use and predates the legally mandated requirements of the USDA and PHS. The *Guide* was first published in 1963 under the title, *Guide for Laboratory Animal Facilities and Care*. It was subsequently revised in 1965, 1968, 1972, 1978, 1985, and most recently in 1996. The *Guide* is intended to assist institutions in caring for and using animals in ways that are scientifically, technically, and ethically appropriate. As mentioned above, the *Guide* incorporates and expands upon many of the requirements of the Animal Welfare Act, and is the primary guidance document for compliance with Public Health Service Policy. Very broadly, the *Guide* addresses both general and specific recommendations and requirements applicable to a wide variety of facilities and programs. Some of the more specific requirements are based on current regulatory requirements. The *Guide* is generally organized into four major parts: institutional policies and responsibilities; animal environment, housing and management; veterinary medical care; and physical plant. Much of what is covered in the *Guide* is addressed in other chapters of this text.

Particularly noteworthy in the 1996 revision of the *Guide* is the clear change in implementation strategy for the recommendations. In the introductory statements, users of the *Guide* are charged with the responsibility of achieving specific outcomes, but the document leaves it up to them how to accomplish the goals. This has represented a shift from compliance with prescriptive engineering-based standards to more flexible performance-based standards.

The application of the concept of performance-based standards requires a great deal of thought and diligence on the part of facility managers. With fewer defined "specifications," each facility is charged with developing its own set of approaches to accomplish the specific outcomes or goals discussed in the *Guide*. In many ways, this flexibility is very desirable because of the great diversity of facilities, programs and species encountered. However, a successful performance-based approach requires considerable professional input, interpretation, and judgement in order to define and achieve the many goals of the program. Investigators, IACUC members, veterinarians, facility managers, and other key program participants need to be involved in decisions regarding animal use. IACUCs play a key role in development, oversight, and evaluation of institutional animal care and use programs.

The *Guide* highlights three areas in which the performance-based standards approach needs to be broadly applied:

- Farm animals
- Nontraditional species
- Field investigations

The use of **farm animals** in research and teaching has often been separated into biomedical and agricultural use categories. The distinction and regulatory requirements have typically been defined by the project category (agricultural vs. biomedical research) rather than by the goals and focus of the project. The *Guide* recognizes that there are circumstances where a more controlled laboratory housing environment might be needed for agricultural research studies or where farm animals used in biomedical research can be appropriately housed in a typical farm setting. Therefore, the *Guide* recommendations apply generally to farm animals used in biomedical research, whether housed in the laboratory or a farm setting. When the standards of performance permit housing in a farm setting, the *Guide* recommends use of ***The Guide for the Care and Use of Agricultural Animals in Agricultural Research and Teaching (Ag Guide)*** (10), which is discussed later in this chapter.

Nontraditional species and **field investigations** present an even broader array of potential decisions regarding animal care and use. In both cases, many of the concepts presented in the *Guide* can be applied, but each situation will need to be separately evaluated. Expert advice should be sought when developing strategies for these types of situations. Because of the uniqueness of these situations and the lack of readily available or recognized guidelines, establishment of performance-based goals, standardized procedures, and valid measurements of outcomes may be even more critical for these types of programs.

B. AGRICULTURAL ANIMALS

The *Guide for the Care and Use of Agricultural Animals in Agricultural Research and Teaching (Ag Guide)* was first published in 1988 and revised in 1999 by the Federation of Animal Science Societies (10). The *Ag Guide* focuses on warm-blooded vertebrate animals used in agricultural research and teaching, for which the scientific objectives are to improve understanding of the animal's use in production agriculture. These studies often require a simulated or actual production agriculture setting consistent with consideration of the animal's well-being.

The type of animal facility used for agricultural species depends on the nature of the research or teaching objective, and may vary from a carefully controlled environment to actual farms and ranches. In many cases a blending of existing guidelines will be necessary, and will require appropriate professional judgement. The organization of the *Ag Guide* is very similar to the NRC *Guide*. The first four chapters provide general guidelines for institutional policies, animal husbandry, agricultural animal health care, and physical plant. The remainder of the publication addresses requirements for specific agricultural animal species (i.e., beef cattle, dairy cattle, horses, poultry, sheep and goats, swine, and veal calves).

The *Ag Guide* focuses on agricultural animals in agricultural research activities. The use of these species in this setting is not specifically regulated by the Animal Welfare Act. Effective March 6, 2000, the U.S. Department of Agriculture adopted both the *Ag Guide* and the NRC *Guide* as official guidelines for the use of agricultural animals for nonagricultural purposes (i.e., for biomedical research) (11). In doing so, the USDA recognized the balance and flexibility necessary in managing and evaluating various types of research programs. Because the AWAR provide little species-specific information on agricultural animals, these two guides represent the most current thinking on appropriate practices for the handling, care, treatment, and transportation of farm animals for nonagricultural purposes. While the USDA has stated that it will not require regulated entities to comply with the recommendations in the two guides, there is clearly an expectation that these guides be used as references.

Both the *Guide* and the *Ag Guide* represent the current best thinking of highly qualified and experienced professionals in these respective fields. The USDA's recognition of user-defined guidelines represents an example of how a regulatory agency has adopted and expanded the concept of performance-based standards in a regulated environment. Goal definition, written procedures, measurement criteria, and documented evaluation will likely be expected for compliance with these requirements.

III. FOOD AND DRUG ADMINISTRATION

In recent years, many more institutions are becoming involved in research, development, and testing activities regulated by the **Food and Drug Administration (FDA)**. Safety studies (sometimes referred to as pre-clinical or nonclinical studies) that demonstrate the safety of a product or therapy are regulated by the FDA under the regulations and standards referred to as **"Good Laboratory Practice for Nonclinical Studies" or GLPs** (12).

More specifically, compliance with GLPs is required for laboratory studies that support or are intended to support applications for approval of products as required by the FDA. Such products include drugs, biologics, and medical devices for human and animal use. These types of studies typically use animals as the test system, although they also include *in vitro* test systems. The GLP regulations do not apply to studies utilizing human subjects or field trials in animals, nor do they apply to basic exploratory or feasibility studies on a potential product.

The GLP regulations address specific test facility, personnel, and recordkeeping requirements for this type of study. These requirements can often be met with little or no significant change in operations for most animal facilities. Compliance may simply involve adoption of written Standard Operating Procedures (SOPs) and more detailed documentation of adherence to the SOPs. Some requirements may, however, involve significant facility, personnel, and operational changes.

Following are examples of GLP requirements that impact directly on animal facility operations. There are many other specific requirements for institution personnel responsible for planning and implementing a safety study.

A. ORGANIZATION AND PERSONNEL

The GLP regulations are very similar to the AWAR in that all personnel involved in the conduct of a safety study or responsible for the supervision of a safety study must have the education, training, and experience to perform the assigned functions. The regulations specify that a summary of training and experience and a job description be maintained for each individual. This information is typically maintained as an individual employee training file. Other requirements are very general, such as sufficient numbers of personnel, use of protective clothing, and exclusion of personnel due to illness that could impact the study outcome. The testing facility management is responsible for several assurances including the requirement that personnel, resources, facilities, equipment, materials, and methods are available as scheduled. Some of these functions and available resources reside in the animal facility and are therefore the responsibility of animal facility management. In the course of a safety study, all activities defined in the study protocol and SOPs must be extensively and accurately documented in order to ensure complete traceability of what was done, when it was done, and by whom it was done.

B. STANDARD OPERATING PROCEDURES

The GLP regulations (12) require that facilities have written SOPs adequate to ensure the quality and integrity of the data generated in a safety study. The regulations specify that SOPs must be established for at least the following animal study activities:

    Animal room preparation
    Animal care

Receipt, identification, storage, handling, mixing, and method of sampling test
and control articles

Test system (e.g., animal) observations

Laboratory tests

Handling of animals found moribund or dead during a study

Necropsy of animals or postmortem examination of animals

Collection and identification of specimens

Histopathology

Data handling, storage, and retrieval

Maintenance and calibration of equipment

Transfer, proper placement, and identification of animals

The SOPs related to the process being performed must be immediately available in the laboratory. A historical file of SOPs and all revisions including dates must be maintained.

C. ANIMAL FACILITIES

Animal facilities used for the conduct of safety studies must provide a degree of separation that will prevent any unrelated function or activity from having an adverse effect on the study. There must be a sufficient number of animal rooms to allow separation of species, hazardous activities, test systems, and studies. Appropriate space must be provided for quarantine of animals. Similar to conditions required by the AWAR and the *Guide,* separate areas must be provided, as appropriate, for the diagnosis, treatment, and control of animal diseases, and for collection and disposal of animal waste and refuse. Storage areas for food and bedding must be separated from the animal housing rooms and protected from infestation or contamination. With one exception, the animal facility features and practices listed above should not be notably different from animal facilities at most institutions. The exception may be the requirement for physical separation (usually by room) of individual safety studies.

D. EQUIPMENT

Use of equipment that supports the conduct of safety studies typically requires testing and documentation not usually part of the standard practices in most animal facilities. The regulation applies to any equipment used in the generation, measurement, or assessment of data, as well as equipment used for facility environmental monitoring and control. All equipment must be adequately inspected, cleaned, maintained, calibrated and/or standardized, and tested. Written SOPs are required and must include sufficient detail of the methods, materials and schedules to be used in the routine inspection, cleaning, maintenance, testing, and calibration and/or standardization of the equipment. The SOP should also specify actions to be taken in the event of failure or malfunction of the equipment. Specific personnel (generally identified by job title) responsible for performing each operation must be indicated.

Records must be maintained of all related operations and must include the date and SOP reference for routine procedures. Documentation of non-routine repairs due to failure or malfunction must indicate the nature of the problem, how and when it was discovered, and action taken to resolve the problem. The requirements above are very general in nature and interpretation of these requirements varies with the type and use of the equipment.

Even for very simple equipment such as thermometers, certain controls may be needed. For example, a thermometer or electronic probe used to monitor or record the temperature of a room or rectal temperature of a study animal, should periodically be tested and calibrated against a standard. Scales and balances used to weigh animals and other study materials should be calibrated periodically using nationally accepted standards such as those published by the National Institute of Standards and Technology (NIST). Test equipment that generates data (e.g., a serum chemistry analyzer) must be calibrated against appropriate standards and should be used with appropriate standardized controls.

Equipment that electronically acquires, stores, manipulates and/or generates data (computerized systems) presents substantive additional requirements. Electronic equipment comes under a relatively new regulation, 21 CFR, Part 11, that became effective in 1997 (13). Briefly, the regulation entails absolute assurance that electronic records be trustworthy, reliable, and generally equivalent to paper records. Applicable electronic records are defined as any combination of text, graphics, data, audio, pictorial, or other information representation in digital form that is created, modified, maintained, archived, retrieved, or transmitted by a computer system. Compliance with this regulation generally requires a formal, documented validation process to demonstrate that the electronically stored data remain unaffected during storage and can be retrieved in the same form (i.e., identical to) as that used for original interpretation of the data. Validation ensures accuracy, reliability, consistency, and the ability to discern invalid or altered records. It also requires that any calculations or data manipulations done electronically have been validated over the expected range of data collected. The stringency of these FDA requirements mandates a high standard for the use of computer software systems. Any system proposed for use in acquisition, analysis, or storage of data for FDA-compliant studies will require careful selection and use.

System security is also emphasized. Limited access, usually via password protection, is expected. The ability to control and document changes to the electronic data must also be assured. This includes documentation of when the change was made, by whom, and the reason for the change.

E. ANIMAL CARE

Subpart E of the GLP regulations, entitled "Testing Facilities Operation," defines the SOP requirements discussed above and deals specifically with the requirements for animal care. Specifically, the animal care SOP should include procedures for the housing, feeding, handling, and care of animals. All newly received animals from outside sources should be isolated from existing populations. The health status of new arrivals should be evaluated in accordance with acceptable veterinary practice. Although an SOP on animal quarantine and conditioning is not specifically mentioned, FDA inspectors will typically ask to see one.

At the initiation of a safety study, animals should be free of any disease or condition that might interfere with the purpose or conduct of the study. Animals that contract such a disease or condition during the course of the study should be isolated, if necessary. They may be treated, provided that the treatment does not interfere with the study. The diagnosis of the condition as well as the authorization, description, and dates of treatment must be documented and retained as part of the data package for the study.

Warm-blooded animals (excluding suckling rodents) should be individually identified if used either in procedures that require manipulations and observations over an extended period of time, or in procedures that require the animals to be removed from and returned to their home cages for any reason. Removal includes cage cleaning, animal treatment, and other routine practices. The listed examples of appropriate identification given are tattoo, color code, ear tag, and ear punch. All information needed to identify each animal within an animal housing unit should appear on the outside of that unit.

Although some types of studies may call for individual housing of animals (e.g., metabolism studies), the regulation does not specifically require that animals be housed in separate cages. However, some facilities typically house animals singly in order to minimize the opportunity for identification and dosing errors. Implantable chip identification systems have greatly facilitated animal identification in group-housing situations and for long-term studies. The electronic systems require initial validation efforts, as mentioned earlier.

Animals of different species are typically housed in separate rooms. Valid study-specific exceptions to this standard would be unusual. Animals of the same species being used in different studies are likewise not ordinarily housed in the same room. Separation by study prevents inadvertent exposure of animals to unrelated test or control articles and reduces the potential for animal misidentification.

Sanitation procedures are not specifically outlined in the GLP regulations. The only statements in this regard specify that cages, racks, and necessary equipment be cleaned and sanitized at appropriate intervals. Bedding used in animal cages should be of a material that will not interfere with the purpose or conduct of the study. It is to be changed as often as necessary to keep the animals clean and dry. It is expected that other regulations such as the AWAR, as well as accepted practice, will be followed. Adherence to the facility's written standard operating procedures is expected.

The GLP regulations require that feed and water be analyzed periodically to ensure that contaminants known to be capable of interfering with the study are not present at levels above those specified in the protocol. The protocol must reference specific SOPs for water and feed quality control. The requirement for water quality assessment is usually met with periodic sampling and analysis of the water and the water distribution system as defined in a facility SOP. For feed, analysis or certification of each lot or shipment of feed may be required. In some cases, reserve samples of feed are kept for potential future analysis. Results of feed and water analyses are documented and retained as original or raw data.

Use of pest control materials should be documented. Cleaning and pest control materials that might interfere with the study should not be used. Typically, FDA inspectors will ask to see a written SOP addressing pest control along with documentation of implementation.

In response to most regulatory requirements, demonstrating compliance relies heavily on sound and conscientious record-keeping practices. The practice of recording what is to be done (protocol, SOP), what was done (data, results), when it was done (date), and who did it (signature) constitutes a good approach.

IV. OCCUPATIONAL HEALTH AND SAFETY

A. OCCUPATIONAL SAFETY AND HEALTH ADMINISTRATION

The United States **Occupational Safety and Health Administration (OSHA)** is responsible for enforcing regulations and standards related to workplace safety. The primary authority for this activity comes from the **Occupational Safety and Health Act of 1970**, amended in 1990 and 1998 (14). The purpose of the act is to ensure safe and healthful working conditions, provide for enforcement authority for adherence to standards developed, and assist states in efforts to ensure workplace safety. The act also provides for research, education, and training in the field of occupational health and safety. The **Occupational Safety and Health Standards** (15), developed pursuant to the Act, include many parts that apply to the research animal laboratory. The discussion below will highlight some of the standards that are key to complying with the requirements of the Act.

The employee "right to know" concept is very generally laid out in the introduction to the standards. Employers must ensure that all employees are thoroughly apprised of all hazards to which they are exposed in the workplace. In addition to naming and describing these risks, the employer must outline relevant symptoms of exposure, appropriate emergency medical treatment, and proper conditions and precautions to ensure safe use. Employers must provide suitable protective equipment and control procedures, and provide for monitoring at locations and intervals as necessary to protect employees. The use of engineering-based standards, work practice controls, and personal protective equipment are stressed. These include the use of gloves, masks and/or face shields, protective clothing, safety glasses with side shields, and additional protection as necessary. Medical examinations, at employer cost, must be provided as appropriate to determine the effect of the hazard on the employee. Each specific standard includes a provision for training programs that must be in place to inform employees of workplace hazards.

The **Bloodborne Pathogens Standard**, Part 1910.1030 (15) is designed to protect employees from disease transmission from bloodborne pathogens and other potentially infectious material. While this standard focuses primarily on human pathogens, the **"Universal Precautions"** outlined are clearly relevant to protection of workers from potential hazards in an animal facility. These universal precautions, including the use of personal protective equipment (PPE), are intended to prevent parenteral, mucous membrane, and non-intact skin exposure to pathogens. These Universal Precautions are clearly applicable for certain animal studies involving infectious agents that are transmissible to humans. All procedures involving macaques are currently subject to implementation of Universal Precautions and other safeguards due to the incidence of zoonotic herpesvirus in the macaque population. (See also Chapter 13.)

The standard emphasizes safe work practices such as hand washing, prohibition of eating, drinking, or application of cosmetics in work areas, and safe transport of laboratory samples. Housekeeping practices such as the use of EPA-registered disinfectants, a written schedule for cleaning, and regulated waste handling are covered. It is in the Bloodborne Pathogen Standard that the disposal of contaminated needles and other sharps is discussed. The standard states that these materials "shall not be recapped or removed unless the employer can demonstrate that no alternative is possible" or that "recapping or needle removal is accomplished through the use of a mechanical device or one-handed technique." The regulation defines appropriate disposal containers and describes their use. The National Institute of Occupational Safety and Health (NIOSH) and the Centers for Disease Control and Prevention (CDC) recently published an alert regarding needlestick injuries in healthcare settings (16). The alert requires employers to implement a program to reduce needlestick injuries. The directive includes eliminating needles where feasible, implementing the use of devices with safety features, and ensuring that workers are properly trained in the safe use and disposal of needles. The features of available safety devices and specific use situations are suggested.

The importance of and requirements for the use of labels and signs are also specified in the OSHA regulations. Depending on the nature of the hazard, specific information is required to be posted in a specific manner. Examples include specific radioisotopes, chemicals, and infectious agents used in the room or area.

The OSHA standard specifically addresses the use of personal protective equipment (PPE) commonly used in animal facilities. In addition to the previously mentioned applicability to the use of hazardous materials, the **Respiratory Protection Standard**, Part 1910.134 (15) is broadly applicable in animal facilities due to the incidence of animal allergy (17). It emphasizes that engineering-based controls (physical and functional containment of the hazard and ventilation of the work area) should be used as extensively as possible before considering the use of respirators. In today's animal facility, the use of such containment is quite prevalent. When the presence of hazards requires the use of respirators, the facility must establish a written respiratory control program. The program must include: selection procedures, medical evaluation of employees required to use the respirator, fit testing, procedures for proper use, procedures for maintaining the respirators (cleaning, storage, inspection, repair), procedures to ensure adequate air quality and quantity for atmosphere-supplying respirators, and personnel training.

Specific hazards are also separately addressed in parts of the OSHA standard. For example, Exposures to Formaldehyde, Part 1910.1048 (15) applies to some activities in most animal facilities. This section requires that employers have a formaldehyde monitoring program in place when employees are exposed to certain levels of formaldehyde. The use of formaldehyde as a tissue fixative in an animal facility typically does not result in exposure levels that exceed threshold limits or the OSHA action level. Facilities should, however, conduct workplace testing to determine the exposure levels of employees under conditions of maximum expected formaldehyde use.

B. NATIONAL RESEARCH COUNCIL GUIDELINES

In 1997 the National Research Council (NRC) published guidelines entitled *Occupational Health and Safety in the Care and Use of Research Animals* (18). This publication was written to provide guidance for protecting the health and safety of workers who care for and use research animals. The need for these guidelines was based on the recognition that the animal research facility presented a broad array of occupational hazards. The NRC also recognized the need for guidance in complying with Public Health Service Policy requirements for an occupational health program. This publication not only addresses the components of an effective program, but also suggests approaches to developing and implementing the program. The recommended approaches to developing a sound program for occupational health and safety are not that different from the concept of performance-based standards that has already been discussed. More detailed information is provided in Chapter 13 of this text.

As with any planning process, it is important to involve individuals and functions that may be affected by the occupational health and safety program. A multidisciplinary team focused on occupational health and safety is typically charged with hazard identification and risk assessment specific to the varied research programs at an institution. The programs and procedures may vary between institutions, but the desired result remains the same – a safe workplace.

One important concept in the NRC safety guideline is that it is not considered appropriate to base employee participation in the program solely on "substantial animal contact." This phrase had been included in the 1985 and prior editions of the *Guide* as the barometer for determining the need for, and extent of, participation of an employee in the occupational health and safety program. While animal contact is an important part of this determination, other factors must also be considered. These risk factors include:

- Exposure intensity
- Exposure frequency
- Physical and biological hazards presented by the animal
- Hazardous properties of agents used in research protocols of the employee
- The occupational health history of employees doing similar work

It is expected that all of these factors will be used during job or project-related risk assessments. The description of the need for hazard identification and risk assessment in the NRC publication mirrors the language use in the 1996 edition of the ILAR *Guide*.

C. CENTERS FOR DISEASE CONTROL AND PREVENTION AND THE NATIONAL INSTITUTES OF HEALTH

For many years the publication *Biosafety in Microbiological and Biomedical Laboratories* (BMBL) has provided guidance for the use of infectious agents in research and animal laboratories (19). The fourth edition, published in 1999 by the CDC and NIH, provides the most current information on the use of infectious agents that may impact the health and safety of employees in animal resource facilities. The BMBL focuses on practices, safety equipment, and facilities required when working with infectious agents at each of the four specific **Biosafety Levels** (BSL). There are four corresponding **Animal Biosafety Levels** (ABSL) for working with vertebrate animals that have been inoculated with infectious agents. The BSL and ABSL for working with some infectious agents are the same. There are some notable cases in which the BSL and ABSL for a given agent differ.

The four ABSL (1–4) represent combinations of practices, safety equipment, and facilities that provide for increasing protection of personnel working with animals in these environments. A well-run animal care facility meets all the standards for ABSL 1. Applicable criteria for working with agents having higher ABSL classification are typically developed on a case-by-case basis through cooperative efforts between the IACUC and the institutional safety office. While the BMBL guidelines provide considerable detail on facility requirements and specific infectious agents, facility managers unfamiliar with the conduct of these types of experiments should seek help in the assessment of facility design and development of SOPs for the activity.

V. CONTROLLED SUBSTANCES ACT OF 1970

Animal anesthesia and analgesia often involve the use of drugs that are regulated by the Controlled Substances Act of 1970 (20), under the Code of Federal Regulations, Title 21, Food and Drugs, Part 1301 (21). Most animal facilities register with the **Drug Enforcement Administration** (DEA) to obtain a registration certificate to enable use of essential controlled substances. Policy strategy for institutional compliance with this Act may vary depending on size, number of sites, types of activities and agents used.

DEA research registration requires annual renewal. The registrant specifies the classification (i.e., Schedule) of drugs that are used. Most animal facilities are registered for the use of drugs in Schedules II – V. Drugs typically used in animals are narcotics such as morphine (Schedule II), and non-narcotics such as pentobarbital (Schedule II), thiopental and ketamine hydrochoride (Schedule III), diazapam (Schedule IV), and buprenorphine (Schedule V).

Use of Schedule I substances such as heroin is sometimes part of valid scientific investigation involving animals. Registration for use of Schedule I agents involves very specific controls by the DEA including approval of the research protocol by the agency. Specific requirements for the use of these substances will not be discussed here.

Once registered, there are specific requirements for the acquisition, receipt, use, and disposal of controlled substances. When ordering Schedule II drugs from a supplier, a pre-printed order form (DEA Form 222), obtained by the registrant from the DEA, must be used. Improperly filled out forms will be returned by the supplier. In addition, pharmaceutical suppliers will request a copy of the purchaser's DEA registration certificate for their files. Upon receipt, the order completion must be recorded on the registrant's copy of DEA Form 222.

Storage requirements for all controlled substances are specified in the regulations (21). The registrant is charged with providing effective controls and procedures to guard against theft and diversion of the controlled substances. The following factors should be considered when evaluating the overall security system:

1. The type of activity
2. The type and form of controlled substances handled
3. The quantity of drugs
4. Location of the premises
5. Type of building construction
6. Type of safe or secure enclosure used for storage
7. The type of closure on the storage area or enclosure
8. Adequacy of key control or lock systems
9. Adequacy of alarm systems
10. Extent of unsupervised public access to the facility
11. Adequate supervision over employees
12. Procedures for handling guests, visitors, maintenance personnel and non-employee service personnel
13. Availability of security personnel or local police protection
14. Adequacy of the system for monitoring the receipt and disposition of the controlled substances during normal operations

These considerations, as stated, are relatively general in nature, and the regulations go on to give examples or expectations of how to fulfill the requirements for Schedule II–V drugs. They state that storage areas should be accessible only to an absolute minimum number of authorized employees, and that key or combination lock access should be controlled in a manner to minimize access. Typically, the drugs are kept locked in a safe or steel cabinet, and within a room or area that can be closed and locked when not in use. When in use, the area should be kept under direct supervision of a responsible employee. Under the Controlled Substances Act and DEA regulations, there is the expectation that the registrant should store and use these substances in a manner to prevent theft or diversion of the drugs. The regulations provide little guidance, other than security requirements, on how to accomplish this goal.

Documentation of the receipt and use of the drugs under control of the registrant is expected by DEA inspectors. The U.S. Department of Justice, DEA has issued a publication entitled *Physician's Manual: An Informational Outline of the Controlled Substances Act of 1970* (22). Although directed at practitioners (i.e., physicians, dentists, veterinarians), many of the recommendations for record keeping can be applied to research activities. Records of controlled substances should enable an investigator to readily trace the disposition of drugs from the time of receipt to use or disposal. An initial inventory of drugs on hand should be conducted at the time a registrant first engages in regulated use of controlled substances and every 2 years thereafter. In practice, it is recommended that inventories be conducted at much more frequent intervals (e.g., monthly or quarterly). Depending on the frequency of use and quantities involved, a more frequent inventory process enables the registrant to ascertain in a timely manner, whether the drugs have been appropriately used and accounted for, or have been diverted for other use.

The guidelines do not specifically address the various circumstances encountered in the use of controlled substances in animal research. It is appropriate to follow the requirements for "dispensing" and "administering" the drugs. Specifically, when dispensing a drug, a record of the transaction must be kept. In animal laboratories, this may involve dispensing of a given quantity of drug from a central safe to a use area (e.g., surgery, necropsy) or to an authorized individual for administration to one or more animals. The record of administration is generally interpreted to necessitate identification of animal(s) treated, drug dose/amount administered, date, and individual administering the drug. Disposal of small remaining or contaminated amounts of drug should also be documented.

In some instances (e.g., expired drugs) it may be necessary to dispose of larger quantities of controlled substances. If the supplier is unwilling to accept return of the expired drugs, it is recommended that the registrant contact their local/regional DEA office to request disposition instructions. In some cases the DEA will request submission of DEA Form 41, "Registrant's Inventory of Drugs Surrendered," with shipment of the drugs to them for disposal, or they may request submission of Form 41 without drug shipment. Following review of the form, they may request shipment of the drugs, but more typically, they will provide instructions for witnessed and documented disposal by the registrant. As has been previously mentioned, response to regulatory requirements and demonstration of compliance relies heavily on sound, conscientious, record-keeping practices.

VI. ANIMAL TRANSPORTATION

There are a number of regulations regarding transportation of animals that may impact on animal facilities. Most relevant are those contained in the AWAR (2). Applicable requirements are included in Part 2, Subpart G and in Part 3. The standards in Part 2 apply primarily to record-keeping requirements for carriers and intermediate handlers. Animal resource managers, however, should review this section as a part of evaluating vendor compliance. In Part 3 of the AWAR, transportation standards, including record keeping, are specified for regulated species (i.e., dogs and cats, guinea pigs and hamsters, rabbits, non-human primates, and marine mammals). A health certificate from an accredited veterinarian may be required. Many animal facilities occasionally ship or transport animal species covered by the regulations to other facilities. The AWAR specify requirements for primary enclosures used for transport, transport vehicles, provision of food and water, care in transit, and general handling. An understanding of these requirements is key to ensuring legal acquisition and transport of animals to the facility.

Occasionally, animal facilities will be involved in the import or export of animals. Several regulations apply to these activities. Much as the AWAR specify requirements for interstate transportation of animals, international air shipments are controlled by the **International Air Transport Association (IATA)** regulations (23). Member airlines of the IATA conform with IATA's **Live Animals Regulations**. These regulations address specific handling and welfare requirements for over 1900 species, and are designed to ensure that live animals arrive at their destination healthy and in good condition. The regulations are published annually in October.

The **Endangered Species Act** (24) also has an impact on transport of animals. Regulatory authority under this Act is delegated to the U.S. Department of the Interior, Fish and Wildlife Service. The Fish and Wildlife Service is the U.S. management authority responsible for compliance with the **Convention on International Trade in Endangered Species (CITES) of Wild Fauna and Flora** (25). The management authorities of participating countries must approve of the import or export activity. Approval depends, in part, on meeting transportation requirements of IATA.

VII. OTHER REGULATIONS

Depending on the types of research, teaching and testing programs, and animal species used, various other federal, state, and local regulations may apply to management of animal resource facilities. For example, the U.S. Environmental Protection Agency and the U.S. Nuclear Regulatory Commission enforce regulations that impact on facility waste management and use of radioactive materials, respectively. In these cases, and others, primary regulatory authority is designated to state and local government agencies. Facility managers should, therefore, contact appropriate safety officials at the institution to learn more about their state and local requirements.

REFERENCES

1. **Food Security Act, Animal Welfare Act, P.L. 99-198**, 1985.
2. **CFR (Code of Federal Regulations), Title 9, Animals and Animal Products; Parts 1, 2, and 3 (Docket No. 89-130)**, Federal Register, Vol. 54, No. 168, August 31, 1989, and **9 CFR Part 3 (Docket No. 90-218)**, Federal Register, Vol. 56, No. 32, February 15, 1991.
3. **Silverman, J., Suckow, M., and Murthy, S., Eds.**, *The IACUC Handbook*, CRC Press, Boca Raton, 2000.
4. **Committee on Dogs**, *Laboratory Animal Management: Dogs*, National Research Council, National Academy Press, Washington, D.C., 1997.
5. **Committee on Well-Being of Nonhuman Primates,** *The Psychological Well-Being of Nonhuman Primates,* National Research Council, National Academy Press, Washington, D.C., 1998.
6. **CFR (Code of Federal Regulations), Title 9, Animals and Animal Products; Part 3 (Docket Number 95-100-2).** Federal Register, Vol. 63, No. 13, January 21, 1998. Humane Treatment of Dogs and Cats; Wire Flooring.
7. **Committee to Revise the *Guide for the Care and Use of Laboratory Animals*,** *Guide for the Care and Use of Laboratory Animals*, National Research Council, National Academy Press, Washington, D.C., 1996.
8. **Health Research Extension Act, Animals in Research, P.L. 99-158**, November 20, 1985.
9. **NIH (National Institutes of Health)**, *Public Health Service Policy on Humane Care and Use of Animals*, Office of Laboratory Animal Welfare, September 1986, Reprinted, October 2000.
10. **Federation of Animal Science Societies**, *Guide for the Care and Use of Agricultural Animals in Agricultural Research and Teaching*, Federation of Animal Science Societies, Savoy, IL, 1999.
11. **Department of Agriculture, Animal and Plant Health Inspection Service (Docket Number 98-116-2).** Federal Register, Vol. 65, No. 23, pp. 5301–5303, Animal Welfare; Farm Animals Used for Nonagricultural Purposes, February 3, 2000.
12. **CFR (Code of Federal Regulations), Title 21, Food and Drugs, Part 58 (Docket No. 83N-0142).** Federal Register, Vol. 52, No. 172, Good Laboratory Practice for Nonclinical Laboratory Studies, September 4, 1987.
13. **CFR (Code of Federal Regulations), Title 21, Food and Drugs, Part 11 (Docket Number 97-6833).** Federal Register, Vol. 62, No. 54, Electronic Records; Electronic Signatures; Final Rule, March 20, 1997.

14. **Occupational Safety and Health Act. P.L. 91-596**, December 29, 1970; P.L. 101-552, amended November 5, 1990; P.L. 105-198, amended July 16, 1998; P.L. 105-241, amended September 29, 1998.
15. **CFR (Code of Federal Regulations), Title 29, Labor, Part 1910, Vol. 5 and 6**, Occupational Safety and Health Standards, U.S. Government Printing Office, Washington, D.C., July 1, 1999.
16. **NIOSH/CDC (National Institute of Occupational Safety and Health/Centers for Disease Control and Prevention)**, *NIOSH Alert: Preventing Needlestick Injuries in Healthcare Settings*, HHS (NIOSH) Publication No. 2000-108, November 1999.
17. **Harrison, D.J.**, Controlling Exposure to Laboratory Animal Allergens, *ILAR J.*, 42, 17, 2001.
18. **Committee on Occupational Safety and Health in Research Animal Facilities**, *Occupational Health and Safety in the Care and Use of Research Animals*, National Research Council, National Academy Press, Washington, D.C., 1997.
19. **CDC/NIH (Centers for Disease Control and Prevention/National Institutes of Health)**, *Biosafety in Microbiological and Biomedical Laboratories*, 4th ed., U.S. Government Printing Office, Washington, D.C., 1999.
20. **Controlled Substances Act, Title 21, Food and Drugs, P.L. 91-513**, 1970.
21. **CFR (Code of Federal Regulations), Title 21; Vol. 9, Food and Drugs, Part 1301**. Registration of Manufacturers, Distributors, and Dispensers of Controlled Drugs, Revised, April 1, 1999.
22. **Drug Enforcement Administration**, *Physician's Manual: An Informational Outline of the Controlled Substances Act of 1970*. U.S. Department of Justice, Washington, D.C., revised March 1990.
23. **IATA (International Air Transport Association)**, *IATA Live Animals Regulations*, 26th ed., International Air Transport Association, Montreal, Quebec, October 1, 1999.
24. **Endangered Species Act**, Title 16, Conservation, P.L. 93-205, 1973.
25. **CITES (Convention on International Trade in Endangered Species of Wild Fauna and Flora)**, Convention of the Parties, Washington, D.C., March 3, 1973, Amended, Bonn, Germany, June 22, 1979.

7 Managing Quality in Animal Resource Units

Robert E. Mueller II, Ph.D.

Definitions of terms will aid in the discussion of quality management. These terms can help determine the differences between the concepts of quality control, quality assurance, quality management, quality planning, and total quality management. Quality management programs have a language all their own; the job of the manager is to bring life and action to the terms, to give them meaning within the workplace.

Quality management is the aggregate of all activities of the overall management function that determine the quality policy, objectives, and responsibilities, and implementation of them by means such as quality planning, quality control, quality assurance, and quality improvement within the quality system. **Quality planning** is the sum of all activities that establish the objectives and requirements for quality and for the application of quality system elements. Quality planning covers product planning, managerial and operational planning, and the preparation of quality plans.

Quality control (QC) is the sum of operational techniques and activities that are used to fulfill requirements for quality. It involves application of techniques to monitor a given process and eliminate causes of unsatisfactory performance at all stages of the quality loop.

Quality assurance (QA) is the sum of planned and systematic activities implemented within the quality system and demonstrated as needed to provide adequate confidence that an entity will fulfill requirements for quality.

A **quality system** is the organizational structure, the procedures, processes, and resources needed to implement quality management.

Total quality management (TQM) is the management approach of an organization, centered on quality, based on the participation of all of its members, and aimed at long-term success through customer satisfaction and benefits to all members of the organization and to society. (1)

I. BASIC THEORY

A. DR. W. EDWARDS DEMING

Deming's Fourteen Points of Management Obligations (2) have served as a guide for the installation of quality programs throughout the world. These 14 points apply to small and large organizations, to the service industry as well as manufacturing. The manager should consider how the principles can be applied to his/her work situation. The 14 points are:

1. Create constancy of purpose toward improvement of product and serv-ice with the aim to become competitive and to stay in business, and to provide jobs. Decide to whom top management is responsible.
2. Adopt the new philosophy: "We are in a new economic age. We can no longer live with commonly accepted levels of delays, mistakes, defec-tive materials, and defective workmanship."
3. Cease dependence on inspection to achieve quality. Eliminate the need for inspection on a mass basis by building quality into the product in the first place.
4. End the practice of awarding business on the basis of price tag. Instead, minimize total cost. Move toward a single supplier for any one item, on a long-term relationship of loyalty and trust.
5. Improve constantly and forever the system of production and service, to improve quality and productivity, and thus constantly decrease costs.
6. Institute modern methods of training on the job.
7. Institute leadership; the aim of supervision should be to help people and machines and gadgets do a better job.
8. Drive out fear so that everyone may work effectively for the company.
9. Break down barriers between departments. People in research, design, sales, and production must work as a team, to foresee problems of production and use that may be encountered with the product or service.
10. Eliminate slogans, exhortations, and targets for the work force, asking for zero defects and new levels of productivity. Such exhortations only create adversarial relationships, because most causes for low quality and low productivity belong to the system and thus lie beyond the power of the work force. In this regard, the manager should:

    • Eliminate work standards (quotas) on the facility floor.
    • Exhibit leadership.
    • Eliminate management by objective, numbers, and by numerical goals.

11. Remove barriers that rob the hourly workers of their right to pride of workmanship. The responsibility of supervisors must be changed from sheer numbers to ensuring quality.
12. Remove barriers that rob people in management of their right to pride of workmanship.
13. Institute a vigorous program of education and training.
14. Put everybody in the company to work to accomplish the transforma-tion; the transformation is everybody's job. Create a structure in top management that will emphasize the preceeding 13 points every day (2).

The above points can help the manager remain focused on the central themes of Deming's philosophy.

Joseph Juran (3) and Phillip Crosby (4) have also suggested guidelines to achieve Quality Improvement, as follows:

B. JOSEPH M. JURAN

Ten Steps to Quality Improvement (3)
1. Build awareness of the need and opportunity for improvement.
2. Set goals for improvement.
3. Organize to reach the goals (establish a quality council, identify problems, select projects, appoint teams, designate facilitators).
4. Provide training.
5. Carry out projects to solve problems.
6. Report progress.
7. Give recognition.
8. Communicate results.
9. Keep score.
10. Maintain momentum by making annual improvement part of the regular systems and processes of the company.

C. PHILLIP B. CROSBY

Fourteen Steps to Quality Improvement (4)
1. Make it clear that management is committed to quality.
2. Form quality improvement teams with representatives from each department.
3. Determine where current and potential quality problems lie.
4. Evaluate the quality awareness and personal concern of all employees.
5. Raise the quality awareness and personal concern of all employees.
6. Take actions to correct problems identified through previous steps.
7. Establish a committee for a zero defects program.
8. Train supervisors to actively carry out their part of the quality improvement program.
9. Hold a "Zero Defects Day" to let all employees realize that there has been a change.
10. Encourage individuals to establish improvement goals for themselves and their groups.
11. Encourage employees to communicate to management the obstacles they face in attaining their improvement goals.
12. Recognize and appreciate those who participate.
13. Establish quality councils to communicate with one another on a regular basis.
14. Do it all over again to emphasize that the quality improvement never ends.

D. QUALITY PRINCIPLES AND PRACTICES

As one might expect, there is no one best book on "quality" or "quality theory." The manager should read from a sampling of references to get several points of view on practices and ideas for implementation. Although one may find the style and jargon difficult at first, it helps to substitute the word "investigator" for "customer" or "administrator" for "customer." In research animal resource management there are many customers. TQM is a dynamic process, placing as many demands on management as on the staff. Establishing a workplace where everyone is engaged in problem solving through the team approach can be stressful, yet ultimately satisfying when the results yield tangible improvements.

The approaches and detailed descriptions of Deming, Juran, and Crosby have been summarized by Scherkenbach (5) into the following three principles and eight practices:

1. Total Quality Management — Three Principles

- Achieve customer satisfaction
- Make continuous improvement
- Give everyone responsibility

2. Total Quality Management — Eight Practices

- Focus on the customer
- Effective and renewed communications
- Top management leadership and support
- Employee empowerment and teamwork
- Reliance on statistical analysis of processes
- Enhanced rewards and recognition
- Long-term commitment
- Commitment to training

The manager's decision to adopt the principles of TQM requires him or her to "walk the talk" in order to involve the organization's employees. TQM offers an opportunity for the manager to change staff attitudes and possibly alter the nature of the employment relationship. This relationship assumes trust and it is up to management to realize that this trust must be developed. The manager needs to sell him/herself and the program, but the effort will be more successful if one has upper level (e.g., Department Head, Dean, Director, Vice-president, Provost, or Presidential) support.

Whether as a result of customer demand, employee expectations, or world market demands, many corporations have established their own quality management policy, following the points of Deming or one of the other quality theorists. One of the challenges presented to management is to establish a management policy. As an example of optimal level of institutional commitment to the TQM program, Agfa Corporation has a quality management policy (published on its Web site: www.agfa.com/about/quality management/ [6]).

The quality movement that started in industry has spread to almost every aspect of our culture. For example, the healthcare industry has adopted a TQM approach to customer service and quality in its efforts to improve patient care. Likewise, many employees expect their workplace to have a quality management policy. The TQM approach has reached veterinary practices and other single-owner businesses where individual control is supplanted by a focus on customer satisfaction. The world has become customer (i.e., investigator) oriented, requiring management to relinquish control over individual employees to the customer. When a laboratory animal technologist helps an investigator with his/her study, the investigator has control over the technologist. This orientation toward quality service emphasizes the need for training and group goal setting within committed organizations.

The workplace is dynamic, changing to meet the needs of both internal and external customers/investigators and markets. Few managers of animal resources predicted the upsurge of transgenic animals, but many facilities are now attempting to adapt to the increased demands placed on their physical plant and staff by this new animal technology while maintaining and improving the quality standards set by the institution.

E.   APPLICATIONS AND IMPLICATIONS FOR ANIMAL RESOURCE MANAGEMENT

Good Laboratory Practice Act compliance is the minimum standard for animal data collection in many situations. All systems for data collection need to be validated. Many animal resource managers need to become proficient in validation of their data collection techniques. Certification of management is as important as technical certification. The wise manager hires new employees with the intent of fitting them into the quality program and teaches quality techniques to his team from day one, setting standards and goals for quality and performance. Monitoring techniques and documentation that affirm compliance is essential to every operation. When the manager wants to hire a caretaker or technician, he or she should always select for quality awareness, ability to document activities, and learning capacity. Committed teams perform quality work, which benefits everyone in the laboratory, department, and institution.

II.   EMPLOYEE INVOLVEMENT AND EMPOWERMENT

Precedents enacted into policy manuals, corporate processes, and training programs often outlive the particular industry context that created them.

The empowerment that counts the most — the freedom to challenge standard operating procedures, workflow design, and bureaucratic procedures — is the freedom that is most often denied to entry-level employees. Although it is one thing to let an animal technician bring the cage wash operation to a halt when a defect is found, it is quite another to let that same technician have a significant voice in task design and facility layout. The pursuit of total quality is the key to management innovation in our field. To the uninitiated this must sound strange indeed. What has quality to do with innovation in management methods? The connection is simple. The foundation of a quality program is a willingness to trace every quality-related problem back to its roots. The fact is that those roots usually reach far beyond the immediate vicinity of the problem. They reach into areas such as vendor relationships, work design, information systems, physical infrastructure, and the like; and it is those closest to the quality-related problems that are best positioned to offer real insight into how corporate processes and systems could be improved. Marginally enlarging the scope of authority for an entry-level employee is not enough; every employee must be given the freedom to challenge anything that interferes with the pursuit of a unit's or institution's strategic intent.

All employees need to be given the tools to contribute toward advantage-building efforts. The tool kit may include information related to statistical analysis, general problem-solving techniques, benchmarking methods, systems modeling, and teamwork disciplines. An attitude of learning how to improve work results needs to be established. Management must be aware that it is not realistic to ask employees to build new products or obtain results with their bare hands. Barehanded (not giving the technicians the proper physical and theoretical knowledge tools) empowerment is really no empowerment at all.

In short, the problems generally lie not in the performance of individual tasks and activities, but in the processes, and how the units fit together into a whole. For decades, organizations have been attacking task-related problems with gusto but haven't laid a glove on the processes (7). For example, one might fix the rack washer, but fail to look at the flow of racks into and out of the cage wash area.

A.   EMPLOYEE INVOLVEMENT AND EMPOWERMENT

The success of the quality management approach is dependent on having well-trained and motivated staff and ensuring that their efforts are focused toward improving the systems that produce the products or services. In this regard, staff must be involved and empowered.

Involvement means that management actively encourages **involvement** of the staff in running the operation and improving the processes. **Empowerment** is something more; it means that management recognizes that when given training and provided with the right information, employees are in the best position to control their own work processes. This being the case, they should be empowered to do it, to become problem solvers.

There are various techniques to solicit employee involvement. Suggestion schemes work well when they are well publicized and when worthwhile rewards are provided. The job design can be improved to be more satisfying. **Continuous Improvement** teams should include staff at the working level so that they become involved in the quality improvement effort.

Empowerment means delegating control to the working level. This needs to be done gradually, as people get used to the idea and as they acquire the skills. Training is needed to provide staff with the skills to control their production processes, and to investigate and solve problems.

B. MANAGING QUALITY AS A PARTNERSHIP

Another way to look at the complex relationships within the work place is to view them as partnerships from the perspective of the participants. Aspects of this relationship include (8):

1. **Commitment** — The desire to continue the relationship and work to ensure its continuance (implies the importance of the relationship to the partners and a desire to continue the relationship into the future).
2. **Communication** — The process of information exchange between the partners. This includes the channels and methods of communication.
3. **Trust** — The belief that one relationship partner will act in the best interest of the other partner.
4. **Cooperation** — The action that firms (departments) take to achieve mutual outcomes or singular outcomes with expected reciprocation over time (also implies the willingness to engage in these actions).
5. **Joint planning/problem solving** — The collaborative planning and problem-solving process that attempts to find mutually satisfying solutions.
6. **Shared knowledge** — The understanding of each other's businesses (work product) and processes. This includes not only where they are, but what they wish to achieve.
7. **Social Bonding** — The degree of mutual personal friendship and liking shared by manager and employee.
8. **Tangible Outcomes** — The quantifiable business/revenue results stemming from the partnership. They include decreasing costs, increased productivity, and improved service to investigators/customers.
9. **Intangible Outcomes** — Those outcomes that stem from the partnership yet cannot be readily quantified (e.g., employee involvement in work assignment, new organizational knowledge, feeling of ownership).
10. **Partnership Satisfaction** — The degree to which the interactions of the partners and the outcomes meet the expectations of the partners.

A sound relationship between supervisor and employees is important because it leads to:

- Increased trust (two-way)
- Open communication
- Pleasant work climate
- Better chance of effective delegation
- Fewer problems that get blown out of proportion
- Greater ease in providing direction, sustaining motivation, and effectively counseling employees
- Generally better productivity and job satisfaction

- Less "crisis" management
- Greater ease in getting cooperation for the "big push" situations
- Greater team cohesiveness

C. BARRIERS TO LEADERSHIP

In fact, real empowerment is a most natural state of affairs; technicians, supervisors, managers, all know what they have to do and simply get on with it, like the worker bees in a beehive. Perhaps the really healthy organizations empower their leaders, who in turn listen to what is going on and by doing so look good. Is TQM really that simple? Frances Hesselbein, President and CEO of the Drucker Foundation, and the former chief executive of the Girl Scouts of the U.S.A. comments on barriers to leadership as follows:

"What are barriers to leadership? The request forced me to shift gears, to consciously distill what I had learned from experience but not yet articulated about barriers to leadership. From this introspection emerged two types of barriers: one personal and self-imposed, the other institutional, structural, or cultural."

Thus, barriers to leadership may be either self-imposed or institutional.

1. Self-Imposed Barriers

a. Lack of formal, articulated personal goals and a road map of how to meet them. These should be written and close at hand, not just rolling around in one's head.
b. Lack of a clear understanding of one's own strengths and weaknesses (this calls for input from others, plus a plan for improvement).
c. Belief that there is something called "professional ethics," that there can be two standards: one for our personal lives and one for our professional lives.
d. Lack of generosity — not sharing ideas, time, encouragement, respect, compliments, and feedback with others — resulting in exactly the same treatment from them.
e. Leading from the rear — being tentative, fence sitting, never taking responsibility.
f. Always stressing what others can't do well rather than building on their strengths.
g. Playing "Chicken Little" instead of "The Little Engine That Could." Lack of a positive approach to serious issues; failure to present suggested solutions along with the problem.
h. Failure to take charge of one's own personal learning and development

2. Institutional Barriers

a. Hierarchical structures that restrict, constrict, and box people in.
b. Corporate cultures that encourage mediocrity and reward "playing it safe."

c. Corporate culture and practice that "kill the messenger."
d. Racism and sexism going unacknowledged and unaddressed.
e. Fuzzy lines of accountability.
f. A lack of sharp differentiation between governance and management, and policy and operations, with no clearly defined roles and responsibilities.
g. No mentorship plan for promising staff members.
h. Failure to see people as the company's greatest asset.
i. Failure to build a richly diverse, pluralistic organization that includes diversity on the board of directors and top management teams.
j. Failure to "walk the talk" — a leadership team whose behavior doesn't match its message.
k. Static staffing structures, with no job rotation or job expansion.
l. Lack of a formal, articulated plan for succession.

It takes courage for a leader to identify and confront self-imposed barriers, and to put in place the personal strategies required to unleash the energy, innovation, and commitment to self-development. It takes equal courage to identify and confront the institutional barriers that limit and inhibit the people of the organization. And it takes real leadership to bulldoze the barriers – frequently time-honored, tradition-bound, deeply ingrained practices. But when the barriers come down, the result is a competitive, productive, and motivated workforce focused on the future. Morale soars, performance rises, and the organization (unit) is liberated to reach its highest potential. Seeking out the barriers demands high intelligence; doing something about them demands managerial courage (9).

III. MONITORING FOR CONTINUOUS IMPROVEMENT

Monitoring is essential for sustaining the momentum toward continuous improvement. Monitoring allows the manager and staff to improve the system, spending time on eliminating the source of problems rather than solving them. When Deming says, "Constantly and forever improve the system," it is accomplished through monitoring. Consultants often spend countless hours teaching about measurement tools used for process improvement. There are tools used for planning, analysis, or interpretation, which when combined give the manager a picture of where the organization is and the progress that is being made toward meeting goals related to quality.

Monitoring can help answer the following questions:

- Where are we?
- Where do we want to be?
- What is the gap?
- What are the causes?
- What are the solutions?

A.   TOOLS FOR MONITORING OF QUALITY

Two of the most commonly used monitoring tools are:

1. Fishbone diagram – A line diagram that ends with a problem (the effect) and branches out into the problem causes. The lines coming off the core horizontal line are the main causes and the lines coming off those are sub-causes.

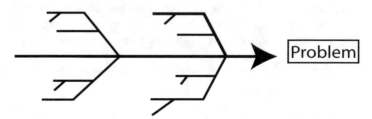

2. Chart – A chart that shows the distribution of items (i.e., problems or causes) and arranges them from the most frequent to the least frequent. This tool can help the manager to determine the relative frequency or importance of different problems or causes, allowing focus on vital issues by ranking them in terms of significance.

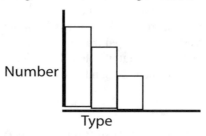

The Pareto chart can help the manager decide what aspect of a problem to tackle first. While working on the problems (investigator complaints, tardy employees, and data recording errors), the manager should continue to investigate. For example, just because a certain problem occurs more frequently than others doesn't necessarily mean it demands the greatest attention. One should ask oneself the following questions:

• What issue makes the biggest difference to the investigator?
• What will it cost to correct this problem?
• What will it cost if the problem remains uncorrected?

With the data that are collected the manager can decide which problem should be tackled first. Charts and graphs can also aid in communicating problem-solving methods and results to employees and investigators, and in creating opportunities to discuss other problems and solutions. Although one will not have the time to chart or graph every problem, the technique is useful when implemented on a limited basis.

IV. HOW LONG SHOULD A QUALITY MANAGEMENT PROGRAM TAKE?

The myth that quality processes take a long time to define and launch has been a major stumbling block for many institutions. In part, it originates from a misunderstanding of what "quality" is. It is not something extra that is to be added to a company's list of tasks, as though the employees will now have to find time to accomplish additional tasks related to quality. Instead, quality deals with how existing tasks are done. Rather than being an add-on, quality management will most likely result in time savings.

Another major delaying tactic (and one whose primary purpose could be seen as enriching consultants) is the idea that everyone must receive extensive training before anything happens. Often, this idea results in sending the executives to an off-site location for their training, and then hiring trainers to train all other employees on location.

The objective of a quality process, however, is not to create a group of chart-ready statisticians—it is to give everyone the opportunity to improve their contributions to the organization's processes, products, and services. At a meeting of 10 people who work together, only one has to know how to construct, use, and explain a Pareto Chart in order for the group to be able to use the results. In other words, one way an organization can both save money and greatly accelerate the quality process launch is by reducing the preparatory training programs.

Even if the intent is (as it should be) to actively engage every single person on the payroll in the quality process, in-depth pre-launch training needs reach no more than 10% of the employees.

Perhaps the most important concept for managers to understand at the outset of a quality process launch is that "Doing quality" carries a cost. That cost can either be the cost of the managers' time, energy, and personal commitment, or it can be the checks that are signed and given to the consultants. The question is whether the managers prefer to spend their personal resources or the company's cash.

The expenditure of time, energy, and commitment yields far greater results, but signing checks is a lot easier, and turning over the responsibility and authority for the quality process to a group of outsiders also means that, when the quality program falls short of explicit or implicit promises, the consultants can be blamed. A team of managers, perhaps guided by a part-time consultant, should be able to very rapidly define and then ensure the availability of the appropriate procedures and mechanical components (e.g., a computer-based idea-tracking program) needed at the outset of a quality process. By explaining to their employees what is going on and why, and by establishing up front their own commitment to the process, the managers can further accelerate the acceptance and implementation of the quality process.

Experience has shown that six to eight months is a reasonable goal for implementation of a quality management program. If it takes any longer than that, one or both of two things can legitimately be called into question: the competence of the quality guru/consultant, and/or the commitment and understanding of the managers (10).

V. CUSTOMER FOCUS

Every animal resource has customers. The customers can be **external** to the animal resource, as in the case of investigators who purchase a service, or **internal**, when one group within the resource needs the service of another group within the resource. A key point for quality improvement is to determine the customer/investigator needs. When the needs are fairly simple, this can be determined merely by communicating with them in a courteous manner. It further means that every work group has to think about providing value to the people who use their product (e.g., cleaning, handling, assisting, collecting data). This involves finding out exactly what the user/investigator needs and wants, and ensuring that the process provides it. For instance, the internal customers of a supplier inspection group will want to receive timely reports on supplier performance, early warning of potential delivery delays and helpful assistance in resolving problems with suppliers.

When dealing with an external customer, determination of the customer/investigator's needs can be quite time consuming and might require a detailed analysis. Determining customer/investigator needs accurately is an important aspect of quality control. Obviously, it is less costly to rectify a mistake in defining customer requirements before a product is produced or before the work done rather than afterward. Thus, spending the time and effort to communicate with investigators to correctly determine their needs prior to the start of a project is time well spent.

VI. PROBLEM SOLVING

Quality management depends on people having good problem-solving skills. It is through the continuous process of identifying problems, and solving and implementing solutions that the business is improved. Problem solving consists of identifying the root causes of a problem and implementing actions to correct the situation. There is a **simple four-step approach to problem solving** that can be applied to many situations:

1. The first step is to **define the problem**.
2. The next step is to **seek the root causes** of the problem. There is a tendency to accept the first cause that comes to mind. This is hazardous as it can focus on the wrong cause or simply correct a symptom. In many

situations the root cause can be identified through brainstorming, just writing out solutions on a piece of paper. More complex problems require more sophisticated techniques, such as cause/effect diagrams or system failure analysis.

3. Once the likely causes of the problem have been found, one should **identify a variety of potential solutions** and implement the best. **There is a ranking order for selecting solutions:**

   • The best solutions are ones that eliminate the problem altogether, making the system foolproof.
   • In some cases the problem cannot be eliminated so one may relax the requirements.
   • When these solutions are not feasible the problem may be resolved by training personnel to control the circumstances that contribute to the problem.
   • A less preferred solution is to resort to inspection and testing to sort good products or services from bad.
   • The worst solution is to use cautions or warnings of possible hazards.

4. The final step in the problem-solving sequence is to **evaluate the effectiveness of the solution**. This is done after implementation to ensure that the solution really does work. It is also a learning experience for the organization so that people can learn from the successes and pitfalls experienced by others.

The manager must also deal with **problem personnel**. Once a facility's TQM program training is under way, careful attention to each person's commitment level and TQM actions is necessary. If problems occur with some individuals resisting or actively sabotaging adoption of TQM, written documentation is recommended for each meeting and counseling session with the problem employee. If the problem is not resolved in a suitable period of time, a decision will have to be made on the future tenure of the problem employee. There is no place to hide a problem employee in a company committed to quality and customer satisfaction.

Allowing the staff to solve problems will allow the manager time to be better informed about customer needs and process improvement. Animal resource management, like most businesses, is a series of problems to be prevented, solved, or minimized. The problem with hands-on management is what occurs when the hands are taken away. It is not uncommon to hear an employee say, "That's not my problem"; however, it is the employee's problem if the manager makes problem solving part of the employee's job. To lead is to set boundaries, expect certain outcomes, and develop measurements for that outcome. Allowing staff members to thrash around and learn more about the alternatives can be a building experience to increase effectiveness in future behavior, especially if followed by face-to-face dialogue. Behavior can be a protection or projection of self, and the management style will make the staff member select the one needed to survive in the facility environment.

VII. WHY ATTEMPTS AT TQM SOMETIMES FAIL

When TQM fails, it is usually a result of faulty implementation rather than anything intrinsically wrong with the concepts. Possible reasons include the following.

1. Improper Planning

Organizations tend to be so anxious to begin doing "something" that they start off unclear as to what they are trying to accomplish and how to get there. There is a time to jump to action and a time to ensure that the actions are properly planned and considered. Jumping in too early creates chaos and cynicism, as expectations are frustrated.

2. Management Confusion

Managers need to lead the organization to quality processes. Too often managers have not considered what this means on a day-to-day level. Many managers will need some coaching on what their roles might be, and how to carry them out.

3. Inadequate Support for Managers

Often, TQM consultants are hired for a brief visit to start the process. This puts incredible pressure on managers since they have little ongoing access to the expert help they need to make TQM work. Also, some activities that are part of TQM are best carried out by "outsiders" who bring a different kind of objectivity to the process.

4. Partial Implementation (Hedging)

Many organizations jump in by implementing only one piece of TQM, usually focusing on the customer, or collecting information from employees. Customer service is only one part of the puzzle, and empowering employees is not likely to bring about change unless other issues are addressed.

5. Inadequate Marketing

Often employees have seen management fads come and go without impact. TQM programs that do not communicate the TQM principles and management intent usually fail. TQM must be explained in ways that show how it will benefit all members of the organization, then management must lead by example.

6. Impatience

Any organizational change requires perseverance and patience. The management that is not willing to work at change over an extended period of time will start backing off the principles and become inconsistent in actions, thereby destroying its own credibility and the credibility of organizational change in general.

Some company employees (e.g., cage washers, shipping and receiving personnel, accounting) who do not have regular direct contact with customers may be confused about what their new roles would be with a TQM customer satisfaction program. The answer is that the more everyone in the facility knows about the customer's business, scientific needs, complaints, and sources of satisfaction with the facility, the more motivated, productive, and efficient they are likely to be.

Managers must commit to sharing and communicating customer information and customer feedback with all their personnel. This information should consist of the customer/investigator's research description, personality, expectations, problems, opportunities, and periodic survey feedback (keeping in mind, of course, that certain information about the customer/investigator should be kept confidential). Managers must also allow employees to share and discuss this same customer information, where confidentiality is not essential, to encourage fellow employees to improve quality and customer satisfaction.

VIII. THE CHALLENGE FOR THE FUTURE

The challenges faced by TQM are never-ending, requiring flexibility and adaptability when approaching operational opportunities.

The organizational champion is the leader, a person who believes in the strength of the individual. Leaders must have followers (people), but managers need only projects (things). TQM requires leaders who incorporate service excellence and caring into daily activities. Six leadership principles apply to the TQM program (11). The manager should:

1. Preach and lead with vision – without it, the staff will lack direction and inspiration.
2. Always practice what he/she preaches, set the standard and the example – actions speak louder than words.
3. Make people accountable – encourage team members to have pride in the outcomes, not in adherence to a process.
4. Empower the staff – support them, ask, listen, inform, act, recognize, and reward; create heroes and superstars.
5. Take risks – opportunity and danger are inseparable. The manager should trigger change, not direct it.
6. Go for the long haul, not the quick fix – never start a plan unless one has the energy to follow through, get the dollars committed, and invest in Total Quality Management.

Management philosophy and commitment set the stage and enable the key players — the facility staff — to move in the same direction, reach for common goals, and be measured by fair standards. By starting with a clear vision of total quality management in service excellence, the manager can set the tone for behavior standards. One can affect behavior, not attitude; a poor attitude is a symptom, not a cause.

The leader's job is to build a responsive animal resource team – responsive to the needs of both the scientist and the research animals. The leader initiates this responsive behavior by being responsive to the staff's needs. Leaders need to communicate clearly and openly to build understanding, commitment, and investment, and to enforce and reinforce high personal values leading to equally high performance standards. With a commitment to TQM, the manager can have a value-driven facility that has strength, focus, and inspiration at the delivery level as well as at the helm.

In their book, *The Leadership Challenge* (12), James Kouzes and Barry Posner set out to discover what it takes to be a leader. Their study analyzed thousands of cases and surveys of how an individual can become a positive leadership force. Their work revealed the following five fundamental practices of exemplary leadership.

1. Leaders challenge the process

Leaders search for opportunities to change the status quo. They look for innovative ways to improve the organization. They experiment and take risks. And since risk taking involves mistakes and failure, leaders accept the inevitable disappointments as learning opportunities.

2. Leaders share an inspired vision

Leaders passionately believe that they can make a difference. They envision the future, creating an ideal and unique image of what the community, agency, or organization can become. Through their strong appeal and quiet persuasion, leaders enlist others in the dream. They breathe life into the shared vision and get people to see the exciting future possibilities.

3. Leaders enable others to act

Leaders foster collaboration and build spirited teams. They actively involve others. Leaders understand that mutual respect is what sustains extraordinary efforts; they strive to create an atmosphere of trust and human dignity. They strengthen others by sharing information and providing choice. They give their own power away, making each person feel capable and powerful.

4. Leaders model the way

Leaders create standards of excellence and then set an example for others to follow. They establish values about how constituents, colleagues, and customers should be treated. Because complex change can overwhelm and stifle action, leaders achieve small wins. They unravel bureaucracy, put up signposts, and create opportunities for victory.

5. Leaders encourage the heart

Getting extraordinary things done in organizations is hard work. To keep hope and determination alive, leaders recognize contributions that individuals make in the climb to the top. And because every winning team needs to share rewards of team efforts, leaders celebrate accomplishments. They make everyone feel like a hero.

Leaders can make a difference, especially in reference to TQM. The role of the leader is essential to improving the process of quality and sustaining the belief that the goal can be achieved. Kouzes' and Posner's evidence suggest that leaders who begin to use the five fundamental practices of exemplary leadership more frequently seen by others as better leaders:

- They are more effective in meeting job-related demands.
- They are more successful in representing their units to upper management.
- They create higher-performing teams.
- They foster renewed loyalty and commitment.
- They increase motivational levels and willingness to work hard.
- They promote higher levels of involvement.
- They reduce absenteeism, turnover, and dropout rates.
- They possess high degrees of credibility.

In addition, people working with leaders striving to abide by these fundamental practices are significantly more satisfied with the actions and strategies of their leaders, they feel more committed, excited, energized, influential, and powerful. In other words, the more the manager engages in the practices of exemplary leaders, the more likely it is that he/she will have a positive influence on others in the organization.

REFERENCES

1. **ANSI/ISO/ASQ A8402-1994**, *Quality Management and Quality Assurance*, 1999.
2. **Deming, E.W.**, *Quality Productivity and Competitive Position*, Cambridge Center for Advanced Engineering Study, Massachusetts Institute of Technology, Cambridge, MA, 1982.
3. **Juran, J.M.**, *Quality Control Handbook*, 3rd ed., McGraw-Hill, New York, 1974.
4. **Crosby, P.B.**, *Quality is Free*, New American Library, New York, 1979.
5. **Scherkenbach, W.W.**, *The Deming Route to Quality and Productivity: Road Maps and Roadblocks*, Mercury Press, New York, 1991.
6. **Agfa Corporation**, *Quality Management Policy* (published on its Web site: www.agfa.com/about/quality management/), 2000.
7. **Hammer, M.**, *Beyond Reengineering: How the Process-Centered Organization is Changing Our Work and Our Lives*, HarperCollins, New York, 1996.
8. **Bantham, J.H. and Bobrowski, P.M.**, Using the Baldrige Award criteria as an organizing framework for exploring buyer-supplier partnerships: a case study, *Proceedings of the Decision Sciences Annual Meeting*, 3, 1996.
9. **Hesselbein, F.**, Barriers to leadership, *Leader to Leader*, December, 1996.

10. **Townsend, P. and Gebhardt, J.**, *How Organizations Learn: Investigate, Identify, Institutionalize*, Crisp Publications, Menlo Park, CA, 1999.
11. **Catanzaro, T.E.**, *Building the Successful Veterinary Practice*, Iowa State University Press, Ames, 1997
12. **Kouzes, J.M. and Posner, B.Z.**, *The Leadership Challenge — How to Keep Getting Extraordinary Things Done in Organizations*, Jossey-Bass Publishers, San Francisco, 1997.

SUGGESTED READING

Aguayo, R. and Deming, E.W., *The American Who Taught the Japanese about Quality*, Simon & Schuster, New York, 1991.

Berk, J. and Berk, S., *Total Quality Management: Implementing Continuous Improvement*, Sterling Publishing Co. Inc., New York, 1993.

Chang, R.Y. and Niedzwiecki, M.E., *Continuous Improvement Tools*, Vol. 2, Pfeiffer, San Francisco, 1993.

Crosby, P. B., *Quality is Free: The Art of Making Certain*, McGraw-Hill, New York, 1979.

Godfrey, A., Quality management, the New Millennium, *Quality Digest*, December, 1999, www.qualitydigest.com/currentmag/html/godfrey.html

Hammer, M., *Beyond Reengineering: How The Process-Centered Organization is Changing Our Work and Our Lives*, HarperCollins, New York, 1996.

Rye, D.E., *1001 Ways to Inspire, Your Organization, Your Team and Yourself*, Career Press, Franklin Lakes, NJ, 1998.

Spechler, J., *Managing Quality in America's Most Admired Companies*, Industrial Engineering and Management Press, Norcross, GA, 1993.

8 Developing Policies and Procedures

Steven M. Kuhlman, V.M.D., Dipl. ACLAM

There are many benefits to having an organized system of written policies and Standard Operating Procedures (SOPs). The requirement for SOPs is stated in several regulatory documents, including the Good Laboratory Practice (GLP) standards, which state, "A testing facility shall have standard operating procedures in writing setting forth nonclinical laboratory study methods that management is satisfied are adequate to insure the quality and integrity of the data generated in the course of a study" (1). Most quality standards indicate the need for written documents stating institutional policies and procedures (2–4). The benefits of written policies and SOPs include:

- Keeping employees aware of their roles and responsibilities
- Reducing the learning curve for new employees and providing continuity
- Supporting the institutional training program
- Serving as a marketing tool, outlining the intention of an institution with regard to customer satisfaction through production of items and/or services that are fit for a specific purpose (2)

The specific requirements of an institution will define the complexity for the system of policies and procedures. Often regarded as a necessary evil produced to appease authorities, there is growing awareness in many laboratory animal resource units that SOPs provide an essential foundation for the production of reliable data for decision making and regulatory purposes (5). Thus, SOPs have grown from efforts to ensure correctness and uniformity of processes and procedures. The resultant compliance with regulations and other requirements reduces human error, and has the secondary benefits of increasing efficiency and reducing costs (6).

I. DEFINITIONS

A. A **policy** is a high-level overall plan embracing the general goals and acceptable procedures of an organization (7). Institutional policies address philosophy, objectives, and authority or responsibility of individuals within the organization.

B. A **standard operating procedure** is a set of instructions that aid individuals, whether working alone or within a complex framework, and which facilitates the correct execution of a function on every occasion (6). These written instructions can govern many aspects of daily activities in a laboratory animal resource facility (5).

II. POLICIES

Institutional policies address the operational intent of an organization. These policies are often a component of a "Quality" program that may have a more formal structure, as in a "quality assurance unit" in a facility conducting nonclinical laboratory studies conforming to GLP standards. "Quality" may also vary also refer to a total quality management program within the institution. Composition of policies will differ from institution to institution, but must always have the support of top management to be successful. The first step in adopting institutional policies is to generate an overall policy by the Chief Executive Officer/ President stating that management will support the institutional policies and will operate in accordance with their principles. There must be mandatory compliance with all policies and procedures (8). See Appendix I to this chapter for an example of an institutional policy statement on Good Laboratory Practice.

There is no defined format or content for policies; it is more a matter of institutional choice. Policies are organized in a logical system that is consistent with the design of the standard operating procedures. All activities or functions covered are collated into the chosen format (2). Responsible personnel who will establish, define, implement, and enforce the policies must be identified. In addition, the policies should address conflict resolution (8).

All policies are formatted in a similar manner. They should be designed for easy updating and be flexible enough to recognize differences among various units of the institution. Policies should be numbered and may contain several subtier sections (8).

The essential elements covered by an institution's policies include:

- Organization chart (best to use titles/functions rather than names)
- Quality program
- Safety program
- Facilities
- Operations
- Maintenance
- Animal care and use standards
- Business ethic
- Human resources

It is desirable to have standardization of these elements. The level of detail gives an understanding of the process, but should not be as detailed as the standard operating procedures. Ideally, the organization of policies will permit the incorporation of the SOPs (8).

Finally, it is important that staff members are familiar with the institutional policies. There should be some mechanism to ensure that all personnel have access to the most recent version of the policies (2).

III. STANDARD OPERATING PROCEDURES

Since laboratory animal resource managers have more responsibility for standard operating procedures than for institutional policies, the remainder of this chapter will focus on SOPs. It is beyond the scope of this chapter to describe the set-up of SOPs for a laboratory facility conducting GLP studies; such an institution requires a **Quality Assurance person** to provide guidance for this task. Instead, this section will focus on developing procedures for use in a non-GLP environment, although many principles will be similar.

Standard operating procedures address a "how to" set of step-by-step instructions. They establish the **who** to do **what, how, when, where,** and possibly the **why** of an activity (2). The primary purpose of SOPs is to guide and standardize working procedures in order to ensure data reliability and integrity. Standard operating procedures also have other purposes.

- SOPs are opportunities for management to analyze existing work procedures and to put better ones in place.
- A historical collection of SOPs enables the reconstruction of workings that were current at any given point of time in the past, and that can assist in routine documentation for an old experimental report, as well as finding reasons for discrepancies between old and new data.
- SOPs reflect the institutional attitude toward data integrity. This can be a significant component of public relations for an institution, especially an organization that performs some contract research.

A. ORGANIZATION OF SOPs

There should be a structured approach to the organization of the collection of standard operating procedures. The manner in which the SOPs are organized is individualized for each institution and ideally reflects the users' perception of how the laboratory or facility is organized. The SOPs are subdivided into logical sections that are easily located by the end user. For example, the method of division into sections could include: species (e.g., rat, dog), activities (e.g., dosing, specimen collection), protocol type (e.g., teratology, antibody production), institutional unit (e.g., cage wash, clinical pathology), or some variation of these sections. If there is a large number of SOPs in a section, they are further divided into manageable subsections.

When main sections are established, it must be decided which SOPs to write and where to place them in a section. Ideally, the numbering of the subsections is consistent between sections. This might be done in the order in which the SOP might be needed. For example, if the sections for the animal facility are organized by species, the first SOP in all sections may be dedicated to receipt of animals, the second SOP to animal identification, the third to housing, etc. The number of SOPs, the arrangement of materials in SOPs, and the level of detail depend entirely on the organization of each individual facility. Obviously, this requires planning by those responsible for organizing the SOPs. It may require several attempts before a suitable system is established.

B.   TOPICS

The Food and Drug Administration (FDA) GLPs state that standard operating procedures shall be established for, but not limited to, the following.

- Animal room preparation
- Animal care (including housing, feeding, handling, and care of animals)
- Receipt, identification, storage, handling, mixing, and method of sampling the test and control articles
- Test system observations (typically for the animal to which the test article is administered)
- Laboratory tests
- Handling of animals found moribund or dead during study
- Necropsy of animals or postmortem examination of animals
- Collection and identification of specimens
- Histopathology
- Data handling, storage, and retrieval
- Maintenance and calibration of equipment (including methods, materials, and schedules to be used in the routine inspection, cleaning, maintenance, testing, calibration, and/or standardization; it shall specify, when appropriate, remedial action to be taken in the event of failure or malfunction of equipment and designate the person responsible for the performance of each operation)
- Transfer, proper placement, and identification of animals

The topics for the SOPs may be different from those listed above according to the needs of the individual facility. Some of these topics may even be used to initially organize the collection of standard operating procedures.

C.   AUTHORSHIP

A standard operating procedure should convey a clear list of instructions. Logically, the people most familiar with the procedure (i.e., those actually performing the procedure) should write the SOP. The authors of the SOP describe the procedure in a manner that is appropriate for operators of the procedure at other institutions to understand. This permits the style and language to be consistent with that of others performing the procedure. Also, if users write the SOP, they are more likely to follow the SOP as written, resulting in improved compliance.

There are some general rules for writing SOPs.

- Use short active sentences.
- Use simple words and terms.
- Write sentences as instructions (e.g., 'do this,' 'do that').
- Write instructions in chronological order, so the operator knows when to do each appropriate task.
- Separate instructions from general information, either typographically or by putting general information in a footnote.
- Limit the amount of information per page (suggested maximum of ten separate actions).
- Limit the number of pages (suggested maximum of four for the procedure).
- Use diagrams when appropriate.

When the SOP is drafted, the director or supervisor of the area should review the procedure. It is important that the SOP be consistent in content and style with related SOPs. The SOP then goes through an approval process where suggested changes go to the original author(s) for review.

D. AUTHORIZATION

Regulations recommend that management approve written standard operating procedures, although the level of management is not defined. The purposes for authorization of SOPs include the confirmation of an appropriate method for a given procedure, standardization of the laboratory's performance of the procedure, and communication of these decisions to all concerned. The most effective authorization is done by an individual with both organizational influence and specialist insight. There may be instances where the specialist who writes the SOP might also approve it. In this instance, it is best to go to the next level of supervision for approval.

Since it is likely that many people might be writing SOPs, it is advantageous to give one individual editorial responsibility. This person is responsible for style and format, edition number, consistency of content in context with relevant SOPs from other departments, and compliance with policies and regulations. This person is also responsible for storing the SOPs in the archives and maintaining an inventory of this collection.

Finally, when the SOP has been reviewed and approved, the requisite number of copies are made. Each of these copies is stamped "DO NOT COPY" with a colored stamp or some other means to distinguish the original from photocopies. This precaution against unauthorized copying facilitates withdrawal of obsolete versions and helps prevent superseded practices from being used. The individual responsible for the distribution and collection of SOPs should be defined for each department.

Many institutions today use electronic storage of SOPs. An official single file copy of each SOP is maintained. A policy that ensures use of the most recent SOP version prevents use of obsolete versions.

E. LAYOUT AND PRODUCTION

Initially, an institution needs to produce a standard operating procedure determining layout, contents, and handling of all SOPs. Items to be included can be found in Scrip Reports on *Standard Operating Procedures* (6). The items included in this template are:

1. The requirements for a proforma / frontispiece. They include:
   - The document code
   - The serial/edition number and copy number
   - The document title

- Signature and date blocks for the drafting of the document
- Signature and date blocks for approval of the document
- A date block for when the document becomes effective
- A date block for when the document will be reviewed (and revised)
- The total number of pages in the document
- A statement to the effect that photocopying is prohibited. Other items that may be included:

  - The storage location of the master document (both hard and electronic copies)
  - The procedure to be followed when replacing or adding (and destroying) individual pages, the individuals responsible for such procedures and provision for double signatures to confirm that correct procedure has been followed
  - The procedures to be followed to ensure that staff have read the replaced/ additional pages
  - The distribution list showing the exact number of copies administered
  - Company name or logo

2. Maintenance of a complete list of existing SOPs with effective and review date
3. Information on the manner in which all SOPs are coded and numbered and the way in which serial/edition numbering is indicated
4. The manner in which pages should be numbered (e.g., 1 of 4)
5. Information on display/layout of SOP (e.g., paragraph numbering method)
6. Policy on authorship, review process, approval process, implementation, and restrictions on access to original SOPs
7. Instructions on circulation to staff, replacement of SOPs or individual pages, procedure for introduction of new SOPs, procedures for integrating new / updated SOPs, and procedures for induction and training new staff
8. Requirement to ensure personnel are complying with current SOPs
9. The requirement for clear and unequivocal definitions of responsibilities
10. Additional instructions on the use of language (e.g., use of acronyms, "shall" / "must" to be used rather than "should," and the use of standardized statements for consistency)

F.   IDEAL SOP CONTENT

All effective procedures will be consistent in presentation and carry a similar list of contents. A commonly used format is a six-section presentation that comprises **purpose, scope, references, definitions, procedure,** and **documentation** (2). These sections are included in every SOP, although not all sections may be pertinent to every SOP. They come after a cover page with the information specified in the proforma / frontispiece discussed in the previous paragraph. Most of the following information is taken from *Quality Assurance: The Route to Efficiency and Competitiveness* (2). See Appendix II for an example of a SOP using this format.

The **purpose** section outlines the objective or intent of the document. The **scope** section outlines the department, group, or personnel to which the procedure applies. The **references** section details other documents that have a bearing on the activities within the procedure. The **definitions** section explains any word not readily understood. The **procedure** section details the actions of those personnel involved in the activity. It states who does what and how, where, when, and possibly why the activity is carried out. The **documentation** section lists any documents referred to within the procedure and generated as a result of implementing the procedure. These documents are attached as an appendix. Published literature may be a supplement to SOPs (1).

The format chosen is followed without variation. If there is no appropriate information to be placed within a section, insert the word "NONE." On each page the document code, title, and page number should be listed.

G. USE OF SOPs

Regulations require that each laboratory area have immediately available SOPs relative to the laboratory procedures being performed (1). Experienced staff may not need to consult the SOPs very often after the first few readings and some practice, but the location and content of SOPs should be common knowledge. A **SOP deviation** is a procedure that does not comply with the written instructions (5). All deviations must be authorized by the study director and documented in the raw data (1). Intelligent analysis of the cause of deviations can lead to many changes and improvements (5). Significant changes in established SOPs must be properly authorized in writing by management (1). Management should evaluate deviations to determine where problems exist in the laboratory, but deviations must not be used as a negative tool. If it is perceived that staff members who incur deviations will be punished, future deviations may be covered up to avoid repercussions. This would defeat the intent of the SOPs.

A historical file of SOPs, and all revisions thereof, including the dates of such revisions, must be maintained (1). SOPs are issued under controlled conditions. The document is given a serial number and allocated to a specific person. The recipient of the document acknowledges the receipt and is automatically provided with reissues (2). Electronic copies are controlled by an institutional policy to ensure use of the most recent version.

H. QUALITY

In an effort to prove that quality is assured, SOPs are the tool of both the operator who carries out the tasks (i.e., by following the SOPs) and the monitor who verifies compliance. Compliance is verified by two methods:

1. Continuous checking of procedures
2. Audit

The presence of clear, precise written instructions (SOPs) assures quality (**Quality assurance — QA**). Monitoring and auditing confirm the quality (**Quality control — QC**) (6).

It is prudent for management to introduce a schedule for automatic review of SOPs and auditing of procedures. Authors of SOPs are requested to perform a formal review of their SOPs at a regular interval. This is frequently done on an annual basis. It is also useful for an audit of the procedure to be conducted by an independent party on a regular basis. The inspection should determine that:

- Appropriate SOPs are available and followed.
- Edition numbers are correct and obsolete editions have been removed from circulation.
- Distribution lists are current.
- SOPs are complete, specifying all actions of the working procedure.
- If transfer of data or materials to another laboratory or area is necessary, the relevant SOPs follow the process the entire way and are consistent with SOPs in the next area.

I.   LIMITATIONS

While SOPs are powerful tools for controlling activities and ensuring data reliability, like any tool, they function best in the right hands. They do not replace training of personnel but are used to supplement training. The repeated correct execution of a procedure in accordance with the SOP can be used to determine when an employee is properly trained. SOPs should be continually evaluated for unexpected interpretations, particularly by people unfamiliar with the procedure. It is expected that there will be successive versions of a SOP as it is refined (5).

IV.   SUMMARY

Standard operating procedures are helpful, but not sufficient in themselves for the production of quality data. Not only are SOPs assets to the institution, they bring the opportunity to clarify working routines and areas of responsibility. A collection of good SOPs shows management's commitment to the production of quality documentation. The SOPs are only successful if they are read, understood, and followed. If users are also authors, the purpose is usually fulfilled (5).

Deviations from SOPs provide insights that the institution can use for optimizing work routines. It is counterproductive for management to allow a judgmental attitude toward deviations, as this will drive them from sight, resulting in compromised data.

The SOPs should be used as practical tools. They have the same limitations as any tool, functioning best in skilled hands. The use of SOPs can entail pitfalls and surprises, and less than critical use can be a danger to data reliability (5).

APPENDIX I: EXAMPLE OF AN INSTITUTIONAL POLICY ON GOOD LABORATORY PRACTICE (5)

The management will ensure work is carried out to the highest standard possible, in terms of good scientific practice, and that research and development work is carried out to the principles of Good Laboratory Practice (GLP). These criteria can be met by:

1. Experiments being properly planned and performed
2. Procedures coming from recognized SOPs and validated
3. Equipment and devices being serviced regularly and fully functional
4. Animals and materials being obtained from accredited suppliers
5. Results being correctly recorded, analyzed, checked, and reported

To ensure that this system is capable of operation, a system of Good Laboratory Practice has been implemented and will be defined in this policy statement.

SCOPE OF GLP

All departments should strive to achieve good scientific practice and those departments required to comply with GLP will ensure that all aspects of their research and development are carried out to these standards. The execution of these practices can only be brought about by discussion with the department managers, the quality assurance manager, and the managing director. Matters such as the nature of the work, staff skills, and experience must also be taken into account.

When work is undertaken to satisfy regulatory statutory requirements for international agencies, the management will aim to comply with these principles insofar as they are practicable and in conformity with the current laws and practices of the country.

No action will be allowed that contravenes health and safety practices or those regulations governing the use of laboratory animals.

OPERATION OF GOOD LABORATORY PRACTICE

The management will assume responsibility for the definition of GLP in accordance with the principles applicable to the country. By meetings and information dissemination, the staff will be made aware of the requirements and their responsibilities. This action will be brought about by senior management and delegated where necessary.

A detailed code of practice, copies of the GLP requirements, and any in-house documentation relating to the subject will be produced and given to the staff.

It will be the responsibility of each staff member to become familiar with the contents of the documentation and to comply with the rules and regulations therein. Likewise, any department specific matters should be carried out in conjunction with the above.

GLP INSPECTION

It is with full management backing that the relevant government inspectors will be allowed to carry out their duties to ensure compliance with GLP is being maintained. The company will make available any information relevant to the study under review or the facilities in general, if that is the case. Any matters of a confidential nature will be covered by the institution confidentiality agreement.

APPENDIX II: EXAMPLE OF A SOP ON PROCEDURES — PREPARATION, STYLE, AND FORMAT (2)

CODE: XYZ-DOC-002 REVISION 2

TITLE: PROCEDURES — PREPARATION, STYLE, AND FORMAT

Author signature and date:
Approval signature and date:
Effective date:
Review date:

CODE: XYZ-DOC-002 REVISION 2

TITLE: PROCEDURES — PREPARATION, STYLE, AND FORMAT

1.0 PURPOSE

1.1 The purpose of this procedure is to describe the method of preparation, style, and format of all procedures established for use by XYZ Institution departments.
This procedure shall be used as an example of such preparation, style, and format.
2.0 SCOPE
2.1 This procedure shall apply to all documents which identify the activities and functions of a department or group and shall be observed by all XYZ Institution departments without exception.
3.0 REFERENCES
3.1 XYZ-DOC-001 Numbering System for XYZ Institution Documents
3.2 XYZ-DOC-003 Procedure for Development, Approval, and Implementation of Activity Documents
3.3 XYZ-DOC-004 Procedures Index

4.0 DEFINITIONS

4.1 Procedure: a document that details the purpose and scope of an activity and specifies how it is to be properly carried out.

CODE: **XYZ-DOC-002** REVISION 2

TITLE: PROCEDURES — PREPARATION, STYLE, AND FORMAT

5.0 PROCEDURE

5.1 Authorization to proceed

The need for a procedure shall be identified by the department manager concerned and the development of such agreed with the appropriate personnel (refer to document XYZ-DOC-003).

5.1.1 Once the requirement has been agreed and an author delegated, the author shall obtain a definitive procedure number from the document control center (refer to document XYZ-DOC-001). This procedure number shall be unique for the procedure to which it is to be applied and shall not be used to identify any other document. In the event that the decision to proceed with the procedure is rescinded, then the document control center shall be so advised and the number reinstated for future use.

5.2 Procedure format

5.2.1 The cover page of the procedure shall be in accordance with the form DOC-0021 (see attachment #1) and completed with the following information: document code, document title, revision number, author and approval box, and effective and review dates. Refer to the cover page (Page 1 of 5) of this procedure for standard format. The cover page shall always be identified as "Page 1 of _" at the bottom of the document and have the statement "Photocopying is prohibited" in colored ink.

CODE: **XYZ-DOC-002** REVISION 2

TITLE: PROCEDURES — PREPARATION, STYLE, AND FORMAT

5.2.2 The subsequent pages of the procedure shall carry appropriate document code, revision number, and document title at the top of the page. The page number and copying prohibited statement shall be at the bottom of each page.

5.3 Procedure content

All procedures shall carry the same content which shall be as follows:

5.3.1 Purpose: outlines the object or intent of the document

Photocopying is prohibited

5.3.2 Scope: outlines the sphere, department, group, or personnel to which the procedure is applicable

5.3.3 References: details other documents which have a bearing within the procedure

5.3.4 Definitions: explains a word or action not universally understood, or may have a specific interpretation in the procedure

5.3.5 Procedure: details the actions of those personnel involved in the activity

5.3.6 Documentation: lists any appendices referred to within the procedure

5.4 The procedure shall always include the content listed in 5.3 above. There shall be no variation. In the event that there is nothing under a heading, the word "None" shall be inserted.

CODE: XYZ-DOC-002   REVISION 2

TITLE: PROCEDURES — PREPARATION, STYLE, AND FORMAT

5.4.1 In the event that additional details are required to be incorporated as a supplement to the procedure, then these shall be incorporated as an appendix to the procedure.

6.0 DOCUMENTATION

None

Photocopying is prohibited

REFERENCES

1. **CFR (Code of Federal Regulations), Title 21, Food and Drugs, Part 58 (Docket No. 83N-0142)**. Federal Register, Vol. 52, No. 172, September 4, 1987. Good Laboratory Practice for Nonclinical Laboratory Studies.

2. **Stebbing, L.,** *Quality Assurance: The Route to Efficiency and Competitiveness*, Ellis Horwood Limited, Chichester, England, 1986.

3. Conference Proceedings, November 18–20, 1985, *Managing Conduct and Data Quality of Toxicology Studies*, Princeton Scientific Publishing Co. Inc., Princeton, NJ, 1986.

4. **Paget, G.E. and Thomson, R., Eds.,** *Standard Operating Procedures in Toxicology*, University Park Press, Baltimore, 1979.

5. **Carson, P.A. and Dent, N. J., Eds.,** *Good Laboratory and Clinical Practices: Techniques for the Quality Assurance Professional*, Heinemann Newnes, Oxford, 1990.

6. Scrip Reports, *Standard Operating Procedures*, PharmaBooks Ltd., New York, 1992.

7. *Webster's New Collegiate Dictionary*, G. & C. Merriam Co., Springfield, MA, 1999.

8. **Roberts, G.W.,** *Quality Assurance in Research and Development*, Marcel Dekker, Inc., New York, 1983.

9 Physical Plant

Gail A. Heidbrink, RLATG

The laboratory animal resource manager must address several major tasks on a daily basis. An area of tremendous importance is the development and maintenance of the physical structure and assessing the effects of that structure on the animals, the technicians, the research program and the institution. Unfortunately, few have received specific training for this endeavor. There is a multitude of issues relating to the animal facilities physical plant. Each facility is in a different stage of planning, renovation, maintenance, acquisition, or closure. This chapter cannot present a recipe to satisfy all situations, but will instead present information and references relating to broad categories of concern that are relevant to the maintenance of a quality animal care facility.

A critical daily requirement is the ongoing assessment of the facility status. The current facility requirements may include in the short term:

- Planning a new facility
- Renovation of an existing facility
- Maintenance of an existing program

Regardless of the stage of growth or decline, the program must be in a constant state of adjustment, adapting to the continually changing requirements of the research and animal care programs. Assessing, reviewing, and reaching out for new ideas present constant challenges for the facility manager.

This chapter presents information relating to assessment, planning, maintenance and the incorporation of new technologies as they reflect changing philosophies and requirements in the field.

I.   Facility Assessment as a Management Tool

The physical plant is only satisfactory if it addresses the needs of the programs and users of the facility. These include, but are not limited to, the animals; the research; veterinary and husbandry programs; the technician, research and veterinary staff; the applicable standards and guidelines; and the plant maintenance program. Assessing the level of congruity these elements have with the current facility aids in the development or maintenance of the facility strategic plan. Facility management is challenged with enhancing the level of satisfaction by exploring and utilizing materials, agents, devices and systems that are current and effective.

A. Physical Properties

Understanding that no two research animal resource programs are alike or have identical requirements, it is still practical to find common ground and utilize the knowledge and experiences of others. Basic standards are set forth in *Guide for the Care and Use of Laboratory Animals* [*Guide*] (1), which is used in part by the Association for the Assessment and Accredidation of Laboratory Animal Care (AAALAC), International as a basis for program assessment. Animal care programs that maintain accreditation status with AAALAC are constantly involved in the activity of self review of the plant status and subject themselves to peer review by AAALAC on a regular schedule. Institutions that are not accredited by AAALAC but desire an assessment can request a program assessment that will not prejudice future accreditation applications.

The AAALAC application form is an excellent tool that can be used to organize an internal assessment effort. The forms are in a downloadable file format on the Web site, www.AAALAC.org. The topics for assessment, with references to the appropriate page location of that topic within the *Guide* are located at that Internet location.

There are several references readily available that provide background information and suggestions to enhance a self evaluation. Additionally, many architectural firms and planning services specialize in laboratory animal care facilities and are available for assistance. When seeking advice relating to assessment of the existing physical plant or when seeking assistance in planning for a new or renovated facility, it is important to identify reliable references, qualified advisors, and other facilities to visit with similar research goals and programs. For example, facilities with programs that focus on toxicology and testing will have needs for basic construction requirements similar to those of a multi-disciplined university. However, the animal care programs and research requirements do not have similar goals and criteria, so the facility design and layout may be significantly different. One should remember to seek advisors and experts that can demonstrate experience relevant to the needs of his/her institution's animal care and use program.

References that are commonly used in assessment and for planning or renovation include:

AAALAC, International Position Statements. 11300 Rockville Pike, Suite 1211, Rockville, Maryland 20852-3035.
Tel: 301-231-5353; Fax: 301-231-8282 accredit@aaalac.org

The Animal Welfare Act of 1966 (P.L. 89544) and subsequent amendments, as promulgated in USDA regulations 9 CFR Chapter 1, Subchapter A, Animal Welfare. Parts 1, 2, and 3. http://www.aphis.usda.gov/ac/awainfo.html; USDA-APHIS-AC Unit 84, 4700 River Rd., Riverdale, MD 20737, 301-734-7833.

Public Health Service Policy on Humane Care and Use of Laboratory Animals. Reprinted 1996. Office for Protection from Research Risks, National Institutes of Health, 6100 Executive Boulevard, MSC 7507, Suite 3B01, Rockville, MD 20892-7507; http://grants.nih.gov/grants/olaw/references/phspol.htm

Handbook of Facilities Planning: Vol. 2. Laboratory Animal Facilities. Ed. T. Ruys. 1991. New York: Van Nostrand Reinhold. ISBN 0-442-23426-0.

Laboratory Animal Medicine. Ed. J. G. Fox, B. J. Cohen, and F. M. Loew. 1984. New York: Academic Press.

Biosafety in Microbiological and Biomedical Laboratories. DHHS Pub. No. (CDC) 938395, 4th edition, May 1999. Division of Safety, NIH, Bldg. 31, Rm. 1C02, Bethesda, MD 20892; 301-496-2801; http://www.nih.gov/od/ors/ds/pubs/bmbl/index.htm

Guidelines for the Prevention and Treatment of B Virus Infection in Exposed Persons. Clinical Infectious Diseases, 1995, 20:421-439. Occupational Health and Safety Administration Standards 29 CFR 1910.1030 - Bloodborne pathogens. Occupational Health and Safety Administration Standards 29 CFR 1910.1450 - Occupational exposure to hazardous chemicals in laboratories.

Criteria for a Recommended Standard Occupational exposure to Waste Anesthetic Gases and Vapors; DHEW Pub. No. (NIOSH) 77-140, March 1977. Occupational Health and Safety in the Care and Use of Research Animals, 1997. National Research Council, National Academy of Sciences. National Academy Press, 2101 Constitution Ave., NW, Lockbox 285, Washington, D.C. 20055; 800-624-6242.

Report of the AVMA Panel on Euthanasia; JAVMA, 202: 229249, January 15, 1993. http://www.nal.usda.gov/awic/pubs/noawicpubs/avmaeuth.htm AVMA, 930 N. Meacham Rd., Schaumburg, IL 60196; 800-248-2862.

Guide for the Care and Use of Agricultural Animals in Agricultural Research and Teaching. Federation of Animal Science Societies, First rev. ed., January 1999. FASS, 111 North Dunlap Avenue, Savoy, IL 61987; 217-356-3182.

Laboratory Animal Management: Rodents. 1996. National Research Council. Laboratory Animal Management: Dogs. 1994. National Research Council. ILAR, 2101 Constitution Ave., MH 372, Washington, D.C. 20418. 202-334-2590.

Guidelines for Construction and Equipment of Hospital and Medical Facilities. AIA Press, 1993. AIA Press, 1735 New York Ave., NW, Washington, D.C.; 202-626-7332.

The Psychological Well-Being of Nonhuman Primates. National Academy Press, Washington, D.C., 1998. National Academy Press, 2101 Constitution Ave., NW, Lockbox 285, Washington, D.C. 20055; 800-624-6242.

Guide to the Care and Use of Experimental Animals. Canadian Council on Animal Care. Volume 1 (2nd ed.), 1993. Canadian Council on Animal Care, 1000-151 Slater Street, Ottawa, Ontario, Canada, K1P 5H3.

Guide to the Care and Use of Experimental Animals. Canadian Council on Animal Care. Volume 2, 1984. Canadian Council on Animal Care, 1000-151 Slater Street, Ottawa, Ontario, Canada, K1P 5H3.

B.   FUNCTIONAL AREAS

A consideration for evaluating the adequacy of a facility for meeting the program requirements is the gross square footage, and how that square footage is utilized for various functions. There are no hard and fast rules in this exercise. For example, rodents have an extreme population density in comparison to primates or small livestock. Therefore, using a "typical" square footage formula for animal holding areas is not practical. In assessing a facility, it is necessary to evaluate whether or not each functional area meets minimum criteria regardless of the square footage assignment.

Other sources have presented areas of a facility and provided sample "Room Data Sheets" for each functional area (2). The data sheets define essential elements to be considered in each functional area. Not every functional area would be required for all programs. There are no recommendations for square footage. This model follows the pattern frequently used as the basis for facility planning: identify the functions and form a logical flow pattern for efficiency, protection of the animals and protection of the research. This model is generally referred to as "Form Follows Flow." The functional areas identified in the outline are:

1. Quarantine
2. Small rodent housing
3. General purpose small animal housing
4. Primate housing
5. Dog housing
6. Farm animal housing
7. Treatment and intensive care
8. Necropsy
9. Diagnostic laboratories
10. Cold storage for animal carcasses
11. Support areas
    • Manager/secretary/records offices
    • Receiving area
    • Storage area (feed, bedding, cages, supplies, etc.)
    • Locker rooms

- Toilets and showers
- Lunch and break rooms
- Cagewash area
- Cage and equipment repair
- Diet preparation

Additional areas that may be required are:

1. Technician workspace outside of the controlled animal area
2. Receiving and loading dock space
3. Transgenic suites
4. Assigned research space
5. Surgery suites and surgery preparation rooms
6. Recovery rooms
7. Controlled substance rooms
8. Detergent and chemical storage

Oversight of the physical plant usually refers to the oversight of the **macroenvironment** of the animal care facility. General guidelines for the macroenvironment are documented in the *Guide*. Legal requirements, enforced by the Animal Plant Health Inspection Service of the USDA are documented in the Animal Welfare Act (PL 89544) Regulations and its revisions (3, 4). A facility must comply with the statutes to be in compliance with the law. The recommendations in the *Guide* should be followed to maintain a quality program.

The macroenvironment is a reflection of the plan, the construction materials, construction quality and the environmental control system. All are elements exterior to the primary cage that impact the animals' well-being. Construction standards have remained relatively constant for decades. Recently, major advances in the science of animal care, ergonomic and safety issues, and the availability of new construction materials have prompted the reconsideration of traditional design and construction standards. In the assessment of the macroenvironment, a facility manager should review the animal housing area, exterior to the primary confinement, with a perspective of what aspects of the environment are controlled and could be enhanced to improve the well-being of the animals and the staff.

C.   EVALUATION PROCESS

In the assessment approach to plant oversight, the functional areas are evaluated in light of meeting the needs of the programs and its users. It is critically important to identify the people responsible for maintaining the oversight process. The people responsible for maintaining the evaluation process must be knowledgeable about the needs of the program and the relationship of the physical plant to the research program. The manager must ensure that the physical plant satisfies the needs of all components of the program. The following are suggested points to be evaluated in the self-assessment of the physical plant.

1.   Animal Housing

a.   *Are the walls and ceilings in good repair?*

- The manager should ensure that the interior surfaces are sealed and impervious to moisture, for a cleanable surface.
- Suggested materials* include:
  - epoxy paint
  - fire retardant, fiberglass reinforced plastic (FRP)
  - hand-laid fiberglass (not to be applied to raw block wall surfaces)
  - sprayed-on fiberglass
  - epoxy flooring coved up the wall
  - stainless steel sheet sealed to the wall
  - ceramic or glazed tile, with sealed grout

b.   *Are the floors in good repair and easy to maintain?*

- Ensure that the floor surfaces are sealed and impervious to moisture, for a cleanable surface.
- Floor drains may be required for sanitation, depending upon the species.
- If the drains are capped, there must be a regular maintenance program of the drain traps to prevent the escape of gases into the room.
- The floor should be an even, skid-resistant surface.
- The floors should be coved up the walls to aid in the ease of cleaning and room hose-down operations.
- The floors should slope to the drains.
- Tile floors must have the grout sealed.
- Tile can be a difficult surface to maintain because dirt and particles will collect in the grouted seams.
- Suggested materials* include:
  - poured epoxy
  - methyl methacrylate (MMA)
  - hand-laid fiberglass
  - urethane-sealed concrete

Floors with grouted seams between tiles (e.g., ceramic tile, terrazzo) present difficulties in long-term maintenance. It is far more desirable for a floor to be monolithic or to have a minimal number of joints.

A vinyl floor surface may not have the strength to withstand the weight load of heavy objects such as large ventilated racks. Also, it is difficult to obtain a good seal in the cove during application. This could lead to an area behind the cove that will harbor vermin. One must be cautious in the selection of floor surfaces and the application process.

---

* Improved materials are constantly being developed. When planning a new facility or when upgrading an existing facility, one should examine all options with the architect and contractor.

c. *Is the lighting appropriate for the species? [Suggested reading (5)]*

- Review the light intensity recommendations for all species in the facility.
- Adjust the photoperiod for the species to be housed in each room.
- Monitor the light cycles for each animal room with frequent physical inspection.
- Use sealed light fixtures to prevent harborage of vermin and use water-resistant fixtures in areas with high water use, such as cage washing.
- If there are windows, examine the impact of natural light on the animals' normal schedule and the research protocol. In some instances, windows in animal rooms have been justified as an enrichment tool for such species as nonhuman primates, dogs and cats.

d. *Is the heating, ventilation, and air conditioning (HVAC) system functioning properly?*

- Review the ambient temperature and humidity requirements for each species. [Suggested reading (5)]
- Adjust the temperature and humidity levels to an appropriate range. If only zonal control is available (as opposed to control for each individual room), animals requiring the same temperature and humidity range can be grouped under the same zonal control.
- Review the needs for containment of each room and determine if the air exchange rate and the pressure differential are appropriate.
- Determine if the air supply and exhaust systems create drafts that will cause discomfort for the animals.
- Determine if the filtration system and the percentage of fresh air supply is appropriate.
- Determine if the room air supply is the only form of ventilation control used, or if ventilated cage racks, isolation cubicles, or vinyl-sided clean rooms are also used.
- Ensure up-to-date evaluation of the HVAC and the filters.
- Evaluate the method and frequency of recording temperature, humidity, and air exchange.
- Evaluate the procedure for cleaning duct work and ventilation systems.
- Are the door sweeps part of the barrier for differential pressure balance? If yes, determine if they in good working order and the frequency of inspection.

e. *What steps have been taken to reduce, control, and monitor noise levels?*

- Review the hearing frequency ranges for each species.
- Evaluate the decibel levels and frequencies within the animal room.
- Determine if the normal ambient noise and frequencies emissions are within a comfortable level for the species.
- If decibel levels are not within a comfortable range, determine if strategies can be developed to reduce noise levels. Possible approaches include:
  - Sound-dampening panels suspended or wall mounted
  - Sound-dampening surfaces within the primary cages

- Use of sound-dampening interior and exterior walls
- Review movable equipment for unnecessary noise generation
- Monitor for excessive noise generated near the animal rooms

2. Husbandry

a. *Ensure that feed and bedding storage and diet preparation areas are appropriate and regularly maintained.*

- Ensure that the feed is stored on elevated platforms that promote rather than hinder sanitation.
- Ensure that the room interior surfaces are sealed and easily cleaned.
- Determine that the temperature is maintained at a level adequate to preserve the integrity of the diet.
- Ensure that the floor base and surface material are adequate to withstand the weight load.
- Evaluate the potential for contamination of diet by vermin and feral animals.
- Determine the pest control plan and implement monitoring procedures.
- Ensure that the surfaces used for diet preparation are sanitizable.

b. *What is the water source and how is it evaluated?*

- Identify how the water is evaluated for quality and the frequency of evaluations.
- Consider if the water is processed through an in-house filtration system or treated.
- Consider the methods used to determine the quality of the treated water.
- Identify any experimental protocols that can be adversely affected by water treatment.
- Establish a program to change filters and sanitize the automatic watering systems.

c. *Are the sanitization procedures and equipment adequate to meet the program requirements?*

- Ensure that there is there sufficient cage, rack, and bottle-washing equipment to meet the needs of the animal care program.
- Cage sanitation equipment may include some or all of the following:
  - Rack and cage washer
  - Tunnel washer
  - Flushing/sanitization system for automatic watering manifold
  - Autoclaves
  - Cabinet washer
  - Sipper tube washer or sanitizer
  - High pressure washer
  - Bedding dispensers
  - Bottle fillers
  - Waste removal equipment
- If amines are added to the steam line, determine if they are affecting the life of the plastic cages.
- Determine if the equipment is efficient and effective and periodically monitor the efficacy of this equipment.

- Determine if the equipment and chemicals might affect the duct work and sewage lines.
- Determine if the floor base and surface are sufficient to hold the weight of heavy detergent barrels.
- Consider installation of a dyking separation between chemical types to prevent accidental mixing of dangerous materials.
- Determine if there is sufficient exhaust ventilation within the cage-washing area to prevent excess steam, moisture, and heat from escaping and affecting the animals.
- Determine if there is sufficient equipment and water access to accommodate the sanitation of the animal rooms and service areas.

3. Technical Staff

a. *Does the technical/caregiving staff have adequate and appropriate tools to maintain and service the program?*

- Ensure that the racks, transport carts, and husbandry and sanitization equipment are ergonomically suitable. If they are not, possible remedies might include:
  - Purchase of improved, tested casters, for ease of rolling
  - Installation of push/pull handles at appropriate heights
  - Obtaining automated equipment to reduce repetitive motion injuries
- Restrict future equipment purchases to equipment that can demonstrate reduced weight features.
- Review processes to reduce the need for heavy equipment transfers.
- Eliminate unnecessary thresholds in egresses and cage entry.
- Add wall and protection devices to protect surfaces from impact of heavy equipment.
- Develop and/or obtain mechanical means for lifting and transport of heavy items.
- Ensure that the sanitation equipment is safe and convenient to use.
- Ensure that there is adequate space for staff training and relaxation.
- Ensure that there is adequate space for the conduct of technical and clerical responsibilities.

4. Research Needs

a. *Does the facility provide sufficient space to accommodate a variety of species?*

- Ensure that there is the adequate space for separation of projects and animal models.
- Ensure that there is adequate space for the introduction of new animal models.

b. *How are the animals accessed by the research staff?*

- Ensure that there is an appropriate means of animal transportation from the animal resource facility to the research laboratories.

- Ensure sufficient support areas have been provided to meet the research requirement. If possible, provide designated research space within the animal resource facility.
- Plan and adapt where appropriate to locate the animals near the research laboratories.

II. MAINTENANCE OVERSIGHT

A. ROUTINE MONITORING

At the conclusion of the evaluation, a format for regular maintenance should be developed. Each facility will have unique requirements, based upon the self-evaluation. However, for facilities that strive to maintain accreditation standards, it would be wise to include the items contained within the "Program Review" document, available at the AAALAC, International Web site. Such an approach will save time when accreditation reports and applications are due. For facilities that will not be seeking accreditation status, the Program Review document still provides an excellent guideline for self-evaluation.

Environmental monitoring systems can be a great asset in oversight and documentation. A variety of parameters can be monitored, such as temperature, humidity, and light cycle. Additionally, monitoring systems can incorporate a security system. It is important to understand that environmental monitoring systems are not environmental control systems. Some environmental control systems also provide monitoring, although a separate monitoring system could be considered as a redundant checking or validation system if there is an existing control system in place.

The manager should prepare a maintenance schedule and assign responsibility for each area. For example, the evaluation and documentation of the HVAC system for a typical animal room may include the following:

Element	Room #105B	Room #116	Room #118
FUNCTION	Bedding Storage	Housing	Housing
PRIMARY SPECIES	N/A	Dogs	Mice
CAGING STYLE	N/A	Kennels	Ventilated cage racks
AIR SUPPLY	Recirculated	100% fresh	100% fresh
AIR TREATMENT	Coarse Filter	HEPA	Coarse Filter
DATE OF RECENT FILTER CHANGE	7 Jul 00	4 Apr 99	7 Jul 00
AIR CHANGES PER HOUR	10	18	10
PRESSURE DIFFERENTIAL	–	–	+
AC/H & PRESSURE ASSESSMENT DATE	15 Sep 00	15 Sep 00	15 Sep 00
INDIVIDUAL OR ZONAL TEMPERATURE	Zonal	Individual	Zonal
HUMIDITY CONTROL	No	Yes	Yes
RECORD DATE	Nov 00	1 Nov 00	1 Nov 00

Each functional component of the facility requires unique maintenance oversight documentation. This is different from, and in addition to, the daily room record log. In addition, maintenance documentation should include areas such as:

- Service corridors
- Stairwells
- Interstitial space
- Receiving dock
- Loading dock and refuse disposal area

B.   SPECIAL AREAS OF CONSIDERATION

There are many areas and functions that require special attention. A few areas of special concern are described below.

1.   Cage-Wash Areas

Washers, dryers, autoclaves, sipper tube washers, bedding dispensers, bottle fillers, chemical pumps, etc., all having unique maintenance requirements. It is important to review the product information supplied by the manufacturer and establish standard operating procedures that follow the recommendations for service. The manager should maintain a secure library for the product information and service manuals.

If a new facility or renovation is being considered, one should obtain all service requirements from each potential product manufacturer prior to completing the plan. Several issues that can affect the long-term maintenance of the cage-wash area include:

a.   *Utility consumption (cost of power consumption)*

- Electrical load — Not all equipment requires the same power load; examine the specification data sheets and match it to the available building service.
- Steam consumption — The building supply must be adequate or supplemental steam generation may be required, and/or more effective and cost efficient.
- Hot and cold water consumption — The water supply and plumbing must meet the requirements of the equipment.

b.   *Weight load of the equipment at capacity*

c.   *The effects of cage-washing operations on the facility and building HVAC system*

- There is significant BTU (British Thermal Unit) impact from the air released when an autoclave or cage-washer is opened after use. This process can affect the HVAC.
- Allow for condensate return. The amount of saturated air must be calculated into the system plan. A vent condenser to cool saturated water may be required. The air discharge will have an impact on all connecting duct work. One should

select appropriate materials, such as stainless steel or glass, and the most direct route for discharge.

d.   Drain and discharge

- One should evaluate the pH level and discharge temperature requirements for the effluent water to determine compliance with local ordinances.
- Neutralizing agents and cooling tanks may be required for some municipalities.
- Drains should be selected that can withstand temperatures of at least 180°F and acid discharges.

e.   Chemical impact

- Floor surfaces will experience a great deal of chemical spillage in cage wash areas. A floor surface should be selected that is acid and alkaline resistant. If the floor surface has been tested for resistance to certain chemicals or detergents, one should not assume that all detergents will utilize the same formulas. A floor surface that is tested safe for one product may not test safe for another. One can conduct a safety test in a small area of the floor by applying a cotton ball soaked in the new product to the floor overnight, and then examining the tested area for degradation and discoloration.
- Chemicals can escape from the cage washer into the duct work. Duct work material must be selected that is chemical resistant, such as stainless steel or glass, and that will not allow for steam or condensate backflow. The mixing of some chemicals and steam may cause the release of potentially hazardous products.
- Facilities that have hard water (i.e., where the domestic water is 7 grains of $CaCO_3$ or higher) typically use acidic products to clean cages and maintain washers. Hard water will cause the internal openings of pipes to gradually shrink as the water leaves deposits in the lines. These deposits, generally calcium and magnesium, create a maintenance problem for the building plumbing system. Some facilities may require an acid backflush to keep waterlines open.
- Steam generation, especially in areas with hard water, usually requires additives such as amine compounds to keep the pipes clean. These products can result in steam that is too alkaline and caustic. Such steam, sometimes referred to as "dirty steam," has been associated with the destruction of polycarbonate cages. Polysulfone cages are generally resistant to this effect (6). The addition of separate, clean steam generators with steam traps to filter out impurities is encouraged.

2.   Chemical Storage

Chemicals for cage disinfection are often purchased in bulk. The storage area floor may not have been designed to carry the weight load of the heavy chemical tanks. Before purchasing bulk tanks, one should review the weight load capacity of the proposed storage area and the freight elevator. If planning a new facility or renovating an existing facility, it is important to provide substantial floor strength to support heavy materials and equipment and to allow for the probable weight loads in the corridors, freight elevators, and receiving area.

a.   Chemicals purchased in large holding tanks should be "dyked" and placed in secondary containment centers. This is also a good rule to

follow for chemicals purchased in barrels. Accidental chemical inter-
play can be a dangerous event. For example, chlorinated products
should not come into contact with any acid product (including vinegar);
ammonia and bleach products should never be mixed. These products
should be stored in separate areas.

b. Chemicals can be very sensitive to temperature extremes. They should
be stored in a separate area with temperature control that will prevent
freezing or over-heating. Appropriate safety precautions for chemical
and inhalation hazards, such as the use of fume hoods and personal
protective equipment, should be observed in this area.

3. Substrate Compatibility with Sanitizing Chemicals

a. Animal rooms should periodically undergo a complete decontamination
with chemical disinfectants. This procedure will expose all surfaces
(walls, floors, ceilings, cages, counters, sinks, etc.) to potentially corrosive chemicals. The chemical agent chosen may be caustic or corrosive,
and some may attack stainless steel, causing rapid degradation of even
high-quality stainless steel. Most stainless steel products used in laboratory animal care facilities are manufactured with either Type 304 or
316 stainless steel. Type 316 is more tolerant of acidic products, but also
more costly. If rust appears on the surface of stainless steel equipment,
it likely represents oxidation of surface particles and is not a reflection
of the quality of the stainless steel. Surface rust can normally be removed by processing through a cage washer. If the equipment is not
moveable, surface rust can be removed by cleansing with naval jelly.

b. Walls and substrates should be tested, prior to disinfection, for potential
degradation. If possible, one might submerse floor and wall samples in the
chemicals at the recommended dilution level for 24 hours. After rinsing,
the samples can be examined for degradation. The manager can also ask
substrate or chemical vendors for results of tests related to degradation.

c. The local water supply can play a major role in the effectiveness of
some chemical products. The manager should obtain an analysis of the
local water quality and compare the water qualities to the manufacturer's
recommendations.

d. Automatic watering lines are susceptible to chemical degradation. Facilities that add hydrochloric acid to the water supply may experience
etching to the water supply lines. Water lines made from Type 316
stainless steel will be resistant to this type of degradation.

4. Air Flow Patterns

a. The placement of the cage racks, the supply and exhaust vents, and the
style of the supply vents all impact on the air flow patterns within a
room (7). Also, the heat production of the animals will affect the air
flow pattern. Computerized analysis suggests that a review of rack

placement and the supply and exhaust vent positioning should be conducted prior to rack placement (7–9).

b. Supplying the recommended air changes per hour does not necessarily
ensure that the animals within the cage will receive an adequate fresh
air supply. For example, unless the air flow is very strong, chilled air has
a difficult time penetrating the heated air barrier, produced by the
animal, inside a closed sided cage. Cages with solid sides (or minimal
air holes), backs, and tops will trap the heated air to a greater extent than
cages using combinations or rods and mesh on the sides and tops. Thus,
when selecting primary cages, it is important to consider the impact of
the air flow patterns of the room and whether or not fresh air will be
accessible to the confined animal within the enclosures. Air flow patterns can be observed within the primary enclosures simply by adding
a heat generating item to the interior of the cage (such as a light bulb)
to simulate the BTUs produced by the animal, and conducting a standard smoke test.

5. Lighting

a. Recommendations for photoperiod and light intensity are available for
most species in reference books (5). However, the recommendations for
general room lighting will not necessarily accommodate all animals in
the room. Animals in the lower tier of cages will not have the same
illumination as the animals in top tiers. An attempt to even out the
illumination between levels should be made to provide the consistency
required for all animals within a protocol. Provision of sheltered areas
within the cage, such as tunnels or tubes, will give animals an opportunity to adjust the light intensity to their individual comfort levels.
Another suggestion is to provide vertical light bars on the room walls.

b. Automatic light systems with slow lighting and dimming, to simulate
sunrise and sunset, reduce the shock impact of abrupt light changes on
the animal.

c. In the past, exterior windows have been discouraged in animal rooms to
prevent seasonal changes from impacting the animals. However, in
some situations, seasonal changes are not considered hazardous to the
protocol and exterior windows are provided for environmental enrichment. For example, flowers and bird feeders have been placed near
exterior windows of cat housing rooms in some facilities to provide
visual enrichment for the cats.

III. ADJUSTING THE PHYSICAL PLANT TO MEET CHANGING NEEDS

The fields of laboratory animal care and biomedical research are growing and
changing at a rapid rate. With these changes comes the responsibility for the

laboratory animal resource manager to adapt the facility to meet new challenges, to anticipate change, and to implement new technologies when appropriate. The following are examples of areas that tend to evolve and change in the research animal resource environment.

A.   ERGONOMICS, HEALTH AND SAFETY

Ergonomics, health, and safety issues touch every aspect of the daily routine within a laboratory animal resource facility. The importance of these issues and guidance in the development of a health and safety program is addressed in *Occupational Health and Safety in the Care and Use of Research Animals* (10). Thorough knowledge of this reference is a vital tool for resource management. A few of the issues that relate directly to occupational health and the physical plant include the changing workforce, equipment materials and designs, material handling, and the emerging technology of robotics. The following section will focus on only a few of the common points of these issues.

1.   Changing Workforce

Over the past two decades more females have entered the field of laboratory animal medicine, technology, and care. Historically, with a more male-dominated workforce, the large, bulky caging systems that required frequent lifting and movement were not an issue.

Equipment should be selected that is of a comfortable size and maneuverability to persons of lower average physical stature. Many facilities select door frames to accommodate the increased height of stacked cages, a change that arises from the recognition of height requirements to accommodate postural adjustments and species-specific behaviors of the animals. The result is cage racks that are much higher and heavier. This change also moves the cage door to a higher position. A short person may experience difficulty in maneuvering these large racks and reaching into the back of the cages over cage thresholds. Maneuvering heavy equipment by staff of smaller stature can be aided by several methods:

- Selection of casters with tires and bearings that are easy to move.
- Elimination of pathways that include ramps or thresholds.
- Provision of stools, safety ladders, or elevated walkways to reduce stretching and reaching on the part of the staff.
- Use of equipment that does not have an egress threshold in a cage that restricts access to the back of the cage by small statured individuals.
- Consideration of the total weight and size of equipment. The pathways that the equipment must travel within the facility and the feasibility of moving the equipment along that path should be evaluated. One should remove obstacles that impede movement or that may cause strain in moving the equipment from point to point.

- Protection of the wall surfaces from impact of moving equipment through use of bumper guards or rails.
- Selection of equipment that can be compartmentalized or sectioned into lighter weight components for ease of handling.

2.   Materials

Traditionally, the common material used in laboratory animal caging has been corrosion-resistant stainless steel. More recently, fiberglass, plastic, and composite materials have come into favor, and these materials are generally lighter in weight. The incorporation of these materials in facility equipment reduces the amount of exertion required to maneuver equipment through the facility.

3.   Material Handling

a.   Receiving

Material handling begins at the time of purchase, long before the arrival of the items on the dock. Equipment and supplies should be categorized into two areas: routine supplies and unusual, infrequent items. Routine items include live animals and the supplies to provide for their care. Unusual or infrequent items include items such as large cages, racks, cage washers, autoclaves, etc. An assessment of access to the facility is advisable prior to purchase of any item, to ensure that entrances and pathways can accommodate the item.

For normal shipments and deliveries, provisions should be made to sanitize the receiving area to prevent disease transmission and contamination of the facility. Equipment that might be incorporated into the receiving area includes sanitization sinks, spray-down areas and cabinets, isolation chambers and cubicles, hydraulic lifts, and mechanical moving devices. The receiving area should be designed for all anticipated deliveries.

When purchasing unusual or infrequent supplies, such as cage washers and autoclaves, the size of the item and the feasibility of entrance of the largest components into the facility must be determined prior to purchase. If necessary, the item can be delivered as smaller components for re-assembly or, preferably, installed in the facility prior to construction.

4.   Robotics

Partly to address ergonomic concerns, robotic assistants are being incorporated into many aspects of sanitization and frequent facility activities. Currently, the principal uses are to assist with the cage loading and unloading processes associated with tunnel-type cage-washers and water-bottle sanitization and filling. Robotic systems can increase the available time for cage sanitization, in that a mechanical system does not require time off for breaks and can be set up for 2 hours of processing time at the end of a normal shift period. This can extend the processing hours to approximately 11 hours vs. 7 hours for a normal human shift period (11). The use of robots can also significantly reduce repetitive motion injuries normally associated with loading and unloading cages and reduce exposure to allergens generated during the dumping and refilling of soiled and fresh bedding.

Robotic systems are not suitable for all situations. Cost, return on investment, and appropriateness for the facility must be determined. Some of the factors to consider when determining the appropriateness of robotics for a facility include:

- Initial investment
- Anticipated cost recovery schedule compared to labor costs
- Health and safety costs and potential savings from the reduction of repetitive task injury claims
- Operational costs (utilities, maintenance, etc.) for traditional vs. robotic systems
- Availability and cost of labor for traditional sanitization positions; in a tight labor market, a robotic system would provide obvious advantages.
- Cost of maintenance and service contracts for traditional vs. robotic systems

A thorough cost analysis and facility impact review should be conducted before investing in a robotic sanitization system.

B.   ENVIRONMENT AND EMERGING TECHNOLOGIES

Based upon established data and the requirement for consistency in the research protocol, the physical plant should be assessed in light of the impact of environmental parameters and steps taken to reduce that impact (12).

1.   Effects of the physical plant on animal well-being

a.   *Sound*

The hearing ranges for animals vary significantly from species to species. Many normal daily operations and standard laboratory equipment can cause stress responses in animals (13). Some harmful noise is relatively silent (e.g., ultrasound emitted from a computer display monitor) (14). More obvious startling sounds include fire alarms or the noise caused by the dropping of metal accessory items in an animal room. The animals themselves can generate decibel levels that are unsafe for the human ear. The loud barking in a kennel area is one example. Another example is the noise produced by nonhuman primates banging on sheet metal cage panels to demonstrate aggression or challenge. The combination of all these sounds creates an environment that can significantly challenge the physiologic consistency on a day-to-day basis. When animals experience the relative calm of the weekend routine and then are challenged with the active sounds during the workweek, physiologic responses can be triggered to the extent that the animals tested on a Monday might not provide the same results as animals tested on a Friday (15).

High-decibel noise levels can be an occupational hazard and cause hearing loss. The *Guide* recommends that noise levels be maintained below 85 dB (1). Areas within the typical animal resource facility that might exceed these levels include dog kennels, nonhuman primate rooms, and the cage washing area. Hearing protection should be provided in these areas and other areas in which personnel are likely to be exposed to loud, sustained noise (10).

The facility manager must complete a thorough analysis of the noise levels, at a broad range of frequencies, to determine if there are noise issues to address. References (12) through (28) provide information related to this issue. Recent publications have documented the effects of infrasound on rats, which will require the facility manager to be cautious with the low frequency ranges as well as the ultrasound ranges in a rodent area (28). The animal resource manager must be aware of all frequency ranges that may impact the species housed within the facility. Steps must be taken to reduce noise levels that are offensive and discomforting for animals and unsafe for humans.

Animal facilities can be categorized as a "semi-reverberant field" containing both reflective and direct sound waves (29). Introduction of sound-dampening panels or barriers into the animals' area will reduce the amount of reflective sound within the room. For example, it is traditional for a kennel area to have a complete row of dog pens placed side by side in an open room. Although placing a "noise barrier panel" from floor to ceiling in several locations within a room will impede visualization, the panels will serve to disrupt the sound waves and halt some of the reflective sound bounce. Noise abatement panels are commercially available and will aid in sound absorption. These panels can be strategically placed within the rooms, mounted to the walls or suspended from the ceiling, to reduce the noise.

Cage and material selection also play a significant role in noise abatement. The noise generated by banging and drumming on sheet metal by nonhuman primates can be reduced by using plastics, fiberglass, or composite materials instead of sheet metal. The costs of these materials may be slightly more than the traditional sheet metal and the life span of the product may be less, but the investment should be rated in comparison to the improvement to the environment. In the analysis of loud noise areas, one should keep in mind that some animals are relatively quiet during normal working hours, only to become noise generators after-hours. For example, rabbits produce significant decibel levels with foot-stomping actions on metal grid floors. Nonmetal floor surfaces serve to reduce the impact of this sound.

b.   *Vibrations*

The operation and movement of heavy equipment both inside and outside of the animal facility can generate significant vibration. While the literature suggests that vibration might affect biologic systems, there is no conclusive evidence in this regard (30–37). Nevertheless, because of the possible influence vibrations might have on research animals, the manager should attempt to control this variable when designing and operating the animal resource facility.

c. *Lighting*

Lighting within an animal facility must be suited to the room use and the species housed within the rooms. Careful planning will enhance the comfort level for staff and animals. The first step in planning for light is to determine the room usage. Lighting for staff work areas should be 100-ft candles. Animal rooms should be illuminated at a level that is set to the comfort level of the species, which is usually not the comfort level for the staff. For example, rodent areas require a lower level of illumination than nonhuman primates (38). Different rodent strains also require a variety of light levels, depending upon strain characteristics and pigmentation (39). When accommodations cannot be made through the room lighting systems, provisions should be made for tunnels or shelter areas within the cage or pen to allow the animals to move away from the direct light. Variable or dual control lighting systems will allow for lighting to be increased to 100-ft candles during work and inspection periods for staff.

Light control systems must also reflect cycles that are consistent with the natural behavioral characteristics of the species. For example, ferrets will breed best when the daylight hours exceed eight per day. Nocturnal animals would be more comfortable with low, red lighting during the normal workday periods. It is more important to remember that light intensity levels during the daylight cycle can be impacted by high illumination from the corridors. Consideration should be made to place corridor lighting on the same day/night light cycle as the animal rooms and to utilize low-level red lighting near the nocturnal animal rooms when possible. Traditional mechanical day/night light cycle clocks are available as well as computerized control systems. The computerized control systems offer variable controls for specific areas and recording systems that previous mechanical clocks did not provide. In this regard, the new systems tend to offer more control than older systems.

Another consideration for the lighting system is the potential use as a tool for animal management. For example, most livestock species have limited depth perception. Animals with limited depth perception will normally move toward a more illuminated area. With planning, light can be used to encourage large animals to move from area to area without excessive force. Conversely, light can also be used to discourage animals from proceeding into unwanted areas by darkening off-limit areas.

Lighting fixtures are a key consideration for proper illumination and long-term care. There is a wide variety of lighting fixtures available, each with unique features. Some offer greater light spectra, others offer more control of the water and vapor seals. One should carefully review the lighting requirements for each area and select the most appropriate fixture. One standard fixture may not be acceptable for the entire facility, and several styles may have to be incorporated into the building plan. It is wise to obtain sample fixture covers prior to final selection and process the covers through normal sanitation practices as a test for durability prior to purchase.

d. *Thermoregulation*

Animals strive to maintain a constant body temperature in response to a variety of factors affected by the HVAC system, including temperature and air flow. Depending upon the cages or pens selected for the species, the animals may not be able to adequately thermoregulate. Additionally, the substrate may not offer the opportunity to avoid chilled or heated surfaces, such as metal and concrete floors and walls.

Surfaces and substrates that are thermoneutral (such as plastics, fiberglass, or composites) and that will not reflect the chilled or heated air provided by the central HVAC system should be used whenever possible. If the entire enclosure cannot be made thermoneutral, providing an area within the pen or enclosure that is thermoneutral will allow the animal to select a substrate that is comfortable.

e. *Control of the environment by the animal*

For obvious reasons, animals within the facility do not have ultimate control of their environment. The animals are subject to the environment that is provided by the animal resource management. Determination of the animals' needs should be based upon thorough, current, literature searches that will maximize the compatibility between species requirements and facility operations.

An example of a way to allow the animals to control a part of their environment is the provision of shelter areas, such as nest boxes, tunnels, and dens, which allow them to protect themselves from drafts and direct lighting.

f. *Construction materials*

Traditional construction materials in animal research facilities include concrete walls and floors with applied sealed surfaces. Many new materials have been developed to meet specific needs. A few examples include:

- Floor surfaces of **methyl methacrylate** (MMA) have a better chemical resistance and a faster curing time than traditional materials. A ceramic floor surface with high chemical resistance has also been used successfully.
- As an alternative to block construction, steel framing with dry walls and a sealed **fiberglass reinforced paneling** (FRP) surface has been used to save on space, reduce construction costs, and provide more flexibility for future needs.
- **Sprayed-on or hand-laid fiberglass** wall surfaces can provide a better seal and longer durability than the traditional epoxy-coated surfaces.
- **Structural insulating panels** (SIP) are a sandwich of sealed OSB (oriented strand board) panels, adhered to styrofoam block. SIP panels provide sound dampening and insulating elements not found in traditional block construction,

yet retain the properties required for strength and smooth surfaces impervious to moisture.

- **Acid-resistant duct and drain materials** are often used to provide a more durable system capable of withstanding acid-based detergents.

C.   PLANNING FOR FACILITIES

The planning of a facility should involve many individuals from a wide variety of backgrounds. Architects, engineers, purchasing specialists, animal care specialists, scientists and administration representatives should all be included. Because each party has a different background and level of expertise, everyone will not agree on all issues, and compromises will have to be made. As examples of areas that often require discussion in the planning process, centralized vs. decentralized facilities, manufactured vs. permanent construction, and room flexibility and control of the environment are examined in detail here. There are many other controversial challenges one faces in the planning stages, and these elements are selected only as representative examples to illustrate the decision-making process.

1.   Centralized vs. Decentralized Facilities

Centralized animal facilities have largely become the standard within the research environment. Of course, there are alternative points of view that do not agree that centralized facilities are the most efficient for all situations. Two common reasons cited in support of decentralized facilities are that decentralized facilities (1) maximize the efficiency of investigators because the laboratories are near the animal facility, and (2) protection of animals from infectious disease outbreaks, because groups of animals are more physically separated.

As a compromise to make groups of animals very accessible to research staff and yet not forfeit control of the animal environment, isolation cubicles with double-sided doors that hold one single rack of animals have been utilized in some situations (Figure 1). One cubicle door will open directly to the research laboratory, thus providing direct access of the research staff to their animal models. The other door opens directly to a service corridor that is maintained by the animal care staff, allowing for daily care of the animals under the centralized program. The animals are maintained in a HEPA-filtered environment, with separate light control and constant monitoring of the environmental conditions. This system maximizes the efficiency of the research staff and maintains quality care of the animals by the centralized program personnel.

When there is concern that some colonies or animals on long-term study may need extra protection from infectious disease, removal of those animals to an isolated or remote area may be desirable. Isolated areas can include specialized containment equipment such as isolators, mini-isolation rooms, or isolation cubicles within the central facility. Alternatively, remote animal housing

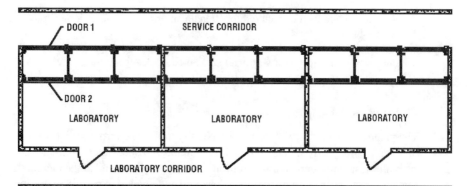

Figure 1. Schematic drawing showing dual-accessed cubicles. Note that Door 1 opens to the service corridor within the animal facility and Door 2 opens directly into the laboratory. This allows isolation of groups of animals and easy access for investigators.

in areas may involve renovation of rooms removed from the centralized facility or temporary, self-contained facilities attached to the existing building or in another campus location. The advantage of the self-contained remote building is that an entirely separate air handling system is used, thus providing total separation from the potentially infectious animals.

2.   Manufactured Facilities vs. Permanent Construction

Pre-manufactured facilities are becoming more popular as a means to quickly accommodate a rapid increase in animal use. Manufactured facilities are generally appropriate when time is of the essence, and program separation is required. Manufactured facilities can provide all of the essential elements available in permanent, accreditable, facility construction, but are more flexible in that the manager has more direct control of the plan, more financing options are often available, and the usage can be planned as either temporary or as a permanent addition to existing space. The modular, manufactured facilities are generally more economical in that construction and space utilization are specific to a targeted need and do not have to incorporate larger building elements, such as stairwells, external corridors, public accesses, etc. Manufactured facilities are suitable in the following circumstances:

- To provide replacement animal housing, cage washing, and laboratory space during periods of new construction or renovation
- To provide additional space for a rapidly expanding program within a shorter time span than is normally accomplished with standard construction
- To provide additional, remote space to accommodate depopulation and disease-control programs
- To provide additional space to accommodate specific research protocols that may be compromised in the centralized facility
- For financial reasons, pre-engineered, manufactured facilities may be more desirable than new construction or renovation

The total program goals must be reviewed when considering new construction, renovation, or the acquisition of a pre-engineered facility. A thorough cost analysis should be conducted prior to making any decision.

3. Room Flexibility and Control Options

Animal rooms must be flexible to accommodate the changing needs of the research program. Planning for flexibility and multiple species use is advisable. Traditional room designs are giving way to standard, plain rooms that utilize equipment that can be moved or relocated as the program adjusts. As an example, it had been very traditional to plan specific rooms for nonhuman primates that included wall-mounted cages and extensive trough and drain systems. Currently, most facilities plan plain rooms that will use racks of cages on casters rather than cages attached to the walls. Sinks and counters fixed to the walls were also considered standard, and required a permanent assignment of that square footage to sink and counter space, even though sinks and counters may not be required on a daily basis. Incorporating quick disconnect utility connections within the wall interstitial space and using mobile sinks as necessary will free up valuable square footage. One more example is the use of soft-sided or rigid class 100 areas within a room, which may reduce the need for constructed ante-rooms, thus making the room more flexible for multi-species use.

Providing a quality environment includes a quality **microenvironment** as well as a quality macroenvironment. Three common methods used to provide a high quality microenvironment are use of (1) ventilated cage racks; (2) isolation cubicles; and (3) flexible film isolators. Each method has advantages that must be calculated into the entire program. Some features include:

- Ventilated cage racks are advantageous in that they provide HEPA-filtered air to each individual cage. A disadvantage is that, in general, cages must be specific to a designated ventilated rack system and existing cages may not be usable or interchangeable. Some ventilated cage systems can operate in either the positive or negative mode. Ventilated cage systems can be mobile or stationary, but with some systems, essential components can be disconnected for sanitization in the cage washer (such as shelves). However, the entire mobile rack is normally very heavy to move and maneuver, and might represent an ergonomic issue.
- Isolation cubicles provide positive or negative HEPA-filtered environments for an entire rack of animals (40). Isolation cubicles are advantageous in that they can be designed to accommodate larger cages for large species or to utilize existing cages and racks for small rodents. Isolation cubicles are stationary; however, egress is enhanced with powered access door operation, thus reducing ergonomic concerns and providing a good seal to maintain differential pressure from the room environment. Constant monitoring of the interior environment (temperature, humidity, air changes per hour, differential pressure, and lighting) can be provided locally on the cubicle front or downloadable to a remote location. Optional air-handling systems control the positive/negative mode,

differential pressure, and air changes per hour. The control is local (at the cubicle) and not dependent upon the building system.
- Flexible film enclosures can be small to accommodate a few cages or large to accommodate several racks of cages. Flexible film isolators can operate in a positive or negative mode and conversion units are available to move the mode from positive to negative. They offer HEPA filtration with 100 or more air changes per hour. They are economical and easily installed for quick operation. The skins are generally made of 16-ml vinyl. Areas of constant use, such as doors and access ports, may have to be replaced after extended use.

Each facility has different needs to address. An evaluation of all systems and applicability to likely situations should be included in the final analysis.

IV. SUMMARY

The physical plant for each research animal resource facility is unique to the requirements of the research program. One set of standards for design and application will not be applicable to the set of standards developed for another facility. Whether the research animal resource is primarily concerned with maintaining an existing quality environment or expanding to meet new needs, thorough research of options and new opportunities should be considered. It is the facility manager's responsibility to keep current and provide the body of knowledge necessary to meet the needs of the research.

REFERENCES

1. **Institute of Laboratory Animal Resources, Subcommittee to Revise the** *Guide for the Care and Use of Laboratory Animals*, *Guide for the Care and Use of Laboratory Animals*, 7th ed., National Research Council, National Academy Press, Washington, D.C., 1996.
2. **Simmonds, R.**, Characteristics of Laboratory Animal Facilities, in *Handbook of Facilities Planning*, Vol. 2, *Laboratory Animal Facilities*, Ruys, T. (Ed.), Van Nostrand Reinhold, New York, 1991.
3. **U.S. Congress, 1966–1985, Animal Welfare Act 7 U.S.C.-2131 et seg.** USDA, Hyattsville, MD.
4. **U.S. Department of Agriculture, 1989, Animal Welfare, Final Rules, 9 CFR Parts 1, 2, and 3,** USDA, Hyattsville, MD.
5. **Fox, J.G., Cohen, B.J., and Low, F.M. (Eds.),** *Laboratory Animal Medicine*, Academic Press, Orlando, 1984.
6. **Novak, G.R.**, Effects of steam sterilization on polymers used to mold plastic rodent cages, platform presentation, Laboratory Animal Management Association, Reno, NV, 2001.
7. **Hughes, H.C. and Reynolds, S.**, The influence of position and orientation of racks on airflow dynamics in a small animal room, *Contemp. Top. Lab. Anim. Sci.*, 36, 62, 1997.
8. **Hughes, H.C. and Reynolds, S.**, The use of computational fluid dynamics for modeling airflow designs in a kennel facility, *Contemp. Top. Lab. Anim. Sci.*, 34, 49, 1995.

9. **Morse, B.C., Reynolds, S.D., Martin, D.G. et. al.**, Use of computational fluid dynamics to assess air distribution patterns in animal rooms, *Contemp. Top. Lab. Anim. Sci.*, 34, 65, 1995.

10. **Committee on Occupational Safety and Health in Research Animal Facilities,** Occupational Health and Safety in the Care and Use of Research Animals, National Research Council, National Academy Press, Washington, D.C., 1997.

11. **Getinge/Castle Scientific Division,** Introduction to robotics and automation in the animal care facility, Getinge/Castle, 2000.

12. **Clough, G.**, Environmental effects on animals used in biomedical research, *Biol. Rev.,* 57, 487, 1982.

13. **Deitert, R.R. and Golemboski, K.A.**, Environment-immune interactions, *Poul. Sci.,* 73, 1062, 1994.

14. **Sales, G.D. and Milligan, S.R.**, Ultrasound and laboratory animals, *Anim. Technol.*, 43, 89, 1992.

15. **Milligan, S.R., Sales, G.D., and Khirnykh, K.**, Sound levels in rooms housing laboratory animals: An uncontrolled daily variable, *Physiol. Behavior*, 53, 1067, 1993.

16. **Anthony, A.**, Criteria for acoustics in animal housing, *Lab. Anim. Care*, 13, 340, 1963.

17. **Pfaff, J.**, Noise as an environmental problem in the animal house, *Lab. Anim.*, 8, 347, 1974.

18. **Pfaff, J. and Stecker, M.**, Loudness level and frequency content of noise in the animal house, *Lab. Anim.*, 10, 111, 1976.

19. **Fowler, M.E.**, *Restraint and Handling of Wild and Domestic Animals*, Iowa State University Press, Ames, 1995.

20. **Besch, E.L.**, Definition of laboratory animal environment, in *Animal Stress*, Moberg, G.P. (Ed.), Williams & Wilkins, Baltimore, MD, 1985, pp. 297–315.

21. **Sales, G.D., Mulligan, S.R., and Khirnykh, K.**, The acoustic environment and its effects on laboratory animals, in *Welfare and Science. Proceedings of the Fifth FELASA Symposium*, Bunyan, J. (Ed.), Royal Society of Medicine Press, London, 1994, pp. 60–64.

22. **Peterson, E.A.**, Noise and laboratory animals, *Lab. Anim. Sci.*, 30, 422, 1980.

23. **Pakes, S.P., Lu, Y.S., and Meunier, P.C.**, Factors that complicate animal research, in *Laboratory Animal Medicine*, Fox, J.G., Cohen, B.J. and Low, F.M. (Eds.), Academic Press, Orlando, 1984, pp. 649–665.

24. **Gamble, M.R.**, Sound and its significance for laboratory animals, *Biol. Rev.* 57, 395, 1982.

25. **Johnson, D.K.**, Facility technology, in *Syllabus: Institute for Laboratory Animal Technology*, American Association for Laboratory Animal Science, Cordova, TN, 1992.

26. **Heidbrink, G.A.**, Incorporating new materials into the enhancement of primary housing areas, in *Proceedings of the 2nd International Conference for Environmental Enrichment*, Copenhagen, 1996.

27. **Fletcher, J.I.**, Influence of noise on animals, in *Control of the Animal House Environment. Laboratory Animals*, McSheehy, T. (Ed.), Laboratory Animals, Ltd., London, 1976, pp. 51–62.

28. **Motzel, S.L., Morrisey, R.E., Conboy, T.A., Lee, S. L., Armstrong, J.H., Barrall, M.D., Segal, M.Y., Buck, J.F., and Klein, H.J.**, Weight loss in rats associated with exposure to infra-sound, *Contemp. Top. Lab. Anim. Sci.*, 35, xx, 1996.

29. **Fox, R.E.**, Noise abatement and evaluation techniques, platform presentation, Laboratory Animal Management Association, Reno, NV, 2001.

30. **Becker Rodgers, J.**, Does building vibration cause reproductive dysfunction in rodents? Correspondence, CompMed, 2000.

31. **Dallman, M.F., Akana, S.F., Bell, M.E. et al.**, Warning! Nearby construction can profoundly affect your experiments, *Endocrine* 11, 111, 1999.

32. **Sumitomo, S., Tsujimoto, S., Maeda, S. et al.**, The influence of the great Hanshin earthquake on human response to environmental vibration due to the Shinkansen, *Ind. Health*, 36, 290, 1998.

33. **Ozkaya, N., Willems, B., and Goldsheyder, D.**, Whole-body vibration exposure: a comprehensive field study, *Am. Ind. Hyg. Assoc. J.*, 55, 1164, 1994.

34. **Montenegro, M.A., Palomino, H., and Palomino, H.M.**, The influence of earth-quake-induced stress on human facial clefting and its simulation in mice, *Arch. Oral Biol.*, 40, 33, 1995.

35. **Soskin, R.A.**, The effect of early experience upon the formation of environmental preferences in rats, *J. Comp. Physiol. Psychol.*, 56, 303, 1963.

36. **Nakamura, H., Ohsu, W., Nagase, H. et al.**, Uterine circulatory dysfunction induced by whole-body vibration and its endocrine pathogenesis in the pregnant rat, *Eur. J. Appl. Physiol.*, 72, 292, 1996.

37. **Slackler, A.M. and Weltman, A.S.**, Effects of vibration on the endocrine system of male and female rats, *Aerospace Med.*, 37, 158, 1966.

38. **Ruys, T.**, Understanding animals as they effect the animal research environment, in *Handbook of Facilities Planning, Vol. 2, Laboratory Animal Facilities*, Ruys, T. (Ed.), Van Nostrand Reinhold, New York, 1991.

39. **Wimer, R.E. and Fuller, S.L.**, Patterns of behavior, in *Biology of the Laboratory Mouse*, Green, E.L. (Ed.), McGraw-Hill, New York, 1966.

40. **White, W.J., Hughes, H.C., Singh, S.B., and Lang, C.M.**, Evaluation of a cubicle containment system in preventing gaseous and particulate airborne cross-contamination, *Lab. Anim. Sci.*, 33, 571, 1983.

ACKNOWLEDGMENTS

The author gratefully acknowledges the assistance and contributions of the following individuals:

Gerard M. Diffine	Schlyer Manufacturing Co. Inc.
Roxanne E. Fox, B.S., LATG	Lab Products, Inc.
Skeeter Georgeson, LATG	Edstrom Industries, Inc.
Amy S. Ingraham, B.A., RLATG	Pharmacal Research Labs, Inc.
Ken Kovar	Bio Bubble, Inc.
William E. (Ned) Leverage, Jr., B.S.	Life Science Products, Inc.
Doug McDonald	Getinge/Castle, Inc.
Gary R. Novak, RLATG	Johns Hopkins Oncology Center
Janet Becker Rodgers, D.V.M.	University of Kentucky
Sally A. Thomas, B.S.	Thoren Caging Systems, Inc.
Jim Tomasine	Schlyer Manufacturing Co. Inc.

10 Fiscal Management

James A. Alford, Jr., M.B.A.

A good program of financial management in a laboratory animal care and use program is no different than in any other business or program. It should tell the financial story in clear terms. It should meet the needs and format of the institution being served, and it should be meaningful. Financial management therefore includes acceptable accounting practices, sound budget planning, and frequent monitoring and adjustments. It is very important to remember that unlike most supplies and services used by the investigators, animal maintenance is usually very close to a monopoly and therefore suspect. The better the accounting practices, the easier it will be for the manager to tell his/her story.

Financial management comprises four processes: **planning, budgeting, cost accounting, and monitoring**. Each of the four steps should be performed on a regular basis for both short-term and long-term management. To ignore any of the steps truly jeopardizes fiscal management in any organization.

I. ACCOUNTING TERMS

A. **Accounting** is the systematic recording, presenting, and interpreting of the financial data to provide information to organizations.

   Information provided by accounting includes the following.

1. **Operating information** is information that is required to conduct the day-to-day operation. This type of accounting would record payroll, supply and service expenditures, revenue received, equipment purchases and inventory balances. The organization needs to know how much it owes, what it needs, and when the debts are due. The organization also needs to know how much money it has to spend and in which categories.

2. **Management information** is a summary of the accounting information used by managers, as they do not have the time to examine all of the details involved in the operating information. The summaries and other indicators allow the manager to carry out his/her function. Managers use the accounting information to **control** (communicate, motivate, attention getting, and appraisal), **coordinate** (look at all areas of the organization simultaneously), and **plan** (budgeting, looking at areas that are over, as well as under, budget).

3. **Financial information** is the information provided to external parties such as other departments within the organization, funding agencies, and the parent organization. It is important that the information is kept in a format that is meaningful to the parent organization, sponsor, or users of the services. The information should be retrievable, reproducible, and meaningful.

B. **Goals** are needed in order have a plan for budgeting. Goals can be set to meet laws and standards or to meet the needs of the researchers being served. Typical goals are accreditation, meeting standards set by USDA, or meeting the animal health requirements of the research being conducted.

C. **Support** for animal facilities comes from grants, contracts, recharges, and institutional sources. The manager needs to be able to understand and account for each of these entities in the format needed. Typically, the terms "**indirect**" or "**direct**" are used for categories of support and costs. **Indirect costs** are not easily attributable to a particular cost center. An example of an indirect cost would be the cost of administering the department or facility. **Direct costs** are those easily attributed to an individual cost center. An example of a direct cost is mouse chow for the cost center "mice."

NIH grants typically have direct and indirect support components. **Direct support** for a grant or contract would be the support for supplies, equipment, and personnel associated with the funded project. **Indirect support** would be the support that goes to the institution and not directly to the department for program support. Indirect support would typically be used to support the institution's infrastructure (i.e., library, security, etc).

D. **Budget** is the monetary plan for the goals being set. Setting the budget should involve everyone responsible for achieving the goals.

E. **Rate setting** is the use of cost analysis to set fee structures for individual cost centers.

F. **Cost centers** are accounting devices for accumulating expenses that have common characteristics. Some examples of cost centers are cage washing, technical services, transportation, mouse husbandry, dog husbandry, and other centers that can stand alone. Cost centers should be as specific as possible and separated into categories that supply information that is truly needed.

Cost centers provide an equitable justification for charging users of services for the service or product provided. Cost centers also provide the director/ manager a means of control and planning. They measure the cost of an activity against its value. Cost centers allow comparison between two or more like units for the cost of a service. They also allow a better justification of service fees to user groups and sponsors.

G.   **Cost Analysis** is the use of all cost information to determine the correct fee for service. It helps identify services that are not needed or are not self-supporting. Cost analysis also assists in planning, decision-making, and the controlling process on a daily, quarterly, or annual basis.

II. PLANNING

The planning process is used to ensure that the animal facility management professionals have a vision and plan for the future. To plan for growth, adding additional services, or eliminating present services requires communication with the administration and investigators. The planning stage can be considered strategic planning in that the management team is looking to meet the needs and wants of the institution and personnel being served. Planning requires attendance at conferences and meetings in order to keep current and knowledgeable of trends in laboratory animal care and use. The needs of investigators have to be met not only today, but also in the future. Most research institutions require years of planning to erect new buildings, increase staff, purchase equipment, or rid the facility of disease. All of these require additional funds that must be generated either through the per diem system or by fund raising, neither of which happens quickly.

Sometimes good practices have to be marketed to the users of the services. Educating and communicating with the investigators and laboratory personnel accomplish marketing best. Marketing is closely linked with planning.

III. BUDGETING

The budgeting process should always be related to the overall planning process of an organization. No one is in a position to plan for the future without a clear sense of what the available resources are. Conversely, sensible budgets and financial plans cannot be put together without knowing the direction the organization will take in the future. Simply allocating money is not enough. Instead, the proper and strategic use of resources is key to the budgeting process. As Thomas Wolf writes in the book, *Managing a Nonprofit Organization* (1), "There are eight steps that an organization should take to complete a successful budgeting cycle."

STEP 1. MAKE A WISH LIST

The first step has nothing to do with numbers or dollars. Rather, it consists of an annual review of the needs of the institution by speaking with senior management and investigators to determine what they want the organization to accomplish in the year or years to come. This is the planning stage previously discussed. The planning stage involves consideration of a number of questions about the upcoming year, such as:

1. What should the organization be doing in the next year or future years?
2. What core activities are essential?
3. What additional activities might be undertaken if cost were not an object?
4. What are the staffs needs associated with these activities?
5. Are there special one-time expenditures that might be considered for things such as upgrading equipment, improving physical facilities, contracting special consultancies in evaluation, or marketing?

STEP 2. Cost Out the List

This involves determining how much it will cost to carry out the activities listed in Step 1. Obviously, there are some basic costs that have to be covered just to keep the organization going. There are the facility expenses, core staff salaries, and expenses related to the basic programs that were established in the past and which are still needed. Each of these programs and activities must be carefully evaluated for cost and impact so that rational decisions can be made about the continuation of such programs. In addition, the expenses and impact associated with new activities must also be evaluated.

There are two approaches commonly used to develop costs:

1. The first approach is called the **incremental budgeting method** and leans heavily on information contained in the previous year's actual expenses and income records. If an organization is carrying out an activity that has been ongoing for several years, then the easiest way to prepare a budget for the coming year is to simply consider a percentage increment for inflation and other cost factors. The percentage increase or decrease added to the figures contained in the previous years financial statement (referred to as *actuals*) then becomes the budget figure for the new budget.
2. The second approach, called **zero-based budgeting**, requires that each line item of a budget be calculated anew. Staff members are told that any item in the budget will be zero unless they can provide a full justification for a new budget figure.

Obviously, some combination of these two approaches is desirable in the budgeting process. It is a waste of time and effort to rely on zero-based budgeting for programs already in place. On the other hand, implementing new programs without a full cost estimate would be irresponsible on the part of management. Costs should always be estimated on the high side. As the costs of new programs and activities are considered, it should be remembered that they will add to the central administrative costs. The simple addition of a program will put added burden on the core staff, supervision, space, and equipment.

STEP 3. ALLOCATE ESTIMATED INCOME

In this process it is imperative to ensure that all "**restricted income**" is placed into the proper program activity. Examples of restricted income would be a grant for a specific activity, a donation for a specific project, or an internal decision to restrict all income for veterinary services to be used for some specified purpose. The restricted income should be allocated into the programs for which it was intended. Other income would be considered "**unrestricted**." The manager should try to cover the most basic administrative costs with the unrestricted income, and then allocate the remaining unrestricted income across all the programs and activities. This process makes it easier to make hard decisions later if the estimated expenses and income do not match.

STEP 4. COMPARE

Comparing the estimated expenses with the estimated income is usually very revealing. It may be clear in the process that some activities will have to be given up if the projected budget does not balance. In fact, if management discovers that income is adequate to cover all expenditures at this point in the budgeting process, there should be concern that the organization is not reaching far enough or being ambitious enough in its planning.

In evaluating one program activity against another, management needs to be careful about using the criterion of cost-effectiveness in the pure sense. Typically we think of cost-effectiveness as the return on investment with a large value gained for a small cost. While cost-effectiveness or breakeven are concerns, the mission may dictate that the organization should carry on certain activities that are not cost effective, at least in the short term. Some activities will have to be conducted in order for the organization to fulfill its mission, even at an apparent loss. An example would be having a small number of one species of animal. As most managers know, the care for a few animals is usually not cost effective and might necessitate cost subsidization until the numbers grow.

It also might be beneficial to spread some costs where specific service charges are hard to allocate, such as animal health, to all animals and not charge on a case-by-case basis. Similarly, one would not want to forego education, certification, and awards simply because income realized from these activities is not readily apparent. Thus, cost-effectiveness is only one criterion but certainly not the only one. The primary criterion should relate to the mission of the organization, its purposes, goals, and objectives.

STEP 5. SET PRIORITIES

Anyone who has participated in a budget-balancing session knows how traumatic it can be. Each suggested activity resulting in expenditures seems to have a defender. In the end, a priority-setting session must relate not solely to dollars and cents, but also to a fundamental assessment of the organization's mission. It is important to seek answers to questions such as:

1. Is this activity really central to what the organization is about?
2. Does it help the organization get where it should be in 1 year, 2 years, or 5 years?
3. Might it be more important to build a reserve to protect the organization over the long term rather than engage in a new activity area?

These are difficult questions, but by asking them the management team is fulfilling a fundamental role in deciding what course is best for the organization and most clearly in the interest of science.

STEP 6. ADJUST AND BALANCE

Once activities have been put in some order of priority, negotiation is still possible as the budget is adjusted and put into balance. For example, an activity that is related to veterinary health could be switched to husbandry if it proves to make husbandry more efficient. Weighing animals and trimming nails are examples that could fall into either category and should be placed where they are most cost efficient. This type of negotiation would be beneficial to both activities and to the mission of the unit as a whole. One must be careful not to move monies into or out of activities that are restricted or to overstate income in order to ease the pain of balancing the budget.

STEP 7. APPROVE

Management should ask hard questions about the budget preparation. They should challenge any documents proposing new activities because they are ultimately responsible for the fiscal health of the organization. Once everyone has agreed upon the budget and the activities to be supported, the budget should be approved. Budget agreement is very important because success depends upon everyone working together to ensure its success. If part of the management team attempts to continue with a program that has been cut, it makes it difficult for the other activities to continue. Nonetheless, the last step gives the budget process some flexibility.

STEP 8. MONITOR AND AMEND

One common mistake in the budget process is to assume it has come to an end once management approves the final document. Two extremes should be avoided:

1. Management should not insist that the approved document is inflexible and force the staff to stick to it without modification throughout the fiscal year.
2. On the other hand, management should not be willing to say the budget document is only a rough approximation and give the staff instructions to "come as close as possible." Management should have final say on any significant changes in the budget figures.

If management or a staff person presents an idea midway through the budget year that is worthy of funding, the idea should be explored. However, the manager must remember this puts him/her back to the first step and he/she will then need to go through the process again. Granted, the process may be abbreviated, but good budgetary techniques require that the eight steps be completed in order to approve funding the new idea.

Each budget activity must be monitored throughout the year. Questions should be asked when budgets are being over/under-spent. Over-spending can suggest ineffective fiscal oversight and under-spending can suggest that the activity is not being performed sufficiently. It is the responsibility of management to ensure that things are going as planned. Cost accounting allows management the opportunity to monitor the activities of the organization.

IV. COST ACCOUNTING

A. BACKGROUND

In order to have good fiscal management there must be a sound accounting system in place. The budget is the financial plan of the organization. Budgeting specifies how much money an organization thinks it will take in and how much it will spend (1). Accounting is the system that is used to record, classify, and summarize the income and expenses of the organization. The information provided is an integral part of the information used in financial management (2). Accounting and budgeting must be recognized as separate systems that interact in complementary manner if managers are to exercise control over the financial resources of their organizations. The budget is the plan; accounting is the record of the plan.

B.   COST CENTERS

The accounting system as stated above records, classifies, and summarizes the business activity of the organization. To break this down further, it records the activity of each cost center. Cost centers should be identified in such a way as to be able to stand alone in respect to the service the cost center provides. The manager should always ensure that the effort and cost of obtaining the cost information is truly needed. Data collection is costly in time and effort. It is recommended that the manager periodically look at the data being collected to see if it is really being used. If it is not being used, the resources used to gather the information have been wasted.

Several benefits can be derived from organizing into cost centers. These are described below.

1. **First and foremost, cost centers facilitate an equitable means of charging users for services provided.** Cost accounting by cost centers also allows the manager a means of analysis, which is useful for organizations evaluating particular programs for cost-effectiveness or for revenue-generating potential.

2. **Cost centers provide the director/manager a means of control and planning**. The activity being accounted for should be as small as possible. The smaller the cost center, within reason, the more accurate will be the expense and income records attributed to the activity. Accurate accounting allows the manager to measure the cost of an activity against its value. It also allows comparison between two or more units for the cost of a service. In addition, it will allow meaningful adjustments of fee schedules. If a manager has two or more cage-washing operations in separate buildings, cost accounting them as different cost centers is one management tool to evaluate the efficiency of each. The information provided could suggest equipment deficiencies, personnel issues, or physical plant designs that need to be remedied. If all cage-washing operations were accounted for under one umbrella, those differences would not show up. Separate cost centers also allow for activities to be dropped or charged differently in times of budget reductions or animal population shifts. For instance, physical examinations and immunizations of animals might be part of the husbandry per diem in a facility housing only dogs and cats. However, if rodent populations start to increase proportionately, physicals and immunizations might be switched to the dog and cat purchase or in-processing charges. Using this same example, labor for cleaning pens may be more of a factor for the dogs, but cage-washing costs would be more of a factor with the rodents and cats. By using dogs, cats, and

rodents as cost centers in this example, it is easier to differentiate the costs to ensure equitable charges.

3. **Cost centers allow better justification of fees to user groups and sponsors.** It is much easier to explain fees to users when actual costs are used. Management should be able to show what cost factors go into each cost center and how that cost was calculated. Cost centers allow the manager the ability to provide and charge for differential services based on need. If an investigator does not need quarantine or cage-washing services, cost center accounting will permit the manager to forgive those portions of the recharges. While the use of all services may be negotiable, some services will be mandatory for legal, humane, or institutional reasons.

The first step in cost accounting is to identify all direct costs. Identifying direct costs is different than using budget figures. Identifying direct costs allow you to assign the budget figures to a particular cost center. Examples of direct costs are labor, supplies, equipment, or facilities used in a specific aspect of the operation such as cage washing, dog husbandry, rodent husbandry, veterinary care, or laboratory support. Second, fair shares of indirect costs need to be assigned to each direct cost center. Examples of indirect costs are supervision, administration, utilities, and general-use cleaning supplies.

C. DETERMINATION OF PER DIEM CHARGES

After the direct and indirect costs have been identified and assigned, the manager is ready to calculate per diem charges.

The following eight steps are useful for determination of per diem charges.

STEP 1. Determine the goals of the organization and the services to be provided.

STEP 2. Budget the direct cost of each service or goal proposed by the organization. Utilities and maintenance could be direct costs depending upon the policies of the institution. It is important to be aware of any pertinent rules and regulations, with respect to appropriate charges for laboratory- and animal-based research, such as policies put in place by the Office of Management and Budget (OMB) (3). In general, the rates will be more accurate if more items can be identified as direct costs.

STEP 3. Determine the total indirect costs that must be allocated to the cost centers identified in the budgeting process. Indirect costs include administration, supervision, benefits, and supplies to accommodate these activities.

STEP 4. Determine how the money will be obtained to cover the various costs. University animal facilities usually receive money from direct recharges to grants and contracts, general support from the university, and their own grants and contracts. Management needs to know how much money will come from each source and how the money can be used, i.e., whether it is restricted or unrestricted. Grants and contracts are usually specific for a particular project. University support may be allocated for faculty, administration, or other specific uses.

STEP 5. Allocate the income money from university sources, grants, and contracts to the total budget in accordance with any specific restrictions. This income is used to cover respective costs according to the restrictions if any are placed on the income. The costs not covered by the income will have to be recovered by recharges to the users of the services supplied.

STEP 6. Allocate the costs that must be recharged to revenue-producing cost centers. For each cost center a "factor" must be included to equitably distribute the indirect costs to each cost center. Examples of costs that would need to be included are animal health activities, administration, and maintenance of non-cost center space such as hallways and supply rooms. This distribution factor could be based on the labor distribution for each cost center, cage/pen space requirements for each species, or some other factor determined by management. It is important that this "factor" is truly representative of the indirect costs included for each cost center, as it has the potential to distribute some very large dollar amounts.

STEP 7. Calculate the number of animal days by multiplying the average daily population by the number of days in the year (365).

STEP 8. Calculate the cost per day (per diem) for each species. This is accomplished by dividing the number of animal days into the total allocated cost for each species.

One of the best sources for cost analysis and rate setting for animal research facilities is a document by that name, *Cost Analysis and Rate Setting Manual for Animal Research Facilities* (4), available from the National Center for Research Resources, Office of Science and Public Liaison. The latest revision was prompted by new technology, use of computers, increased regulation, and an increased need for consistency in cost accounting and rate setting. As research dollars become more scarce, and the cost of maintaining research animals increases, management needs to have good cost containment and accounting practices to attract scientists to their institutions.

Some institutions feel that per diem surveys of other facilities' recharge schedules are equivalent to cost analysis and rate setting. Typically they use these surveys to prove that their costs are reasonable. If used for comparison, and only comparison, the surveys could be meaningful. If used to set per diem charges at your institution, the information is meaningless. Only cost analysis will truly prove what is a reasonable rate for a particular institution.

V. MONITORING AND REFLECTION

Monitoring the animal resource facility by using cost analysis is very important. The reports, if properly used, can be very effective management tools. An example would be if the animal census reports that the canine population has been decreasing for the past 2 months, but the cost of dog food and labor involved in caring for the dogs has not been reduced proportionately. In this case, the manager might suspect that the labor has become inefficient and either the food is going bad or is being used inappropriately. In both cases, the cost analysis reports should give a warning, and appropriate steps should be taken.

Several key questions with respect to monitoring financial management include the following.

A. WHAT DOES A GOOD PROGRAM OF FINANCIAL MANAGEMENT LOOK LIKE?

The organization's finances should show prudent management, appropriate oversight and controls, and proper systems for predicting and tracking revenue and expenses (1).

The management team should keep accurate records that allow prediction of the organization's needs in the future. The management team should review the records and reports on a regular basis. It is wise for the management team to invite others to review the reports and records in order to help ensure a fair audit of the finances.

The budget should be monitored on an ongoing basis to ensure that expense and income are balanced. The cost of each service should be reasonable for the service provided. All costs need to be monitored and recharges justified for all species to ensure that charges applied to one species are not used to subsidize another.

The program should meet the needs of the community being served. All services should be well administered. The management team should continually question the users of the services to ensure that the programs are needed and adequate. The management should periodically determine what would happen if a particular service or program were stopped. It should be determined if anyone or anything suffers and how services and programs might be improved.

As stated in the budget development and review section, a good financial program allows management to position the organization for the future. Management should consider space and equipment needs for present and future users. Management should be involved in recruitment programs and be part of the research planning effort so that they are aware of future institutional needs. Except in extreme circumstances, an animal program should not be reactive in building space and purchasing equipment, but instead be proactive. Being proactive allows management the opportunity to put in place additional programs as the organization grows.

B. How Does One Incorporate Sound Financial Management If It Has Not Existed?

Building a sound financial program where one has not existed depends on strong support from the institutional administration. In all cases it will take time to collect costs, predict income and expenses, and develop budgets. The administration and the users of the services must be patient and supportive. The management team must use the eight-step approach that was discussed under budgeting. This approach will work even if good financial reports and records are not available. The less accurate the data is that is being used in the beginning of the process, the more the budget will need to be changed as the information and data become more precise. It is important for those starting out to remember to have a defensible plan for implementation and to stick to that plan. Change is inevitable as budgets and programs are developed, but if no plan is being followed, the change could be the result of pressure, rather than good decisions. It is the responsibility of the administration and the management team to ensure that the changes are made for the right reasons.

C. What Are Some Milestones or Indicators of Sound Financial Management?

Sound financial management is first measured by the ability of the organization to generate income that equals expenses. A more critical evaluation of sound financial management is to ask the question, "How are we serving our clients?" Breaking even in the income and expense categories is not relevant if management has to overcharge or cut programs that are truly needed. If investigators are not able to conduct research because of lack of facilities or disease in the animal population, then the program is not being managed soundly. The problems that appear in the financial management are better understood as symptoms rather than as disease. The lack of funds or space is usually caused by lack of support of the program from the administration and/or the faculty, or by a lack of vision and understanding of client needs on the part of the facility management. Therefore, a good milestone or indicator of sound financial management is the existence of the resources needed to provide the investigators with the animals and technical capability required to conduct their research in an uninterrupted fashion.

It is important to remember that sound financial management is the same in both academic and industrial animal facilities. The costs must be contained whether the institution is non-profit or for-profit. The big difference is in how the cost is recovered. Typically the cost in academia is recovered through the per diem system of recharges. In industry, depending on the company, cost could be recovered through recharges to the research department or project, or could be assigned to other departments such as engineering, research support, services or some other department. However the costs are covered, they are very important to the success of the institution. The per diem charged in academia is usually the equivalent of the project costs in industry. The labor, equipment, supplies, animals, and facility costs still have to be accounted for and the income to cover the costs has to come from some identifiable source.

Finally, it is important for the manager to take time to reflect. Managers are paid to get things done. Periodically, the manager should take a reflective moment to jot down answers to a few questions, such as: "What are we doing?" "What should we be doing?" "What should we not be doing?" "What should we be doing next?" This informal exercise, when linked with the budget planning and monitoring process, can serve to highlight areas of strength and areas needing improvement.

REFERENCES:

1. **Wolf, T.S.**, *Managing a Nonprofit Organization*, Simon & Schuster, New York, 1990.
2. **Garner, C.W.**, *Accounting and Budgeting in Public and Nonprofit Organizations*, Jossey-Bass Inc., San Francisco, 1991, p. 10.
3. **Office of Federal Financial Management, Office of Management and Budget**, CIRCULAR A-21 (Revised 10/27/98), Washington, D.C., 1998.
4. **Office of Science Policy and Public Liaison, National Center for Research Resources/NIH**, National Institutes of Health, *Cost Analysis and Rate Setting Manual for Animal Research Facilities*, 6705 Rockledge Drive, Suite 5140, Bethesda, MD, http://www.ncrr.nih.govnewspub/CARS.pdf.

11 Acquiring Grants and Contracts

Howard G. Rush, D.V.M., Mary S. Freer, B.B.A., and Patricia A. Ward, LATG

The ability to conduct biomedical research depends on the availability of funds to perform the work. Without a source of funds, investigators cannot hire personnel, purchase the equipment and supplies, purchase the animals, or conduct the experiments. An investigator must identify a source of funds in order to do research. In the private sector, companies set aside research and development funds to conduct research as a normal part of business in order to discover and evaluate new products that have the potential for success in the marketplace or to further develop existing products. In public institutions and research institutes, funds to conduct research are acquired primarily through grants, contracts, or gifts from sources outside the institution. In academic institutions in the United States, the five main sources of funds for biomedical research are the National Institutes of Health, the National Science Foundation, the military, private industry, and private foundations (1).

I. DEFINITIONS

A. **Grants** are types of sponsorship to a scientist to support his/her research. Generally, investigators initiate the process by applying to a granting agency for the funds needed to conduct the studies. The investigator, not the sponsor, determines the subject of the research. The granting agency determines if the subject of inquiry is one worthy of support (2).

B. **Contracts** are other forms of sponsorship for research. Companies interested in a particular area of study initiate most contracts and the sponsor specifically delineates the research to be conducted (2). A company usually has a particular objective in mind when issuing a contract. There may be restrictions placed on the investigator who obtains the contract with regard to publication of results and ownership of data and ideas.

C. **Gifts** are funds given to investigators or institutions, often without restriction placed on their use.

II.   GRANT PROCESS

A variety of grants are available from government sources including training grants, postdoctoral fellowships, individual research grants, program projects, center grants, small business grants, etc. In the United States, the most common source of government funds for biomedical research is the Public Health Service (PHS) National Institutes of Health, which has many subdivisions that award grants. Perhaps the most common grant is the Investigator Initiated Research Grant or R01 grant, which is an hypothesis-driven grant awarded to an individual investigator for the study of a well-defined scientific problem (3).

A.   APPLICATION STRUCTURE

The Application for a Public Health Service Grant (PHS 398) has a very specific format that must be followed in order to apply for a grant (2, 4). **The sections of the PHS 398 include:**

1. Face Page
2. Description, Performance Sites, and Key Personnel
3. Research Grant Table of Contents
4. Detailed Budget for Initial Budget Period
5. Budget for Entire Proposed Period of Support
6. Biographical Sketch
7. Other Support
8. Resources
9. Research Plan
10. Appendix
11. Checklist
12. Personnel Report
13. Personal Data

Detailed instructions are provided for completing each section (5). The **Research Plan** is the section of the grant application that explains why the problem is important to study, what questions the investigator wishes to pursue, and how the questions will be answered. **The Research Plan is further broken down into the following sections:**

1. Specific Aims
2. Background and Significance
3. Preliminary Studies
4. Research Design and Methods
5. Human Subjects
6. Vertebrate Animals
7. Literature Cited
8. Consortium/Contractual Arrangements
9. Consultants

The use of animals in the proposed research is described in detail in the Research Plan, specifically in Section D, Research Design and Methods. In addition, the investigator must complete Section F, Vertebrate Animals, which contains a detailed description of how the animals will be used; justification for the use of animals; the species and numbers to be used; a description of the veterinary care program; the procedures for ensuring that discomfort, distress, pain, and injury will be limited to that which is unavoidable; a description of the use of analgesic, anesthetic, and tranquilizing drugs and/or comfortable restraining devices; and methods of euthanasia.

B. PEER REVIEW

When a grant application is submitted to NIH, the **Center for Scientific Review** assigns it to an **Integrated Review Group (IRG)**, a cluster of study sections that review grants in related scientific areas and to a specific study section, or **Scientific Review Group (SRG)**, within the IRG. The SRG comprises scientists from outside NIH with experience in the area of proposed research. In addition, the proposal is assigned to an Institute or Center with a funding mission that incorporates the subject area of the proposal (6).

The SRG is responsible for determining whether the grant has scientific and technical merit. The five criteria that are evaluated to determine merit include **Significance**, **Approach**, **Innovation**, **Investigator**, and **Environment** (3). The review conducted by the SRG is termed **peer review** because peers of the scientist submitting the proposal conduct it. The SRG assigns a **priority score** to the proposal and forwards it to the **Advisory Council** of the Institute or Center for the next level of review. The proposals are ranked according to priority score and a **percentile rank** is then determined (6).

At the time the proposal is submitted to the PHS or soon thereafter, the investigator must also submit the proposal or some portion of it to his/her Institutional Animal Care and Use Committee (IACUC). Activities involving animals must be reviewed and approved by the IACUC before the studies can be conducted. Some study sections will not review the application until a letter has been received from the IACUC indicating that the project has IACUC approval. If the study section does conduct the merit review without the IACUC approval, a letter must be forthcoming before an award is made.

After the SRG has reviewed the proposals assigned to it, those with sufficient merit are referred to the Advisory Council of the Institute or Center to which the proposal has been assigned. The Advisory Council then performs a second level of peer review. It is this second level of review that determines which proposals will be funded by the Institute or Center. The percentile ranking is paramount for determining funding. The Advisory Council also must consider whether the proposal is relevant to the mission of the Institute or Center. Only proposals with a percentile ranking sufficiently high will actually be funded. This cut-off is termed the **payline**. In general, only about 25% of proposals submitted to NIH are actually funded.

Once a decision has been made by the Center or Institute to fund a proposal, the award is made to the institution, not the investigator. Thus, if an investigator leaves an institution, the grant remains at the institution, unless specific permission is granted by NIH to transfer the award. The award is made for a specific period of time ranging most commonly from 3 to 5 years. At yearly intervals, the investigator must submit a progress report or **non-competing renewal** application to inform the funding agency of progress made on the proposal, changes in personnel, new directions that will be pursued, etc. At the end of the grant period, the investigator must submit a **competing renewal** application to obtain funds to continue the studies.

III. CONTRACTS

A substantial amount of financial support is available from private industry for conducting research. Industry often approaches scientists in academia because they have expertise with a particular model system or substantial depth of knowledge in a particular subject area. Such funds are usually provided in the form of a contract in which a specific study or group of studies is conducted by the investigator for the company funding the project. Contract research is very goal oriented and the company specifies the nature of the studies to be conducted, often in great detail. Generally, there is no peer review conducted in the case of contracts. Unlike the case with grants, funds remaining after the completion of the contract do not have to be returned to the company unless specified in the contract.

Although industry funding of research can present many benefits to investigators, there can be many pitfalls as well. Many issues can arise in conducting contract research that relate to ownership of the data, publication of the results, and patent rights (3). Conflict of interest issues can also arise. An investigator must negotiate the details of the contract in advance before agreeing to perform the studies. Similarly, the company awarding the contract will specify in detail their expectations for the studies to be performed. It is imperative that the institutional legal department reviews the contract before the investigator agrees to the contract.

IV. OVERVIEW OF THE FINANCIAL PROCESS OF A SPONSORED PROJECT

Once an investigator is granted an award to fund the research project, **a budget is established with the following direct cost categories:**

1. Personnel (wages and benefits)
2. Tuition and Fees
3. Supplies
4. Travel

5. Equipment
6. Animal Care
7. Consultants
8. Consortium
9. Other

Direct costs are those specifically attributable to the performance of the project. The award also will include a calculated budget line for **Facilities and Administrative (F&A) costs (indirect costs)**. **Indirect costs** are those costs incurred by an organization that cannot be assigned to a specific project. Examples would include facilities operation, maintenance costs, equipment and building depreciation, and administrative expenses. F&A cost rates are negotiated between the institution and the sponsor. They are assessed on the expenditures in the direct budget. Not all direct categories are assessed indirect cost; examples of exempt categories would be equipment and tuition. The indirect cost charged to a grant is a percentage of the direct expense. For example, if the allowable direct costs on a grant were $100,000, and the institution's indirect cost rate were 52%, then the institution would receive $52,000 for indirect costs in addition to the $100,000 that was received for the performance of the work.

There are rules that govern what expenses are permitted in each category. **OMB Circular A-21** is the rulebook that determines what types of expenses may be incurred on federally sponsored grants (7). For example, a research grant should not pay for clerical help. The personnel budget line of a grant application applies specifically to personnel that are directly performing the research. Some expenses may be "A-21 questionable" but are allowable on the grant. For instance, if a secretary spends part of his/her time entering data into a database specifically for the research project, that part of the clerical salary devoted to the research may be allowed if a written justification is provided.

As expenditures are incurred, the institution will draw from a **Letter of Credit** to cover the direct and indirect expenses on a monthly basis. Note that technically the award is made to the institution and not to the investigator. Hence, as the investigator incurs expenses, the institution draws from the Letter of Credit to pay them. At the end of the reporting period for the grant, the institution must report to the sponsor how the awarded funds were actually spent. Since most of the grants are awarded for a multiple-year period it is possible to carry forward an unspent balance into the next period. If there are unspent budget lines in the final year of a grant, the funds are returned to the funding agency. On the other hand, if there are overruns on the grant, then institution will have to pay the shortfall back to the funding agency.

A.   ANIMAL CARE COST RECOVERY

There are three categories of costs associated with operating an animal research facility (ARF): **ARF direct costs**, **ARF indirect costs**, and **institutional indirect costs**. The ARF direct and ARF indirect costs are recovered by directly charging the research sponsor for goods and services. The institutional indirect costs are usually recovered from the sponsor by a central finance office at the University. For NIH grants, the institution negotiates the indirect cost rate every 3 years with the Department of Health and Human Services.

1.   **ARF Direct Costs** — This category represents the expenses that can be directly attributed to caring for animals or providing some other direct service related to animal use. Examples of this type of expense include direct husbandry labor, animal food, bedding, protective clothing, etc. In general, ARF direct costs are easily assignable to specific per diem categories.

2.   **ARF Indirect Costs** — This category represents the expenses associated with providing the animal care services but cannot be easily attributed to specific per diem categories. This type of expense would include salaries of the ARF support staff (e.g., administrative and clerical support for the husbandry staff), office supplies, cleaning supplies, and maintenance contracts on equipment.

3.   **Institutional Indirect Costs** — This category represents the expenses associated with having the animal research facility on the university campus. These expenses include utility costs, central accounting, purchasing, grounds, building maintenance, etc. The two types of institutional indirect cost rates associated with an ARF are **Facility and Administration Indirect Cost (FA) Rate** and **Special Service Indirect Cost Rate (SSIC)**.

   a.   **Facility and Administration (F&A) Indirect Cost Rate** — All federal grants pay F&A indirect costs. The rules that govern what expenses may be included when calculating the indirect cost rates are outlined in OMB Circular A-21. Most other sponsors pay F&A indirect costs as well. The specific rates are negotiated with each sponsor. In some cases, the sponsor will request an indirect cost waiver.

   b.   **Special Service Indirect Cost Rate** — If the facility meets certain criteria for direct billings, such as having recharge activity greater than $1,000,000 per year, DHHS will probably designate the ARF as a special service facility and will develop a special indirect cost rate for animal care in lieu of the normal F&A indirect cost rate. Federal sponsors pay the SSIC rate as a direct expense budget line on their grants. The rate is calculated using formulas that include the extra cost of utilities, equipment, and central services specifically attributed to the ARF.

4.   **Systems Needed To Track Expenses** — There are two types of accounting systems that should be in place to help manage an animal research facility: one is financial and the other is a cost accounting system.

   a.   **Financial** — A financial accounting system provides profit and loss information and is useful for trend analysis on expense and revenue. In the private sector there are usually three components that make up a complete set of financial statements: an Income Statement, a Statement of Change in Cash Position, and a Balance Sheet. For the purposes of this chapter, only the Income Statement and Statement of Change in Cash Position will be addressed.

An **Income Statement** lists revenues and expenses and determines net income or loss for a specific timeframe. In order to produce an income statement, the research animal resource facility should have a general ledger and general journal in place to process transactions.

A **Statement of Change in Cash Position** is a simple report that tells the manager what the cash balance is in the facility's account at a given point in time.

b. **Cost** — The starting point for a cost accounting system is a reliable financial system. A cost accounting system is needed in order to set a fair per diem rate. The NIH Cost Analysis and Rate Setting Manual (8) gives a full explanation of how to set up a cost study. This manual is available on the Web at www.ncrr.nih.gov/newspub/CARS.pdf.

5. **Setting Special Service Rates** — When setting up rates for special services such as technician time, there are several factors that should be in place. Below is an example of how to create an hourly rate for an employee's time:

Cost of technician's wage and fringe benefits:
$27,000 annual wage,
$11,583 in fringe benefits.

Number of hours available to work:
1,912 hours calculated as follows:
2080 hours in a year
minus vacation: 80 hours
minus sick time: 48 hours per year
minus educational time: 40 hours per year

Amount and cost of effort spent supervising employee:
10% of supervisor's salary plus fringe benefits = $4,205.
Hourly rate = $27,000 + $11,583 + $4,205 divided by 1,912 hours = $22.37 per hour

6. **Research Personnel** — Whether the research team is small or large, a single **principal investigator** heads it. The principal investigator is responsible for the direction of the research project, and is accountable to the sponsor for the project's proper conduct. In addition to the principal investigator, other "**key personnel**" are likely to make substantive contributions to the scientific development or conduct of the research project. These individuals typically hold a doctoral or professional degree, but could include personnel at the master's and baccalaureate level. While most sponsors (notably the NIH) do not recognize co-principal investigators, key personnel other than the principal investigator can serve in any of a variety of roles, including investigator (in addition to the "principal" investigator), research associate or assistant, laboratory technician, post-doctoral fellow, graduate student, and consultant (e.g., statistician), among others. Grant applications to sponsors typically include a section for describing

the personnel requirements and arrangements of the proposed research project, and a biographical sketch for each individual meeting the definition of key personnel. This section must list all of the personnel required to conduct the proposed research, and indicate the percentage of each person's full-time effort that will be needed for the project. For each individual listed, the total percentage of time spent on the proposed project plus other projects on which the person works may not exceed 100%. Biographical sketches need only be provided for key personnel, and describe the education and training, research and professional experience, and pertinent publications of each person. Grant proposal reviewers use this information to assess whether or not the research team is capable of successfully conducting the proposed project. Grant applications may also request optional personal information (e.g., date of birth, Social Security number, gender, race or ethnic origin) about the principal investigator and other key personnel to assist the sponsor in managing and monitoring the award and to ensure that grants are not awarded on a discriminatory basis.

V.   DATA OWNERSHIP AND PUBLICATION RIGHTS

Generally, research institutions own the data resulting from grant-supported research activities conducted under their auspices. However, special considerations may apply with regard to the rights of sponsors and investigators.

A.   **Publishing and Copyrighting** — Investigators conducting publicly supported research are expected to make the results of their research available to the public through reports, presentations, and publications. Such presentations of the research results should always acknowledge the sponsor as the source of support for the research project. Research institutions and investigators are usually encouraged to copyright data, publications, and other copyrightable works, provided the sponsor is granted a royalty-free, nonexclusive license to use the material for its own purposes.

B.   **Patents and Licenses** — Research institutions have rights to inventions developed in the course of government-supported research conducted under their auspices, and may protect inventions through the patent and/or licensing process in accordance with the Bayh-Dole Act of 1980 (37 CFR Part 401). If research institutions waive their rights to an invention, the investigator(s) developing the invention may use the same processes to protect their interests. These processes require research institutions and/or investigators to follow specific requirements for reporting and patenting inventions.

C.   **Unique Research Resources** — In the course of conducting a research project, a unique research resource may be developed. Examples include synthetic compounds, cell lines, viral products, transgenic animals, and computer programs. If the research was supported by public funds, the research institution is expected to make the resource available, after publication, to the general scientific community so that additional scientific inquiries may be pursued.

D. **Freedom of Information** — Federal law requires that federal government information be released to citizens upon request. This requirement also applies to information about federally sponsored research grants. Information subject to release includes grant applications and reports associated with research projects that have received federal funds. Information not usually subject to release includes proprietary information and personal private information submitted on federal grant applications, grant applications not funded (pending or not receiving an award), and findings and recommendations of site visit and research review groups (45 CFR Part 5).

VI. INSTITUTIONAL CERTIFICATIONS AND ASSURANCES

Grant applications must be reviewed and signed by the research institution's officially designated **Institutional Official (IO)**. The IO is typically a vice president or high-level official of the institution with oversight responsibility for the institutional research program. The signature of the IO on a grant application certifies that the research institution will comply with applicable regulations and policies, and abide by the terms of an agreement, called the "**Assurance Statement**," previously negotiated between the research institution and the sponsor. The IO is accountable for both the way that the sponsor-provided funds are used and the manner in which the research activities are conducted. The institutional official must ensure that the institution has administrative systems, policies, and procedures in place to identify, manage, reduce, or eliminate common concerns about the conduct of research. Among these concerns are several that are of particular interest to animal facility managers:

A. **Financial Conflict of Interest** — Research personnel may not use or appear to use their positions for private financial gain for themselves or others with whom they have significant ties (42 CFR Part 50 Subpart F).

B. **Drug-Free Workplace** — The institution will maintain a drug-free workplace and comply with federal reporting requirements (45 CFR Part 46).

C. **Occupational Safety and Health** — The research institution and investigators will manage the research project in a manner that minimizes the risk of illness or injury related to the research activities. Areas of concern include biological (including recombinant DNA), radiological, chemical, and physical threats to the health and safety of personnel and others (29 CFR Part 1910, CDC Publication No. 93-8395, and others).

D. **Lobbying** — Federal funds cannot be used to attempt to influence federal or state legislation (45 CFR Part 93).

E.   **Scientific Misconduct** — Research investigators may not engage in fabrication, falsification, plagiarism, or other practices that seriously deviate from those commonly accepted within the scientific community for proposing, conducting, or reporting research. The term does not include honest error or honest differences in interpretations or judgments of data (42 CFR Part 50, Subpart A).

F.   **Seat Belt Use** — The institution will implement programs that promote the use of seat belts by employees, particularly during on-the-job transportation activities (Executive Order 13043).

G.   **Smoke-Free Workplace** — The institution will provide smoke-free work and public areas for employees and the visiting public, and implement programs to discourage use of tobacco products, in accordance with the PHS mission to protect and advance the physical and mental health of the American people.

H.   **Controlled Substances** — The use of controlled substances in research projects must be in accordance with the regulations of the Drug Enforcement Agency (45 CFR 76).

I.   **Animal Welfare** — The use of vertebrate animals in research projects must be reviewed and approved by the Institutional Animal Care and Use Committee (IACUC), and animal care and use procedures must be performed in accordance with applicable regulations, policies, and nationally accepted standard (9 CFR Part 93; U.S. Government Principles for the Utilization and Care of Vertebrate Animals Used in Testing, Research, and Training; PHS Policy on Humane Care and Use of Laboratory Animals; Guide for the Care and Use of Laboratory Animals).

J.   **Civil Rights** — The institution will not discriminate against qualified persons based on age, sex, race, color, national origin, or handicap under any program or activity receiving Federal financial assistance (Age Discrimination Act of 1975, 45 CFR Part 91; Civil Rights Act of 1964, 45 CFR Part 80; Title IX of the Education Amendments of 1972, 45 CFR Part 86; Rehabilitation Act of 1973, 45 CFR Parts 84 and 85).

K.   **Metric Usage** — Federal policy requires that values and measurements be indicated in metric in applications, reports, publications, and other documents associated with federally funded research projects (Executive Order 12770 and 15 CFR Part 19, Subpart B).

REFERENCES

1. **Ogden, T.E. and Goldberg, I.A.**, *Research Proposals: A Guide to Success*, 2nd ed., New York, Raven Press, 1995.
2. **Reif-Lehrer, L.,** *Grant Application Writer's Handbook*, Boston, Jones & Bartlett, 1995.

3. **Roberts, J.A. and Kaack, M.B.**, Grantsmanship. *J. Urol.*, 163, 1544, 2000.

4. **U.S. Department of Health and Human Services, Public Health Service**, PHS Grants Policy Statement, Publication No. 99-6, October 1998.

5. **U.S. Department of Health and Human Services, Public Health Service**, Instructions for PHS 398 (Public Health Service Grant Application), 1998.

6. **Center for Scientific Review, National Institutes of Health**, Policy, Procedure & Review Guidelines, http://www.csr.nih.gov/REVIEW/policy.htm, 2000.

7. **Office of Management and Budget**, Circular A-21-Cost Principles for Educational Institutions, Revised 8/8/00.

8. **Cost Manual Revision Committee**, Cost Analysis and Rate Setting Manual Animal Research Facilities, National Center for Research Resources, National Institutes of Health, Bethesda, MD, www.ncrr.nih.gov/newspub/CARS.pdf, 2000.

12 Utilization of Information Technology

Farol N. Tomson, D.V.M., Dipl. ACLAM

I. INTRODUCTION

In many ways, every business is an information business. Research animal resource units are no exception; they depend upon information to function properly. The better the information, the more effectively the goals of the organization can be reached. Information and the technology to receive and deliver it can be viewed as the glue that holds organizations together. With massive amounts of information available to more and more consumers via electronic networks, organizations have had to adapt to this technology. **Information Technology (IT)** is a rather new discipline that supports and studies this transfer of information.

Organizations, including animal care service units, are reacting to the expansion in IT. Traditional means by which management controlled the flow of information between individuals in buildings and behind department walls have given way to network administrators controlling the flow of information through userIDs and passwords.

A. INFORMATION

Information is a far-reaching term that includes all facts, data and opinions. Unlike data, information has meaning. **Knowledge**, on the other hand, is information that is put to work. As one can imagine, there is much more information than knowledge. **Facility knowledge**, as the term is used here, is a mix of experiences and values that are embedded in working documents such as standard operating procedures (SOPs). SOPs typically represent the working knowledge that governs the animal care business.

B. TECHNOLOGY

Newer versions of hardware and software are coming to the market almost daily. The acquisition of new technology lies within the mission of the animal resource program. Goals and missions of animal resource units generally are to provide service to others; therefore, the manager needs to demonstrate how newer technology will improve service. It is easy for a program dealing with a few animals and several investigators to adapt and change to a new technology. It is not so easy for an animal resource program dealing with hundreds of investigators and thousands of IACUC protocols to do the same. The benefits of new technology must be of clear value to the users of the facility.

The most common components of information technology are **computers**, **e-mail programs** and the **World Wide Web**. These are rather easy to use and relatively inexpensive to maintain, at least on a small scale. When the number of computers expands beyond the manager's ability to manage them, an IT infrastructure is needed. Most institutions maintain an IT support group, which generally includes computer hardware and software technicians knowledgeable about the advantages, disadvantages, and compatibilities of different programs and equipment. Decisions to change or upgrade to newer technologies must not be made in a vacuum, but rather with the input of the IT group.

C. MANAGEMENT

Animal care and research programs process huge amounts of information. While some organizations, including animal resource programs, struggle to cope with increasing amounts of information, the successful ones do not lose focus on their external environment. Peter Drucker is often quoted as stating, "The purpose of an organization resides outside the organization" (1). In this regard, the purpose of an animal resource program lies outside the animal care environment and within the animal research environment of the scientists. Managing information involves getting the right information to the right people (i.e., scientists, employees, regulators, members of the public, and institutional administrators) at the right time. Animal resource personnel, who provide the right information to the right people at the right time, do not have to worry about competition.

Competition resides with those persons or units providing animal care service more efficiently. The business of providing animal care will not disappear as long as institutions continue to use animals. One major threat to those providing animal care occurs when scientists, employees, or regulators complain or think that the current service can be improved. Institutions often react to these issues by making personnel or management changes. In this sense, the manager's competition resides with his/her successor if he/she is replaced. Therefore, the better one understands the competition and their information, the more effective he/she will be in delivering animal care service to the customers.

II. ORGANIZING INFORMATION

There is no one perfect way to organize information. Understanding the origin of the information one needs is the first step in understanding information management. Whenever possible, whoever "owns" the data and information, should be responsible for entering and updating it. For example, IACUC personnel should know what information they need to get from others and what information they actually create or "own." Other units within the animal resource unit should be encouraged to understand their information this way, too.

Identifying each unit that "owns" its data is helpful. If one does not "own" the information, he/she should find out who does and how to get it. If one can obtain or borrow this information, then he/she won't have to enter it, thereby reducing errors by data entry. Several common units (or owners) of information can be identified. Examples of units and information each might "own" include the following.

A. IACUCs

1. Protocols (active and inactive)
2. Approval and expiration dates
3. Procedures
4. Animals assigned to a protocol
5. Personnel training
6. Facility and program reviews and inspections
7. Compliance

B. PERSONNEL DEPARTMENTS

1. Employees (e.g., name, address, phone number, e-mail address, etc.)
2. Salaries
3. Position descriptions

C. PHYSICAL PLANT UNITS

1. Buildings
2. Rooms
3. Work orders
4. Floor plans
5. HVAC data

D. RESEARCH GRANT OFFICES (SPONSORED RESEARCH, GRANTS AND CONTRACTS)

1. Grant titles (pending, active and inactive)
2. Funding agencies
3. Award approval and expiration dates
4. Principal Investigators (PIs) and Co-PIs

E. ENVIRONMENTAL HEALTH AND SAFETY OFFICES

1. Hazardous substances
2. Radiation Safety
3. Personnel training
4. Occupational health

F. ANIMAL RESOURCES

1. Species (e.g., animal models, animals ordered, animals used)
2. Vendors
3. Supplies, equipment
4. Health and training records
5. Financial (e.g., revenues, expenses)
6. Animal purchasing, billings, orders
7. Regulatory reports (e.g., USDA, OLAW)

G. SECURITY OFFICES, PUBLIC RELATIONS UNITS, ACADEMIC DEPARTMENTS, ETC.

1. Alerts and notices
2. Students
3. Grades
4. Curricula

The above items could also be organized according to who uses the information. For example, information might be divided either into "caring for" or "using" animals. The strategy used here is to organize the information by the users of the information. For example, the IACUC and vivarium could list the information items they use, while investigators could list items they use.

Another way of organizing information is from the standpoint of information movement. Information can be considered "one-way" if it collected, used once, and stored. In contrast, information is considered to be "two-way" if it is collected, distributed, and returned. Common examples of one-way information include:

- Inactive or expired IACUC protocols
- Reference documents
- Historical documents (e.g., accounts receivables, expired animal records)
- Regulatory reports (e.g., annual reports, semiannual reports)
- Newsletters, memos, correspondence
- Material safety data sheets

While technology may be present that could theoretically eliminate all forms of paper, in many cases the paper copy still remains the permanent form. Electronic documents can be easily edited and actually falsified, so until the technology is available to secure the identity and stability of official documents, actual paper documents are still preferred by many.

Efficient organization of information comes from an understanding of how the information originates or how it is used. Once this is done, information becomes easier to manage and the selection of the desired technology becomes easier to make. State of the art technology is not useful if it cannot be used effectively. Information management is the process of using the right technology to get the right information to the right people at the right time.

III. INFORMATION

A. SOURCES

The development of the World Wide Web and the various networks (i.e., internets, extranets and intranets) has presented vast information at the touch of a finger to those persons with computers. One of the dilemmas facing organizations is that more information is being retrieved from the Web than is coming from within their own organizations. Some of this information is "**rich**" (i.e., valuable) and some of it is of no value. For example, information regarding the USDA inspections of research facilities is now available on the Web to anyone with an Internet connection and a browser. While this information may not have value to some, it may be quite rich to others.

Web sites and Web pages are now available that provide information on many aspects of laboratory animal resource management (see Table 1).

Other sources of information for animal care and use activities include regulatory sites (e.g., sites for USDA, OPRR, FDA), agency sites (e.g., NIH, AHA, etc.), and sites of many major medical research universities. Various other related organizations maintain home pages that yield valuable information. For example, the Electronic Zoo home page (**netvet.wustl.edu/e-zoo.htm**) lists thousands of Web sites with information related to animal care and use. In addition, there are numerous electronic bulletin boards, veterinary information networks, and electronic newsletters providing discussion formats regarding many informational topics.

Messages posted on the electronic bulletin boards, mailing lists, and e-mail messages from peers may contain information that could be used by animal resource units. However, this electronic information may reflect personal opinions and even misinformation. There is no 'merit' or scientific review requirement of anything posted on the Web. Not all information obtained in this way is useful or "rich," so the reader needs to beware.

Those with sufficient travel funds can attend national or regional meetings and conferences to acquire and exchange information. Still, with the increasing use of electronic media, conference calls, chat rooms, telecommunication, and distance learning, some of this rich information is becoming available in one electronic form or another without having to physically attend these meetings.

TABLE 1. GENERAL INFORMATION WEB SITES

AALAS — American Association for Laboratory Animal Science: http://www.aalas.org/
AALAS is the premier forum for the exchange of information and expertise in the care and use of laboratory animals. Their membership consists of more than 9,300 clinical veterinarians, technicians, technologists, educators, and business people, researchers, administrators, animal producers, national and international experts.

IACUC.ORG — Institutional Animal Care and Use Committees: http://www.iacuc.org/
IACUC.ORG is an information resource for members and staff of institutional animal care and use committees. It is a link archive where online resources are organized by menus and submenus. Many who browse the Internet for IACUC resources may find it overwhelming to randomly sift through the enormity of Web sites and their online materials. IACUC.ORG was developed as an organizing tool to quickly point to a topic of interest, such as example protocol forms or disaster plans used by other institutions.

LAMA — Laboratory Animal Management Association: http://www.lama-online.org/
Dedicated to enhancing the quality of management and care of laboratory animals throughout the world. LAMA promotes the dissemination of ideas, experience and knowledge; encourages continuing education; and actively assists in the training of managers.

USDA APHIS — Animal Care Home Page: http://www.aphis.usda.gov/ac/
This USDA home page provides legal information and policies regarding the Animal Welfare Act and other rules and regulations governing the use of animals in research.

OLAW — Office of Laboratory Animal Welfare (formerly OPRR): http://grants.nih.gov/grants/olaw/olaw.htm/
OLAW: (1) develops and monitors, as well as exercises compliance oversight relative to PHS Policy on Humane Care and Use of Laboratory Animals involved in research conducted or supported by any component of the Public Health Service; (2) coordinates appropriate PHS regulations, policies, and procedures both within PHS and in coordination with other Departments and Agencies in the Federal Government; (3) establishes criteria for and negotiation of Assurances of Compliance with institutions engaged in PHS-conducted or -supported research using animals; (4) conducts programs of clarification and guidance for both the Federal and non-Federal sectors with respect to the use of animals in research; (5) directs the development and implementation of educational and instructional programs; and (6) generates educational resource materials.

ASLAP — American Society of Laboratory Animal Practitioners: http://www.aslap.org/
ASLAP promotes the acquisition and dissemination of knowledge, ideas, and information among veterinarians and veterinary students having an interest in laboratory animal practice.

AAALAC — Association for Assessment and Accreditation of Laboratory Animal Care, International: http://www.aaalac.org/
AAALAC, International is a voluntary accreditation organization that works with institutions and researchers to ensure the highest standards of animal care and use. AAALAC also offers independent assessments of animal research programs to help institutions continue to improve their animal care and use practices.

ACLAM — American College of Laboratory Animal Medicine: http://www.aclam.org/
ACLAM is an organization of board-certified veterinary medical specialists who are specialists in the humane, proper, and safe care and use of laboratory animals. ACLAM establishes standards of education, training, experience and expertise. ACLAM actively promotes the advancement of knowledge in this field through professional continuing education activities, the development of educational materials and the conduct of research in laboratory animal medicine and science.

No matter where the information is coming from, the problem facing today's manager becomes one of deciding which information is worth saving and using, and which information can be ignored.

B.   USELESS INFORMATION

The amount of information (much of which can be useless or incorrect information, i.e., "noise"), in animal resource units can be overwhelming. When there is a lot of informational "noise," managers and organizations must learn how to review and filter it before it enters the workplace.

The term **"InfoSmog"** has been used to described the situation of having so much information that it is difficult to make an effective decision (2). Navigating through this smog requires that someone read, evaluate, and filter the information. Employees or groups of employees can be assigned the task of filtering the electronic smog for potentially rich information. This process does not generate new knowledge, but simply filters information before entry into the workplace. Employees who read electronic bulletin boards (e.g., CompMed) can provide such filtering by extracting only that information that they think may be useful by the institution (see Figure 1).

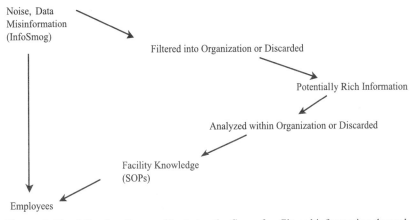

Figure 1. The following diagram illustrates the flow of unfiltered information through the organization and transformation to the employee in the form of an SOP.

C.   STORAGE

Once information is collected, it must be stored. The permanent storage of records is costly because it uses valuable space. Computer records and databases are usually backed-up onto disks, tapes or network drivers in the event of workstation or computer failure. Microfiche storage of documents can be used whereby the original documents are photographed and then destroyed.

More commonly, document storage is achieved by the use of hardware and software products that will 'scan' documents onto a storage tape with an index of key words for retrieval.

Information not requiring storage by the institution or an outside agency should not be stored (3). After the expiration of the required storage time, information can be shredded or otherwise disposed.

IV. INFORMATION TECHNOLOGY

Several good texts and Web sites discuss information technology in detail (4–6) (Table 2). The process of providing the right information to the right people at the right time begins by filtering through the electronic smog to retrieve new information. The effort continues by processing and implementing that new information into action.

A. DATABASES

The basic purpose of a **database** is to organize data so it can be processed into meaningful information and transported to those who need it. While there are different database products for management of a laboratory animal resource unit on the market, the individual charged with managing a small facility could use just about any one of them without much difficulty.

TABLE 2. INFORMATION TECHNOLOGY WEB SITES

Web sites are valuable sources of information. Internet browsers are the tools used to search the Internet for information. Web sites are used to either share information or to sell something. While it is not possible to list all the Web sites relating to information technology or animal research, some suggestions are offered here.

Institutional Information Technology — Most universities and community colleges will offer home pages with Web sites relating to information technology and the tools to develop and use these programs. For example, after finding home pages of major universities, use their search engines to find "information technology" links. At the University of Florida (www.ufl.edu) this search yields more than 50 links ranging from help desks, courses, training, and ethics regarding information technology. Searching the indexes of local community colleges can also yield useful information. For example, searching the index of the Santa Fe Community College (http://www.santafe.cc.fl.us/) offers Web pages on Information Technology Services and Information Technology Education.

The Complete Intranet Resource: http://intrack.com/intranet/
Billed as a complete intranet resource, this site has much useful information. The site includes 10 Intranet Myths (e.g., myth number one: intranets are cheap; myth number three: intranets are for big organizations), a free spreadsheet application to help calculate costs, a mailing list, FAQs, white papers, a bibliography, and important firewall resources.

In contrast, with larger facilities that have larger volumes of information, the concept of relational databases must be emphasized. **Relational databases** are important because they save memory space and reduce chances for data entry errors. A relational database is a collection of relations. Primary and secondary 'keys' identify relationships between information.

An example of a relational database would be a vivarium office that maintains one database table with all the departments in the organization. Another database table would include all the names and addresses of the employees. The two tables are linked together by a primary key so that when a name is selected, his/her department information would automatically be displayed. If the department changed address or phone number, one would only need to change one record in the department table, and not all the records of employees in that department.

Examples become numerous and challenging. Primary and secondary keys can link tables of animal species, vendors, IACUC protocols, and research procedures. When a new IACUC protocol record is started, a new IACUC number is assigned, and items in linked tables are selected to complete the rest of the record without any new text being entered.

Most commercial database programs marketed for animal research facilities use relational database designs. Unfortunately, unless one has a strong interest in doing database programming, he/she will need some help to develop the facility's relational databases.

B.   DATABASE WAREHOUSING

If the information needed is kept in databases maintained by someone else, then one must either make arrangements to obtain it or decide to go without it. Whether it is on a mainframe or another network workstation, database warehousing is the technology that allows one to get the information and download it for one's own use.

A **database warehouse** is a collection of databases with information extracted (or imported) from other databases. In some cases, one cannot access certain databases for security or legal reasons. In other cases, related information may be obtained. Database warehouses operate on a simple principle: take information from one set of databases and put it in another. Database warehousing provides end users with easy access to large amounts of institutional data.

For example, an employee database from the Personnel Department could be the database used to develop the IACUC list of researchers, technicians, and employees to choose from. This IACUC database of employees would be modified to contain only the information needed. All the private information, such as salary and benefits, would most appropriately remain secure in the Personnel Department database.

Database warehousing requires expert planning and performance maintenance for continued success. Database programmers should be available to assist animal resource personnel in the implementation of this technology. There are commercial products available to build one's own data warehouse, but one must work within his/her own institutional infrastructure to link the various network administrators and their databases together.

C.   E-Mail and Attachments

E-mail is a rich source of information and the most pervasive form of electronic communication. It is fast, easy to use, and user-driven. When there is too much mail and it is unfiltered, valuable information and knowledge can be lost. Therefore, e-mail messages should be retained and organized by subject so that others can search and find what they are looking for. An important part of this communication system is the creation of networks that put employees in touch with one another. List servers and other mail services organize these messages for easy retrieval. Too often, employees do not have the resources to search previous or archived messages to review what has already been written on a subject. This causes tremendous inefficiency in the use of the technology.

While electronic mail is quick and appears to save lots of paper, the recipient may not be using compatible software and may see messages in skewed formats and truncated sentences. As a result, although the message may have been sent in one form, it may not appear that way to the recipient. To avoid these format problems, files and documents can be sent as **attachments** to the message. The e-mail may contain a short message like "See the attached file." The recipient has to know a little more about his/her computer and how to retrieve and view the file. If he/she does not have the same software that was used to make the file, he/she may still not be able to view the file. However, with the common use of popular software products, this is becoming less of a problem.

For text documents, there are generic text formats that are well suited for all word processing programs. **General text formats (txt)** and **rich text formats (rtf)** are used to save documents in this way. Recipients of these formatted files can use any word processor to open and edit them.

File documents containing graphics can be saved in a **pdf format** (Adobe; Adobe Systems, Inc., San Jose, CA) and then downloaded and used by anyone having an Adobe® reader program. The reader program is available free of charge, but to covert a document to a pdf file, the Adobe® Distiller writer program must be purchased.

Sending large documents (e.g., IACUC protocols) via e-mail has some drawbacks. Large documents are difficult to read because one must scroll down the computer screen. Recipients can be instructed to print out a hard copy and then read it. Of course, this assumes that they have printers attached to their computers. It is a mistake, however, to assume that everyone has a printer. Again, one should use the technology to get all the information to the right people at the right time. If there are employees or customers who do not have or do not use this technology, then the manager should either provide training, hardware, and the necessary software, or continue to distribute information to them with conventional technology.

D. NETWORKS

After personal computers found their way into common business use, they were quickly hooked up or connected to **networks**. These networks standardize the software applications and make standard programs and procedures available for their many individual 'stations.' Unfortunately, when the networks 'go down,' users often find themselves doing nothing while waiting for the service to be restored. While the downtime can occur on non-networked computers, it is frustrating for entire offices to be paralyzed during downtime of networks.

The **intranet** is a term used to describe a system in which all the computer stations on a network or sharing different networks within an organization or department are connected. Sharing information on the network is easy, because all the users of the network have common access to public directories or areas of the network drives. Now large databases, documents, special printers, software programs, and other devices can be made accessible to everyone on the same network.

TABLE 3. REVIEW OF WEB TERMS

Internet: The Internet is a worldwide "network of networks" that use the TCP/IP (Transmission Control Protocol/Internet Protocol) protocol suite for communications. The Internet was created initially to help foster communication among government-sponsored researchers. Throughout the 1980s, the Internet grew steadily to include educational institutions, government agencies, commercial organizations, and international organizations. In the 1990s, the Internet experienced phenomenal growth, with connections increasing faster than any other network ever created (including the telephone network). Millions of users are now connected to the Internet.

Intranet: An intranet is the use of Internet technologies within an organization (or company) to achieve better results than the conventional means of data access and transfer. Intranet helps in cutting costs. It is easy to use and provides fast accessibility to day to day information. An intranet is a network within the organization whereas the Internet is a worldwide network. An intranet has access to the Internet but not vice versa.

Extranet: Loosely defined, an extranet is an intranet extended beyond the corporate boundaries. When selective access is provided to entities outside the organization an intranet becomes an extranet. For example, if a company allows its suppliers, clients, etc. to have access to its intranet, it now becomes an extranet. Access would of course be restricted by security means like userids, passwords, or encryption techniques.

Firewall: A firewall is any one of several ways of protecting one network from another "untrusted" network. The actual mechanism whereby this is accomplished varies widely, but in principle, the firewall can be thought of as a pair of mechanisms: one that exists to block traffic, and the other that exists to permit traffic. Some firewalls place a greater emphasis on blocking traffic, while others emphasize more on filtering traffic leaving the network.

The intranet may be the ideal solution for an animal resource program where the customers and employees are all part of the same network. This is usually the case when the organizations are small. However, within larger organizations having multiple networks, it becomes more difficult to share information. Network administrators may or may not share the same missions and goals of the organization as individual users, including the manager of the laboratory animal resource unit.

At the author's institution, the animal care database program is placed on one network out of the Vice President's office. There are approximately 50 other networks within the university. While some network administrators may make it easy for 'outsiders' to gain access to their stored information files, others do not. In the latter cases, one is forced to use e-mail and e-mail attachments or conventional methods (i.e., mail, hand delivery) of distributing documents. Thus, while the intranet is a quick and easy way to share information among its members, many managers still have customers and employees that are not on intranets, and they must make sure they are reaching all of their customers.

Unfortunately, using e-mail and networks to communicate forces customers to use similar or compatible hardware and software. The technology that overcomes this incompatibility is "html" formatting used on the World Wide Web.

E.   THE WORLD WIDE WEB

The **World Wide Web** has captivated business and home users alike largely because it is easy, fun, and relatively inexpensive. Consumers can browse through virtual stores, place orders, pay with credit cards, and in a few days products are delivered to the doorstep. Individuals and businesses with Web pages can post information for everyone to see. Documents, graphics, movies, soundtracks, telephones and television can all be viewed on the Web, and with very little computer literacy on the part of the consumer.

Web pages are designed and placed on a network computer that has some capabilities to handle the Internet traffic. A Web page is given a unique address called a **URL (Uniform Resource Locator)** and that address is linked to the rest of the Internet for millions of other users, networks and search engines to use. **Web masters** (a name given to those who manage Web pages) often use electronic counters to keep track of how many times (hits) their Web page is visited.

The main reason Web pages are designed and used is to share information and/or to conduct business. There is no editorial board or ethics review board governing the Internet. Information and data taken off the Internet may be very rich, or it may be totally false and misleading.

The **"html" format** is what all the current Internet browsers interpret. If one decides to post anything on a Web page (newsletters, graphs, tables), he/she must convert the information to html format and transfer the information to the network server site for use on his/her Web page. Most of the current software word processors and database programs save their files in html formats.

The advantage of using the Web (or a Web page) is that anyone on the Internet can view it. It makes no difference what type of software or computer or browser they have, they can all see the information; they can save it, download it, and print it. The Internet extends beyond the boundaries of the intranet. All that is required by the recipient is a computer and access to the Internet.

The future of electronic media and information management rests with Web applications. With more computers coming into use and more computers going online with the Internet, the Web and Web-based programs become the common denominator. All research animal forms, requisitions, surveys, billings, animal orders, etc. could be planned for Web distribution and for Web data collection. The information technology (IT) service group in the organization can help animal resource personnel to use this technology.

F.　INFORMATION MANAGEMENT

Getting proper information to employees at the right time begins with someone who understands what information employees need. This requires leadership and supervision to provide them with the documents they need. Whether hard copy or electronic (i.e., e-mail, Web-based application, or multi-media), the focus is on moving information quickly for employees to easily retrieve. Large-sized animal units are more likely to use Web-based technologies than smaller units because of the higher installation costs.

When employees leave an organization, they in effect take all their information and knowledge with them (7). As a result, one often finds large gaps in the remaining "facility knowledge" after valuable employees leave. These gaps surface when newly hired replacements are put on the job. If the facility knowledge is shared and made more easily available to others, then employee loss will not lead to any appreciable decrease in service or product quality.

It is often desirable to have front-line employees make front-line decisions. In this regard, employees need to act and react quickly to demands made upon them by customers (animal users), and the best way to do that is to make sure they have the information they need quickly and in easily accessible formats (8). Use of newer electronic technologies will not be solutions in themselves for improving animal care and use practices. The real challenge is deciding how to use these technologies to collect information and transfer it into a working facility knowledge base. The following guidelines have been suggested and modified as a means to facilitate functionality of a new information technology system (9–11):

1. **The manager must understand the organizational purpose of the animal resource unit**. Basic to all successful organizations is a statement of purpose or mission.
2. **The manager should determine if the current technology can be updated or if newer technology must be purchased**. Working with

local IT or computer support staff helps. Having one's own local network of computers may have to be justified vs. using someone else's network of computers. When networks of computers are used, additional employees who provide maintenance and security of the hardware and software will be needed.

3. **The manager should organize the information content.** Information technology benefits from some degree of structure. Standard operating procedures are the building blocks of informational content.

4. **One should design Web pages or applications for easy use, making them user friendly.** Courses, seminars and references are available to demonstrate how to build effective Web pages.

5. **The organization should facilitate universal access and universal use.** The technology should be made available to everyone who needs it, and in the language they use. Some information may be distributed to everyone, while other information may be limited to a restricted few.

6. **The manager should consider all costs so budgets can be prepared and supported.** Software, hardware, training, security, maintenance and management are some of the costs to consider. The possibility of occasional downtime and associated lost productivity are other costs to consider.

There are some common errors made in adopting new information technology systems. Over-investing in computer hardware, software, modems, faxes, cellular phones, etc. without having employees trained to use them effectively often occurs. There is no question that these devices can assist knowledge transfer. The danger here is in placing technology ahead of the ability or desire of the employees to use it, or by expecting technology to solve problems that only people can solve. In contrast, under-investing also occurs. There is a delicate balance between over- and under-investing, and good leadership is needed to help make technology investment decisions. Another common error occurs with the idea that an intranet or other electronic media can largely eliminate the need for staffed "Help Desks." This already has been shown to be generally false. Person-to-person contact remains crucial (10).

Many examples exist that show how information can be transformed and mobilized into action. For example, an easy method to communicate changes in regulations might be to simply copy pages from the Federal Register and send them to employees or customers to read. This type of document contains information without action or "facility knowledge." Turning that document into action is the start of information management. Managers could study the new regulations to determine if any of their SOPs (best practices) need to be changed. If so, then a revised SOP is produced and shared with employees and customers. Such an effort would, in effect, translate the information into facility knowledge.

G. Introducing New Technology

Anyone who has purchased items off the Web has likely experienced the convenience and quickness of this process. No longer do you need to talk with anyone, or to have the departmental order form in front of you; no longer do you have to search for the item number or the price; and no longer do you need a signature to verify your identity.

Credit cards can be used with vendors to purchase animals and supplies, thereby easing the animal resource unit of the fiscal responsibility for these transactions. Some animal resource units and IACUCs are already using "interactive" Web pages to conduct business (3), and once quorum and personal security issues are addressed, virtual IACUC meetings might be feasible. It is likely that more IACUCs and animal resource units will begin using such "interactive" technologies as the software and hardware become more useable and secure. These Web-based systems can be used for capturing, archiving and providing information to employees and to the customers (i.e., investigators). Web sites can also be used for entering data into databases, searching and retrieving full texts, and storing file systems for both employees and customers (12). Managers need access to the IT support groups, including trained programmers, and must have the required financial support to use this technology.

Some organizations have already tried introducing new technologies and have learned some hard lessons (10). Suggestions for the introduction of new technologies to employees include the following.

1. **Match the system with your objectives.** There is no single correct way to do this. It is important to figure out what you want to share, how often and with whom, and for what reasons. Using this information will help one to build the system.
2. **Create a structure for defining and classifying your information.** Most animal resource units already list their SOPs in manuals and other formats. Similar organization can be used in an electronic format.
3. **Market your system and applications to ensure they meet the customers' needs.** "If the customer uses this application, how will it improve his/ her day?" is a question that should be asked for every application that is developed and marketed. If it doesn't make their job easier, they won't use it. Make sure you use the customer's language and not your own jargon of information technology. If they understand it, they will be more likely to use it.
4. **Remain flexible.** All things change including information technology. More important is to understand how customers are using the technology. The key is to deliver functional, well-performing applications and solutions to customers. This means careful planning and occasional trade-offs. Stay focused on what works, rather than perfection.
5. **Keep people first.** Information management should be people oriented. It is a social process that uses technology to communicate. Get as many

employees participating as possible. View every employee as an information provider and consumer. View everyone outside as a potential
customer. Improving facility knowledge will result from focusing more
on employees and less on information technology.

6. **Try to measure the impact or result of the technology and information management.** This is difficult to do in all forms of business. The
   common approach is to look at customer satisfaction and see how well
   the service unit fares.

It is important to avoid over-emphasizing the importance of depending on
higher technology to solve problems. Four-fifths of the productive "value
added" by technology change will continue to result NOT from technology
itself, but from the new arrangements of organizations, management, and
people who can make the best use of it (10).

H.   ROLE OF INFORMATION TECHNOLOGY (IT) SUPPORT GROUPS

Currently at the author's institution, there are over 5700 computers on hundreds of networks, serving thousands of employees, customers, faculty, and
students. They have different e-mail systems, calendars, software programs,
security access systems, and passwords. It is not uncommon for faculty members to have to remember multiple passwords to access various programs.
Having IT support groups to assist with standardizing these hardware and
software issues will prevent or eliminate most common problems.

In much the same way animal resource units want to control the quality of
incoming animals and to have lists of approved vendors, IT units would like
to control the quality of the incoming hardware and software.

IT centers vary from institution to institution but the IT services often include:

- Application development
- Mainframe services
- Report generation
- Web-enabling applications
- Database applications
- Security and virus protection
- E-mail
- Web hosting
- Calendars and scheduling

Depending on the size of the organization and the needs of the animal
resource program, the manager should contact the IT support group as soon as
the use of any new technology is considered. They may likely have experience
with some of the hardware and software that will be needed.

V. ROLE OF A LEADER

It takes unique leaders to introduce and nurture information technology into the workplace and to transform it into facility knowledge. Two characteristics of such leaders are described below (13):

1. **A "facility culture" must be created that reflects the mission to gather and share information among the employees.** Employee trust and customer satisfaction become main ingredients. It is a "culture" that defines the unit; it is the unique creation of the leadership. If the leaders do not show and participate in this sharing and learning, others cannot be expected to participate (14).
2. **A strategy to adapt to the changing technology must be developed.** This strategy becomes most apparent when big decisions have to be made. In animal resource units, big moves relate to the expansion or reduction of the physical plant, whether to hire consultants to develop programs or whether to use in-house programmers, when to adapt newer caging (barrier housing) or to stay with the status quo, etc. The difference between a successful and a failing unit depends upon the leaders' ability to make these critical decisions, second only to building a supportive facility culture.

Encouraging employees to participate in this electronic information network and to share their information can be difficult. Several suggestions to help involve employees include the following (10).

1. **Allow all employees access to the system.** Provide them with the hardware and the training to use it.
2. **Allow all employees to make contributions.** Make it easy for them to contribute ideas and to share them with others.
3. **Keep the number of transfer steps between sender and recipient to one.** This avoids the potential for any distortion of information by others.
4. **Make the system available from any location, 24 hours a day.** In this way, employees with computers and Internet access at home are still able to access the system.
5. **Have a user-friendly system able to search on every important word.** Common words used in financial reports, pathology reports, animal diseases, biohazards, management, husbandry, etc. should all be easily entered and searched.
6. **Allow native languages to be used, and provide translators if needed.**
7. **Provide a system that updates automatically when new information is presented.**

The best modern technology will be ineffective if the leadership fails to develop the needed culture and teamwork. Likewise, good managers may fall behind if they are not using information technology effectively.

A. FACILITY CULTURE

Facility culture (i.e., the work environment) is an important key for successful information management. The collection of information and its transfer into effective action take place between people, not machines. How people communicate, posture themselves, write and speak are complex and beyond the scope of this chapter, yet they are vital to understanding any culture. This culture of learning and sharing does not happen by accident. In fact, hoarding knowledge is so deeply ingrained in some businesses that changing this culture is a major challenge (15). Making personal knowledge available to others is the central activity of a knowledge-creating company (8). Organizations have learned valuable lessons regarding the development of their facility culture (16). Some basic principles include:

1. **People want to share.** People like to share ideas, practices, stories, etc. with others. People want to help their colleagues.
2. **Leaders must lead by doing.** If the leaders do not share, do not expect employees to share.
3. **Employees want to develop collaborative relationships with other employees, vendors, customers, etc.** It is important for the manager to encourage such interactions.
4. **Instill personal responsibility for creating knowledge and sharing it.** Employees must want to seek out new information. In this regard, the organization is responsible for providing them with the opportunity and the tools for growth. Management styles will vary on how best to identify and instill this responsibility.
5. **Leaders must create a collective sense of purpose.** Everyone should easily understand "Why are we doing this work?"

There are, of course, barriers working against a change in facility culture. It is important not to leave change to chance (17). Common pitfalls include:

1. **Unknown knowledge.** In many cases, employees, managers and administrators alike do not realize how much information and knowledge they already have, or they do not realize that someone else needs their information. This often happens when certain employees leave an organization, and others soon realize that information or knowledge has been lost.
2. **Unaware employees.** Established SOPs may exist in one area of the organization, yet down the hall, other employees may not know about it. Either they do not search, or they do not know how to search for the information.

3. **Expressing on-the-job knowledge**. On-the-job know-how and judgment accounts for most of the valuable information of the organization. Yet, this is often hard to express or to convey. When the job knowledge is incompletely documented (by poorly constructed SOPs), it should come as no surprise that it will often fail when used by others.
4. **Parochial Pressures.** People often reject valuable knowledge just because it comes from someplace or someone else. Research faculty, veterinarians and technicians all have something to contribute regarding animal care and use. One should not reject valuable information from any source.

The above barriers make change difficult to implement. Even if all the above barriers were overcome, success may still not follow because there are so many other variables and intangibles, such as insufficient money, fear of change, and lack of effective leadership.

B.   CUSTOMERS

One of the most important informational glues in business is the link to the customers (18). Whoever captures customer loyalty is usually guaranteed a long business life. Customers of animal resource units are the animal users (i.e., researchers, faculty, students, etc.). The more information the manager has about them, and how their needs change over time, the better they can be served. Indeed, it sometimes seems as though there is nothing more dynamic than the needs of researchers, faculty, and students.

Customers in the past had to deal with conventional pyramid structures to search for information in organizations, i.e., go to the highest in command where the information resided. Now, businesses often use electronic networks to put information where consumers can easily access it (i.e., on their computer screens). It is important that managers know the animal users well enough to know what they want and when they want it. Sharing "facility knowledge" with the animal resource customers increases their satisfaction and retention. They use this information to improve their own research or teaching objectives, and as they improve the quality of their work, the overall quality of the institution improves as well. Some suggestions to facilitate information management with customers (1) include:

1. **Provide one-stop shopping for the convenience of the customers.** A single phone call, or single Web site, or single office should be able to handle all their needs. Information should be available centrally even if there are many scattered satellite facilities.
2. **Give employees the information and knowledge they need to respond to customers.** Let employees answer questions and solve problems quickly, and on the first call.
3. **Allow or help all the support groups in the animal resource unit (e.g., surgery, laboratory, pharmacy) to become more efficient and**

effective at marketing and selling their services. If customers are no longer using the surgery, laboratory, or pharmacy, find out why. Help the employees sell and resell these services.

A good example of what different customers want can be seen in the protocol forms that IACUCs require. Investigators doing field studies with wildlife, or using agricultural animals in an agricultural setting are often required to submit the same protocol form that biomedical research investigators use. Developing unique IACUC forms for different groups of customers, along with the items mentioned above, may increase customer satisfaction and might be welcomed by the IACUC members as well. Users maintaining only breeding colonies might also be offered unique protocol forms. This can be expanded to protocols dealing with antibody production, and most other non-invasive types of projects. Developing quick and easy links for animal users make it easy for them to submit the appropriate information quickly to the IACUC. In addition, such links can improve the overall knowledge base, thereby facilitating quick review and efficiency of the IACUC.

VI. SUMMARY

On the one hand, information technology has increased the speed of transferring information, while on the other hand it has resulted in too much information to comprehend. Even though technology is becoming more sophisticated, it is not the solution by itself. People remain the solution to the accumulation and transfer of knowledge; technology is just an aide.

Which system works best? Questions like this have been asked and answered by managers who have studied it, and their responses are not profound. One author suggests that, "Even after years of re-engineering front-line employees, middle managers and top management, most companies still achieve higher production from their existing staff; not by firing people, not by buying big new machines, or not by forcing longer workdays, but by simply allowing employees to learn by themselves what works best in other areas and then letting them try it out" (19). If the employees have the information, knowledge, and experience, they can determine the best practice. Each animal resource unit can evaluate its own needs and can determine the best fit for its own employees.

REFERENCES

1. **O'Dell, C. and Grayson, C.J.**, Customer intimacy, in *If We Only Knew What We Know: The Transfer of Internal Knowledge and Best Practice*, The Free Press, New York, 1998, chap. 6.
2. **Applehans, W., Globe, A., and Laugero, G.**, Strategy, in *Managing Knowledge: A Practical Web-Based Approach*, Addison-Wesley Information Technology Series, Reading, MA, 1999, chap. 1.

3. **Tillman, P.C.**, IACUC records and their management, in *The Care and Feeding of an IACUC: The Organization and Management of an Institutional Animal Care and Use Committee*, Podolsky, M.L. and Lukas, V.S., Eds., CRC Press, Boca Raton, FL, 1999, chap. 4.

4. **Evans, P. and Wuster, T.S.**, *Blown to Bits: How the New Economics of Information Transforms Strategy*, Harvard Business School Press, Boston, 1999.

5. **Applehans, W., Globe, A., and Laugero, G.**, *Managing Knowledge: A Practical Web-Based Approach*, Addison-Wesley Information Technology Series, Reading, MA, 1999.

6. **O'Dell, C. and Grayson, C.J.**, *If We Only Knew What We Know: The Transfer of Internal Knowledge and Best Practice*, The Free Press, New York, 1998.

7. **Brooking, A.**, The knowledge based company, in *Corporate Memory: Strategies for Knowledge Management*, International Thomson Business Press, New York, 1999, chap. 1.

8. **Brooking, A.**, Generating knowledge within the organization, in *Corporate Memory: Strategies for Knowledge Management*, International Thomson Business Press, New York, 1999, chap. 7.

9. **Davenport, T.H. and Prusak, L.**, Knowledge roles and skills, in *Working Knowledge: How Organizations Manage What They Know*, Harvard Business School Press, Boston, 1998, chap. 6.

10. **O'Dell, C. and Grayson, C.J.**, Using information technology to support knowledge transfer, in *If We Only Knew What We Know: The Transfer of Internal Knowledge and Best Practice*, The Free Press, New York, 1998, chap. 10.

11. **Leonard, O. and Straus, S.**, Putting your company's whole brain to work, in *Harvard Business Review on Knowledge Management*, The Harvard Business Review Paperback Series, Harvard Business School Press, Boston, 1998.

12. **O'Dell, C. and Grayson, C.J.**, Sequent computer's knowledge slingshot, in *If We Only Knew What We Know: The Transfer of Internal Knowledge and Best Practice*, The Free Press, New York, 1998, chap. 17.

13. **Evans, P. and Wuster, T.S.**, Monday morning, in *Blown to Bits: How the New Economics of Information Transforms Strategy*, Harvard Business School Press, Boston, 1999, chap. 11.

14. **Argyris, C.**, Teaching smart people how to learn, in *Harvard Business Review on Knowledge Management*, The Harvard Business Review Paperback Series, Harvard Business School Press, Boston, 1998.

15. **Allee, V.**, Culture, mapping, technology, and measures, in *The Knowledge Evolution: Expanding Organizational Intelligence*, Butterworth-Heinemann, Boston, 1997, chap. 15.

16. **O'Dell, C. and Grayson, C.J.**, Culture, the unseen hand, in *If We Only Knew What We Know: The Transfer of Internal Knowledge and Best Practice*, The Free Press, New York, 1998, chap. 9.

17. **O'Dell, C. and Grayson, C.J.**, Creating the knowledge infrastructure, in *If We Only Knew What We Know: The Transfer of Internal Knowledge and Best Practice*, The Free Press, New York, 1998, chap. 11.

18. **Evans, P. and Wuster, T.S.**, Competing on reach, in *Blown to Bits: How the New Economics of Information Transforms Strategy*, Harvard Business School Press, Boston, 1999, chap. 6.

19. **O'Dell, C. and Grayson, C.J.**, Achieving operational excellence, in *If We Only Knew What We Know: The Transfer of Internal Knowledge and Best Practice*, The Free Press, New York, 1998, chap. 8.

13 Hazard Identification and Control

Christian E. Newcomer, V.M.D., Dipl. ACLAM

Safety concerns are of paramount importance in the management of the contemporary animal resource facility. These concerns require ongoing vigilance in the detection of hazards through workplace surveillance and animal health profiling, the careful planning of policies, procedures, and practices to minimize exposures, and the training and education of personnel to ensure that they understand and comply with safety precautions. In the creation of a safe and healthy workplace, there are a number of academic, technical, and regulatory issues involved in meeting the institutional obligation to personnel and the community. The successful navigation of the regulatory concerns alone can be challenging, and the failure of compliance can place the financial health and public profile of the institution at risk in addition to having potentially serious consequences for worker health, confidence, and morale. Most institutions have recognized that in order to achieve a safe work environment, teamwork involving diverse areas of expertise is necessary, but the team participants vary with the size and type of the institution and the nature of the its research, testing, and teaching activities. Also, since institutions and their research programs may change over time, the provisions that are in place to ensure workplace safety should be reviewed and refined periodically to ensure that the institution is making a sound investment resulting in a workforce that is fully engaged in the safety program.

There are a number of excellent general references available to managers that address the important considerations for the development of animal facility safety programs of high quality beginning with the 1996 NRC *Guide for the Care and Use of Laboratory Animals,* hereafter referred to as the *Guide* (1). This reference provides the reader with a quick and thorough orientation to the many important facets of occupational health and safety of personnel working in laboratory animal facilities. The growing interest and concern about this topic within the communities of laboratory animal science/medicine, safety professionals and health care professionals stimulated the 1997 NRC publication dedicated solely to this topic entitled, *Occupational Health and Safety in the Care and Use of Research Animals* (2). This publication provides the reader an expanded discussion, and institutions with a broad template for developing the process of program organization and implementation. This document also contains useful factual information about many of the specific hazards involved in research animal care and use (e.g., zoonoses) as well as references to many other definitive resources.

I. THE SAFETY TEAM: MEMBERSHIP, ROLES, AND RESPONSIBILITIES

A. THE SENIOR OFFICIAL AND OVERALL ORGANIZATION

The organization of an effective institutional program in occupational health and safety for personnel involved in animal care and use usually requires a multi-disciplinary team approach. This entails the commitment of financial and human resources, and although the latter may occasionally be invested with a spirit of volunteerism, in most institutions the former usually is not. Accordingly, *Occupational Health and Safety in the Care and Use of Research Animals* (2) clearly identifies that, ultimately, the senior official is accountable and bears the responsibility for a safe and healthy workplace. This individual has the ability and authority to provide the essential resources (financial, facility, and human) and to provide guidance to the program managers responsible for establishing operating policies. Although this document does not carry the force of regulation, it does serve as a primary reference document by the Association for Assessment and Accreditation of Laboratory Animal Care, International (AAALAC, International) in the peer review process. The senior official may (and usually does) delegate or assign responsibility for the program components to other appropriate persons, but should be aware of technical and management issues and be routinely advised on the status of issues in the program. The actual reporting structure and mechanism may vary according to the type of institution. A health and safety professional, veterinary director, or laboratory animal facility manager might be the focal point for interaction with the senior official in this area. Thus, these individuals may be in the position of being the bearer of bad news if there are deficiencies in the program such as a lack of necessary resources or an ineffective team for addressing these matters. The periodic critiques provided by the IACUC in the semi-annual reviews are an important source of information in this area for the senior official and can be an effective way to garner additional institutional support for health and safety initiatives in the research animal facility.

The types of professional expertise that may be involved in the development and operation of a complex occupational health and safety program include:

1. Health professionals
2. Safety professionals
3. Veterinarians
4. Animal facility managers or supervisors
5. Research scientists
6. Laboratory supervisors
7. Human resource and financial personnel
8. Legal advisers
9. Environmental experts
10. Facility engineers

This section addresses only briefly the roles that are played by these individuals, and the reader should refer to other sources for additional detail (1, 2). If scientists are conducting animal studies involving experimental hazards in animals, then their participation also is critical either directly or by proxy through other scientists knowledgeable in the area or through formal institutional review committees composed according to institutional and federal mandates. However, in institutions with smaller and more focused research programs, the resident core of expertise may be much smaller, consisting of only a safety professional, veterinarian, and facility manager or supervisor with the availability of individuals with other areas of expertise on a consulting or as needed basis. As in other areas of the animal care and use program, team composition is not dictated as an engineering standard, rather it is assembled according to a performance standard where positive health and safety outcomes serve as the salient measure of success. It is important to realize that as the institution's size decreases and its research portfolio diminishes, the use of external reviewers for studies involving unique hazards may become more important to ensure a fair balance between the scientist's vested interests and the adoption of best health and safety practices.

B.   A ROLE FOR THE IACUC

As noted above, the IACUC plays a key role, through its review and monitoring of animal use, in ensuring that appropriate interactions are occurring among the various health and safety functionaries in an animal care and use program. Some IACUCs accomplish this by evaluating the review process and documents of other committees and by monitoring how the information from the review is translated into practices through assessments in the animal facility or animal user's laboratory. To buttress the IACUC review of these activities, institutions sometimes appoint a health and safety member to the IACUC to provide prompt information on the status or approach to safety review and communication. In addition, this individual may be valuable in identifying new trends and problems associated with routine animal care practices as well as in the proposed use of experimental hazards within animal studies (3).

C.   THE VETERINARIAN

In association with the IACUC or independently, the veterinarian also plays a key role in the institution's health and safety oversight process. In most circumstances, the veterinarian is the professional most knowledgeable about the zoonotic diseases (i.e., diseases that are transmitted from animals to man) and other hazards intrinsic to the laboratory animal species being used. The veterinarian, therefore, must play a prominent role in the design of prevention and control measures in the animal colonies, the training of personnel about these hazards and provide input for the preventive medical and response plan for humans who may be at risk of exposure. The veterinarians, health professionals, and others who may be involved in these processes can refer to any of several compilations of the literature on zoonoses and animal related hazards for information useful in addressing these matters (2, 4, 5).

D. HEALTH AND SAFETY PROFESSIONALS

The environmental health and safety group (or individual) usually plays a central role in the coordination of the overall occupational health and safety program for the institution. This group also contains diversified expertise to plan appropriately for the various hazards and challenges faced by the work force. Relevant disciplines include industrial hygiene, chemical safety, health physics (radiation safety), biosafety, and ergonomics, and are responsive to federal OSHA regulations or recommendations covering hazardous and toxic substances, carcinogens, personnel protective equipment, radiation hazards, laser hazards, blood-borne pathogens and other infectious hazards, recombinant DNA, latex and occupational allergies, various physical hazards, and ergonomic conditions (6–18). From this partial listing of topics requiring health and safety oversight, it should be clear to the reader why most institutions invest in a group of individuals to handle this enormous institutional obligation.

The environmental health and safety group often also contains or coordinates the institution's occupational medicine function. Many of the areas of concern related to the risks associated with the care and use of laboratory animals involve a medical component that must be addressed by an occupational medicine unit. For example, the blood-borne pathogen, tuberculosis screening, hearing conservation, respiratory protection, allergy prevention (latex and animal), routine vaccination and post-exposure response programs are elements that are integrated into the occupational medicine function (2, 9, 10, 12–14). In many programs, the occupational medical unit functions without a full time physician, and often, the physician is not a specialist in the occupational medicine discipline. In other circumstances common to small institutions, the occupational medicine functions may be available on an external consulting or contract basis and involve only a knowledgeable non-physician health care provider (e.g., a physician's assistant or nurse) as the primary patient contact. Institutions entering into these kind of relationships should ensure that they have appropriate expert input (either from institutional members or external consultants) to structure the relationship appropriately to meet programmatic needs and to address the full spectrum of issues that are relevant to the program. For some areas of research entailing the possibility of high-risk exposure to personnel (e.g., B virus from nonhuman primates), fluid, efficient communication and action would be required; if the institution could not arrange an effective plan for post-exposure management, it simply should disallow the protocols involving these species.

E.   RESEARCH STAFF

The research investigators and their staffs need to be actively engaged in the design, management, and implementation of the health and safety program, particularly as it pertains to the unique features of experimental hazards used in their research efforts. Interactions with the IACUC, veterinarian, and health and safety personnel are essential to safety before new projects are started and the necessary approvals should be acquired. In addition to communicating with the veterinarian and facility managers or supervisors, laboratory personnel should be encouraged to share relevant project and safety information directly with the animal care and use staff. This action can foster a sense of partnership and allay animal care staff concerns while confirming their preparedness to undertake project support in a safe manner.

F.   FACILITY MANAGERS

Monitoring of animal use involving hazards, regardless of the type of hazard, is a two-directional process that must be performed continuously. All personnel have the responsibility to be aware of potential hazards and to follow established policies, rules, and procedures at all times, identifying new hazards when they occur, using safe work practices and promptly reporting accidents and injuries. Management has the added responsibility of assuring that staff is adequately trained in these matters as the first step of work plan development and performing periodic monitoring to ensure that staff remain in compliance. Training should emphasize the active and preventive nature of the successful safety program. Virtually all of the OSHA regulations governing the creation of a safe and healthy workplace contain a mandated training element precluding the opportunity for staff members to plead ignorance in instances of noncompliance in the properly implemented program.

Managers and facility supervisors need to be prepared (and forewarned) that a few employees in the extreme who are vested with a sense of invulnerability or their own standards of acceptable risk will neglect to adhere to important safety practices. These employees are potentially a great risk to the institution. Moreover, a larger employee cohort can become recalcitrant in safety matters if the procedures implemented are perceived to be unnecessarily cumbersome or too rigid for the nature of the hazard involved. Both of these situations strike against an important central tenet of a successful occupational health and safety program: **there must be consistency in the rules, and their enforcement and application to all workers** (2). Inconsistency can undermine a program, and all personnel should be expected to comply equally. Leadership by example is an effective catalyst for the cooperative spirit in the health and safety venture. In contrast, it is particularly damaging to the program when managers, supervisors, facility veterinarians, or research staff fail to adhere to the procedures and practices they have specified. Managers of the various specialty areas involved in setting policy and establishing procedures and practices should base their planning efforts on scientific data and sound professional judgement. This process should be discussed with employees during training to encourage employee buy-in and deter renegade action. Personnel should be clear on the difference between a "rule" that must be followed vs. a "guideline" or "recommendation" that suggests a prudent course of action but allows for some personal judgement. Training in these matters should be repeated periodically to ensure that employees stay current in these issues; annual training is mandated for some topics in the OSHA standards. Also, it is useful to integrate safety conformance measures into the employee's work plan and performance review to re-emphasize the importance of the active, prevention-minded approach to safety.

The occupational health program provider should maintain records for aspects of the occupational health and safety program related to their areas of responsibility and authority. These include medical history/examination records, training and compliance records (especially for training mandated by OSHA) and event logs for accidents, exposures, and work-related illnesses. In particular, it may be necessary for the environmental health and safety personnel to record some incidents on the OSHA 101 Form — Supplementary Record of Occupational Injuries & Illnesses. Knowledge of these events and their pattern over time can aid the institution in monitoring program success and progress and in decision-making about the allocation of time, effort, and money in the program. For example, the author is aware that the use and analysis of accident/injury logs in several institutions revealed that a majority of the incidents recorded occurred in only a small minority of the personnel involved. This event clustering was independent of either facility location (in a physically decentralized program) or of the nature of the work assignment (e.g., mix of animal species, work volume, or shift worked). This pattern suggested that the best return on management's effort would be achieved by a more intensive effort concentrated on the specific work habits and work environment awareness of these apparently "high risk" employees rather than repeating a general overview of the problem areas for the entire group.

II. HAZARDS: IDENTIFICATION AND CONTROL

A. THE HAZARD IDENTIFICATION AND RISK ASSESSMENT PROCESS

The 1996 NRC *Guide* placed a new emphasis on health and safety in research animal facilities. The health and safety provisions that are envisioned in the *Guide* characterize an approach that is comprehensive and seamless but that acknowledges that institutions have resource limitations. Earlier editions of the *Guide* were not considered comprehensive and all-inclusive in the treatment of health and safety issues because institutions were required to extend program coverage only to those individuals deemed to have "substantial animal contact." There was an obvious pitfall in this approach: institutions could arbitrarily decide what constituted "substantial animal contact" and remove a large segment of the animal user population from consideration. Under this approach the mosaic of coverage varied significantly from institution to institution, and more importantly, some persons with potentially significant exposures were not covered adequately. The 1996 NRC *Guide* extended program coverage to all individuals while acknowledging that not all persons need to be covered in an identical manner. The operating principle for coverage in the 1996 NRC *Guide* indicates that the "extent and level of participation of personnel in the occupational health and safety program should be based on the hazards posed by the animals and materials used; on the exposure intensity, duration and frequency; on the susceptibility of the personnel; and on the history of occupational illness and injury in the particular workplace."

Hazard identification and the risk assessment process are important first steps in establishing a program that is cost conscious while meeting the health and safety needs of the personnel involved with animal care and use. Hazards are of a diverse nature and will be discussed in further detail later. Two features are important to the characterization of a hazard: the **severity or seriousness** of the hazard and the **prevalence** (or frequency of occurrence at a given point in time) of the hazard. These are used together to formulate a **hazard factor** that helps in scaling the importance of hazard. For example, rabies virus would result in serious consequences for personnel if they contracted the disease, but in most animal populations used in the laboratory, this disease is extremely low prevalence (essentially it is unrecorded). In contrast, monkey B virus has a high prevalence in macaques and the consequences of human exposure are particularly dire since several deaths in laboratory personnel have occurred in the last decade. Thus, B virus would be accorded a higher hazard factor than rabies virus in the laboratory animal facility housing susceptible animal species.

Personnel often confuse the hazard factor with the level of risk involved in working with a particular agent or substance, and there is a hazard-risk relationship but a high risk does not ordinarily result from a high hazard. Simply stated, **risk** is a product of the hazard factor as modified by a (potential for) exposure factor. The risk assessment process takes both the hazard and opportunity for exposure into account, and risk reduction is aimed at reducing these two factors where possible. Therefore, if the hazard factor can be reduced significantly (e.g., by controlling or eliminating a disease in an animal population) the risk associated with the hazard will also be reduced. Similarly, if the opportunity for exposure can be reduced significantly through control measures (e.g., personal protective equipment and revised work practices) then the risk associated with the hazard also will be reduced as a consequence.

As noted above, it is important for institutions to establish a credible team to conduct the risk assessment process. This team, or some of its members, should also be responsible for the selection of safeguards to curtail risks. Typically, this team has representation from health and safety, occupational medicine, research staff, veterinary medicine, and facility management if warranted by the hazards involved. The team should be prepared to discuss its rationale and decision-making process to explain how the policies, procedures, and practices implemented will result in risk reduction. This is an important step for management because occasionally there are personnel who arrive at their own risk assessment choosing to focus only on the seriousness of the hazard while ignoring the efficacy of the control efforts. Patient and tactful coaching may be necessary to restore the trust and confidence of these individuals that the institution is indeed looking out for their health and safety interests.

B.   A SURVEY OF THE HAZARDS IN THE CARE AND USE OF LABORATORY ANIMALS

There is a rich diversity of hazards that might be encountered in the laboratory animal resource facility resulting from the work environment of the animal facility, the animals involved in the studies, or the protocol-related (experimental) hazards. Physical and chemical hazards in the animal facility work environment constitute the biggest proportion of workplace incidents in the experience of the author. Hazards in the work environment include physical injury by sharps or mechanical equipment, heat, electricity, lasers, UV and ionizing irradiation, pressure vessels, housekeeping (sanitation) practices, noise, ergonomically deficient practices, and chemical exposures. Hazards intrinsic to the animals include exposure to sensitizing allergens, the prospect of bite, scratch, or other bodily injury (particularly with large animals), and zoonotic infections or parasitic infestations. The hazards associated with experimental protocols are scientifically driven and include infectious agents, chemicals (including some that may not be adequately characterized from the hazard standpoint) and other types listed under the work environment above. These hazards are summarized below along with a brief description of the steps institutions should take to control the hazards and minimize the employees' risk of exposure. The reader should refer to other sources for more detailed information (2, 4, 5, 19). The laboratory animal industry has been responsive to the need for specialized equipment for the containment of hazards in a variety of research animal applications, and the strategies for hazard containment and the protection of the animal from external contamination have merged in many research applications. This has helped stimulate the development of individually ventilated rodent cage systems and the resurgence in the use of hard wall and flexible film isolators. It is therefore advisable that animal facility management and staff carefully evaluate the equipment options available when replacing equipment or building inventory to meet scientific needs and to optimize the safe working environment whenever possible. It also is important for management and staff to understand the limitations of equipment. For example, biosafety cabinets are often used as a component of the containment and infection control strategy, but these vary widely in performance according to their design (20).

1. Animal-Related Hazards

a. *Trauma*

Animals are recognized as sources of physical and biological injury. Their bites and scratches can inflict severe physical harm and personnel involved in the care of large domestic animals can sustain crushing injuries when animals kick, fall, or simply shift their body weight. Animal bites can cause severe mechanical damage to tissues resulting in permanent disfiguration. In addition to physical trauma, bites and scratches can inoculate the wound with microbial pathogens or opportunists from the animal's oral cavity or on its skin that may result in localized or systemic infection. The medical management of even localized infections can be problematic, but the potential for the development of systemic illness from an animal bite (such as B virus, rabies virus, hantavirus, or bacterial septicemia) should place personnel on high alert in some circumstances.

The training of personnel in proper animal restraint techniques is critically important to the prevention of animal related trauma in the laboratory. This training should ensure that personnel have an appreciation for the importance of using properly designed and functional equipment for animal restraint, the influence and control of environmental factors that may upset the animal and the ability to properly interpret the behavioral cues of the animal. These conditions should be central to the humane handling of the animal. Most laboratory animals are reasonably tractable; however, the possibility of unpredictable events should not be overlooked especially if the animals are frightened or in pain. Cats and rabbits are two common laboratory animals likely to scratch their handlers as a defense mechanism. Nonhuman primates, particularly the larger nonhuman primate species, warrant special training considerations due to their great strength, dexterity, intelligence and tenacity. Although procedures must sometimes be conducted in awake nonhuman primates, and with careful training, nonhuman primates may become willing participants in some routine procedures (e.g., venipuncture), chemical restraint or immobilization to facilitate the ease of nonhuman primate handling and reduce the risk of injury to personnel is often warranted. The personal protective equipment requirements that should be in effect to prevent B virus exposure from macaques are discussed below.

All bite, scratch, or other animal-related injuries should be logged by the institution. Furthermore, incident review by the institutional trainers or a member of the veterinary staff should be performed in an effort to identify possible predisposing conditions for the event. The determination should also be made whether retraining of personnel may be necessary.

b. *Allergens*

Laboratory animal associated allergy is manifested by allergic respiratory and skin reactions to proteins originating from shed dander and hair or those contained in animal urine, saliva, serum, or tissue. This is a serious and common occupational health disease of laboratory animal care staff and biomedical research personnel estimated to eventually affect 10% of those with laboratory animal contact (2). Hypersensitivity reactions include nasal drainage and congestion, sneezing, itchiness and asthma. Skin manifestations include redness, itchiness, welts, hives and eczema. In addition to the laboratory animal allergens, aerosolized mold spores and proteins found in animal feed may also act as allergens. Recent studies indicate that dispersal of urinary protein from animal litter may be a possible cause of sensitization in laboratory personnel. A similar mechanism of sensitizing laboratory personnel to other allergens is plausible. Laboratory animal allergy also carries the risk of a serious acute anaphylactic reaction in some individuals characterized by generalized itchiness, respiratory compromise, vomiting, nausea, diarrhea, and collapse.

Persons with known allergies to a particular animal species should avoid contact with these animals and their products. Reduction of exposure to animal allergens is recommended for all personnel working with animals. This is why the wearing of particle facemasks is routinely included in the personal protective equipment plans for personnel working in laboratory animal facilities. In addition, the use of protective clothing (e.g., gowns, gloves, and hair bonnets) to prevent skin contact should be encouraged. Once an individual becomes sensitized, disposable particle masks are no longer effective, but HEPA-rated masks (NIOSH designation N95) or respirators may be of some use (2). These also may be warranted for personnel involved in procedures such as the dumping of bedding, which causes the release of large amounts of potential animal allergens into the air. Engineering controls to reduce environmental accumulation and the exposure of personnel to allergens include increasing the air exchange rates in animal-holding rooms, use of ventilated (exhausted) caging systems, housing of animals in exhaust hoods, and utilizing cage filter tops. Allergens from laboratory animals provide an excellent example of a hazard that has a low severity factor, in general, but that are ubiquitous. The technology is already available to eliminate the risk of exposure and prevent laboratory animal allergy through a combination of the use of positive pressure HEPA respirators, protective clothing requirements, and facility engineering controls. However, the cost benefit analysis as well as the resistance of personnel to the excessive use of PPE probably explains why a more moderate course of action has prevailed in most institutions. Queries about the development of laboratory animal allergy should be included in a periodic medical history for all persons with laboratory animal contact. Occupational medicine and health and safety professionals should be engaged to determine the best course of action for personnel that have developed allergies to laboratory animal species, and in some cases, alternate work assignments may be warranted.

c.   *Laboratory Animal Zoonoses*

There are many potential zoonotic hazards associated with the introduction of animals into the laboratory, but the transmission of zoonotic disease in this environment has now become rare. Most research facilities in the United States categorize research animal species by a hierarchy of potential hazard based upon the animal species, its source and the quality and continuity of veterinary oversight and treatment that the species or individual animal has received. According to this hierarchical scheme first generation wild caught animals, and especially nonhuman primates due to the diseases they have in common with and their close phylogenetic relationship to man, are accorded the highest index of suspicion as a potential source for zoonotic hazards. Trailing the wild caught animals are random source animals or known source animals that have not been raised in a controlled, disease-limited environment under a program of veterinary care. In both of these cases, it is important to consider the source of the animal and factors contributing to the likelihood of their exposure to zoonotic pathogens through contact with other animal populations or conspecifics with endemic infections. Research programs involved with the maintenance of wild caught or random source animals require veterinary support sufficient to ensure effective programs of disease detection, diagnosis, treatment, control, and prevention. These programs may also have a special need for quarantine and isolation housing and laboratory management procedures that protect personnel during the health characterization of the animals. Programs using wild mammals or birds, or their fresh carcasses have a special obligation to investigate the health status of these animals and develop appropriate exposure prevention procedures. Hantavirus, West Nile encephalitis virus, and a newly described arenavirus in North America are all zoonotic agents that have caused human fatalities and should serve to sensitize the institutional leadership to realize the gravity of this matter.

Animals bred specifically for research over a number of generations generally represent a reduced hazard with a few notable exceptions that will be discussed later. In the United States, the vast majority of small laboratory animals (e.g., mouse, rat, hamster, guinea pig, and rabbit) used in research have been produced commercially for decades in highly controlled environments under the oversight of comprehensive and rigorous veterinary and animal care programs. By virtue of this history, these animal species now have none or extremely few of the zoonotic diseases associated with their wild animal counterparts. This situation contrasts with that seen in other countries where investigators still must contend with research animals that have multiple, and zoonotic, infections (5).

Although zoonotic agents are now rare in most contemporary research animal colonies, several specific agents have persisted, and there are instances where organizational, procedural and facility design, construction and equipment (physical plant) deficiencies have made reintroduction of zoonotic pathogens into the laboratory environment possible. Specific examples of agents that have continued to persist in part due to ineffective elimination efforts are B virus in macaque monkeys, Q fever among small ruminants, and cat scratch fever among domestic felines. Lymphocytic choriomeningitis virus is a zoonotic agent that has been introduced into healthy animal colonies through contaminated tumors and cell lines and through entry of feral animals. In the contemporary research animal environment that is dominated by expensive, sensitive, and often irreplaceable, genetically manipulated mutant mice, the impact of colony contamination of this type would be devastating. However, even with high quality veterinary support, the technical difficulty and expense of detecting chronic subclinical or latent infections and other factors may impede the progress toward the establishment of research animal populations that have a zero incidence of zoonotic infections. This emphasizes the need for institutions to establish a team approach involving laboratory safety, occupational health, research, veterinary and facility management personnel to achieve an optimal program for reduction of risks associated with zoonoses in the laboratory animal facility environment. The key zoonoses and parasitic infestations transmissible to man from laboratory animals are available in tabular form in many other sources and only a brief narrative discussion for the agents deemed most important is provided here. The reader should refer to other sources for more information on this area (2, 4, 5, 19).

d.   Viral Diseases

Cercopithecine herpesvirus 1 (CHV1, B Virus)

Cercopithecine herpesvirus 1 (CHV1) stands alone as a serious, potentially lethal zoonosis for humans contacting infected animals with human fatalities from this infection occurring during the past decade. This virus is still widely distributed among colonies of macaques used in biomedical research, posing an imminent threat to research personnel who work with these animals. B virus infection in the macaque generally produces a mild clinical disease similar to human Herpes simplex virus infection. Macaques become persistently infected and have periods of latency when the virus is hidden in regional nerves and is not being shed from the typical oral or urogenital lesions that it produces. Asian monkeys of the genus *Macaca* should be considered infected unless they have been obtained from specific breeding colonies known to be B virus-free. Although primarily an infection of macaques, B virus can also cause fatal infection in several species of New World monkeys and other Old World monkeys.

B virus transmission to humans primarily occurs through exposure to contaminated saliva through bites and scratches. However, airborne exposure, exposure of ocular mucous membranes to biological material (possibly feces), needlestick injury, exposure to infected nonhuman primate tissues, and human-to-human transmission have resulted in human infections.

Humans may develop clinical signs within 2 days to (more commonly) 2 to 5 weeks following initial exposure. In one case, an individual developed severe clinical disease from B virus 10 years following his last known exposure to the agent suggesting that human B virus infection may be asymptomatic for many years. The disease produced by B virus in humans has a progressive course and devastating outcome without appropriate intervention. Humans initially develop lesions at the site of exposure with progressive disease characterized by muscle pain, fever, headache, and fatigue, which are later followed by progressive neurological deterioration, paralysis, and death.

A key provision to prevent B virus exposures within an institutional animal care and use program concerns the decision of whether or not the studies proposed warrant the use of macaques. Macaques should be used only when there are no suitable alternative animal models, and efforts to acquire macaques that are free of B virus infection and to maintain them appropriately to preserve this status should be pursued whenever feasible. However, all macaques must be handled as though they are potentially infected because viral shedding is intermittent and viral serology does not adequately reflect the viral status of the animal.

Extensive guidelines have been promulgated for the prevention of B virus and institutions should adhere strictly to these guidelines. Briefly, these recommendations emphasize the need for nonhuman primate handlers to conform fully with a written comprehensive personal protective equipment (PPE) program based upon a thorough hazard assessment of all work procedures, potential routes of exposure and potential adverse health outcomes (20, 21). Protective clothing including leather gloves or full length sleeve garments for hand and arm protection and protective goggles designed for splash protection along with a mask to protect other mucous membranes from exposure to macaque secretions are considered essential equipment. The use of a faceshield is insufficient as a sole method for protection against ocular exposure because droplet splashes to the head may run down into the eyes and infectious materials may enter via the gap along the margins of the shield, and personal eyeglasses are not PPE. The use of latex gloves alone for hand protection should be reserved for the handling of monkeys under full chemical restraint. Chemical restraint or specialized restraining devices should be used whenever possible for nonhuman primates to reduce personnel injuries by alert monkeys. The CDC recommendations further specify that institutions should be prepared to handle patients with a suspect exposure promptly, and the patient should have direct and immediate access to a local medical consultant knowledgeable about B virus. This consultant should be available at any time the worker is concerned that potential occupational exposure to B virus may be relevant to worker symptoms. The wound should be cleansed thoroughly, and serum samples and cultures should be obtained for serology and viral isolation from both the patient and the monkey. Physicians should consult the Viral Exanthems and Herpesvirus Branch, Division of Viral Diseases, Centers for Disease Control and Prevention, Atlanta, Georgia for assistance in case management. Additional information

about the B virus diagnostic resources is available through the B Virus
Research and Resource Laboratory, Georgia State University, Atlanta.

SIMIAN RETROVIRUSES

HIV-1 and HIV-2 are known to have originated as zoonotic infections on
the continent of Africa. These findings have heightened the concerns about
zoonotic retroviral transmission, particularly with regard to the use of
nonhuman primate organs as human xenografts. Only a few cases of
retroviral transmission from their natural host to humans under laboratory
conditions have been documented, both involving nonhuman primates as
source species. Simian immunodeficiency infects a variety of Old World
nonhuman primates and produces a clinical syndrome in rhesus monkeys
and other susceptible macaque species paralleling human AIDS.

Monkeys usually transmit SIV through direct inoculation of open
wounds or mucous membranes with infectious secretions during activities such as fighting. The blood, secretions, and tissues of SIV-infected
monkeys should be presumed to be infectious for persons potentially
exposed to these materials. Human infection with SIV occurred in a
laboratory worker who had dermatitis on the hands and forearms and
who handled SIV-infected blood specimens without wearing gloves. In
this case, evidence of illness or immune deficiency syndrome has not
been recorded.

The simian foamy viruses are complex retroviruses that have been
isolated from a number of New and Old World nonhuman primates and
are similar to their human-origin counterparts. These viruses have not
been demonstrated as the cause of any disease entity in humans or in the
nonhuman primate but have been linked to a number of human disor-
ders. The transmission of simian foamy viruses to humans accidentally
exposed or occupationally exposed to non-human primates (African
green monkeys and baboons) has been reported. Nonhuman primates
infected with these simian retroviruses should be handled according to
OSHA provisions for bloodborne pathogens to protect personnel from
transmission.

VIRAL HEPATITIS INFECTIONS

Nonhuman primates are important experimental hosts in viral hepatitis
research and have been used to study hepatitis A, B, C, D, and E
infections (22); of these, however, only hepatitis A has proven to be an
important zoonosis in the research animal laboratory. The pig is also a
natural host for hepatitis E infection and has been incriminated as a
zoonotic reservoir for this agent, but no instances of transmission have
been reported in the laboratory animal facility setting. Mouse hepatitis

virus, a coronavirus, and infectious canine hepatitis, an adenovirus, are not transmissible to man. Also, there are other natural hepadnavirus infections of animals (woodchuck, ground squirrel, and duck) that are used as animal models of hepatitis B virus, but none are transmissible to humans.

Man is the primary reservoir for hepatitis A virus (HAV) with non-human primate infections resulting from contact with infected humans or other infected nonhuman primates. Infection results from a fecal-oral transmission of the agent. However, more than 100 cases of HAV infection in man have been associated with newly imported chimpanzees. Other great apes, marmosets, owl monkeys, cynomolgus monkeys, and patas monkeys are naturally susceptible and could serve as a source for human HAV infection. An outbreak of HAV infection in young domestically reared rhesus monkeys demonstrated that this zoonotic agent continues to be important in the laboratory animal facility environment. A safe, effective hepatitis A vaccine is now available in the United States and is recommended for individuals at high risk for exposure to HAV infection such as persons involved with the care of nonhuman primates being used in experimental HAV infection studies.

Measles (Rubeola) Virus

Measles is a disease of humans that nonhuman primates usually contract by coming into contact with human populations with endemic infection; however, spread in the reverse direction has also be seen in laboratory animal facilities. With the current emphasis on and success of domestic nonhuman primate production, it has become more likely that institutions would develop large populations of susceptible nonhuman primates who could contract measles and then transmit the disease back to man.

Measles is a highly communicable disease that is transmitted by infectious aerosols, contact with nasal or throat secretions, or by contact with fomites freshly contaminated with infectious secretions. Measles presents with fever, conjunctivitis, and cough in the early phase of the disease, followed by the development of a skin rash and the possibility of serious complications such as secondary bacterial bronchopneumonia or viral encephalitis.

Vaccination for measles is recommended for all nonhuman primate handlers to break the potential human–monkey–human cycle of infection.

Poxviruses

The poxviruses involved in zoonotic transmission in the laboratory animal facility represent three genera, Orthopoxvirus, Parapoxvirus, and Yatapoxvirus, with the nonhuman primate serving as a host for the majority of the potentially zoonotic poxviral species. With the exception of human orf virus infection from small ruminants, these infections are now mostly of historical interest in the laboratory setting. In humans, these infections usually are characterized by the development of proliferative (fleshy) cutaneous or subcutaneous self-limiting lesions, but humans occasionally manifest the clinical signs of systemic disease. Orf, a disease of sheep, goats, and wild ungulates, continues to be prevalent in the United States and worldwide and causes human infections associated with occupational exposures including research animal contact. All age groups are potentially affected but young animals are most frequently and severely affected. However, external lesions on the lips or urogenital area or in the mouth are not always apparent to alert animal handlers to the presence of infection. Personnel should wear barrier clothing as defined in Vertebrate Animal Biosafety Level 2 (ABSL 2) should be sufficient for the prevention of orf virus transmission to humans (20).

RABIES

Rabies is an acute, almost invariably fatal disease that occurs worldwide, but historically it has not been a problem in the laboratory animal facility setting. The main reservoirs are wild and domestic canines, cats, skunks, raccoons, bats, and other biting mammals. Among the rodent and lagomorph species maintained in the laboratory, the wild-caught groundhog and the rabbit appear to represent some risk of carrying rabies; however, rabies transmission from wild animals to dogs, cats or other species with uncertain vaccination histories originating from an uncontrolled environment must be considered. The bat should be regarded as an important reservoir species because most of the recent fatal U.S. exposures have involved strains from two insectivorous bat species: the eastern pipistrelle bat (*Pipistrellus subflavus*) and the silver-haired bat (*Lasionycteris noctivagans*).

Rabies should be regarded as the potential diagnosis in any wild-caught or random source research animal of unknown vaccination history exhibiting encephalitic signs. Vigorous first aid and wound care procedures for bites and scratches inflicted by animals are crucial first steps against the transmission of rabies virus to humans. Whenever possible, animals brought into the laboratory should have histories that preclude their exposure to rabies or ensure that they have been vaccinated for this disease. However, due to the potential for a long incubation (up to a year in some species) in the natural history of the disease, the types of animal models utilized or the prospect of vaccination failures, most institutions are likely to encounter situations where a rabies-free environment cannot be absolutely ensured. For this reason, many institutions elect to offer pre-exposure immunization to rabies to personnel working in high risk categories such as veterinarians, and to people who are working with or involved in the care of high risk or inadequately characterized animals.

LYMPHOCYTIC CHORIOMENINGITIS VIRUS (LCMV)

Lymphocytic choriomeningitis virus (LCMV) is in the family Arenaviridae, which also includes other important zoonotic viruses (e.g., Lassa fever and Argentine and Bolivian hemorrhagic fevers), but LCMV stands alone as a natural infection of laboratory animal species. There are many published reports of human LCMV infection associated with laboratory animal and pet contact, particularly mice and hamsters. Humans usually develop a flu-like illness following an incubation period of 1–3 weeks. More serious manifestations such as systemic and central nervous system involvement can also occur. Also, infections during pregnancy pose a risk of infection for the human fetus.

LCMV is widely distributed among the wild mouse population throughout most of the world. Mice, hamsters, guinea pigs, nonhuman primates, swine, and dogs are among the laboratory animal hosts that sustain natural infections. The mouse has remained the species of primary concern as a zoonotic reservoir in the laboratory as evidenced by a recent outbreak of lymphocytic choriomeningitis in humans, and athymic and other immunodeficient mouse strains may pose a special risk of harboring silent, chronic infections and present a hazard to personnel. The virus is readily transmitted to naïve animals by viral-contaminated transplantable tumors or cell lines. LCMV normally is transmitted via infectious aerosols from secretions and excrement of infected mice. However, ectoparasites and insect vectors in animal facilities have also been incriminated in transmission, making their control in the animal facility an important part of the overall scheme for disease prevention and control. Due to the potential for infection by the aerosol route, research animal facility personnel should observe ABSL 3 precautions and practices when this agent is known to be present (20). Work re-assignment should be considered for pregnant employees working in areas known or suspected of housing LCMV-infected rodents.

HANTAVIRUSES

The hantaviruses are widely distributed in nature among wild rodent reservoirs and numerous deaths from fatal hantavirus pulmonary syndrome have occurred in persons whose outdoor activities and occupations place them in close proximity with wild infected rodents and their excrement. No cases of hantavirus infection associated with laboratory animals have been reported in the United States, but cases have been reported in other countries. The recent cases that have occurred in the laboratory animal environment have involved infected laboratory rats. In this environment, the possibility of transmitting the infection from animal-to-animal by the transplantation of cells or tissues also should be considered. Hantavirus infection is transmitted through the inhalation of infectious aerosols from animal respiratory secretions, saliva and excrement, and extremely brief exposure times (5 minutes) have resulted in human infection.

INFLUENZA VIRUS

Man is considered to be the reservoir for human influenza virus infections. However, influenza virus infections from different antigenic strains occur naturally in many animals including avian species, swine, horses, mink, and seals. In the laboratory, ferrets are highly susceptible to human influenza and often are used as experimental models of influenza infection (23).

The transmission of animal influenza strains from animals to humans is an uncommon occurrence. However, pigs and ferrets experimentally infected with influenza virus in the laboratory have been shown to have directly and readily spread this agent to persons working with these animals.

e.　Bacterial Diseases

TUBERCULOSIS (MYCOBACTERIUM TUBERCULOSIS)

Tuberculosis in animals and man is caused by bacteria in the genus *Mycobacterium*. Many research animals including nonhuman primates, swine, sheep, goats, rabbits, guinea pigs, mice, dogs, cats, ferrets and frogs are susceptible to infection. The nonhuman primate is the most important zoonotic risk for personnel in the research animal facility. Nonhuman primates contract the infection from humans and animals during capture and confinement during holding in regions of the world where the disease is prevalent. Macaques are considered to be particularly sensitive with infection to *M. tuberculosis*, but all nonhuman primate species should be included in periodic tuberculosis screening programs. Suspect animals should be quarantined promptly in a housing zone under negative air pressure.

M. tuberculosis is transmitted from infected animals primarily by the aerosol route, although oral and cutaneous routes of exposure are also possible. The most common form of tuberculosis presents as pulmonary infection, but infection can be widespread throughout many other organs. Accordingly, personnel should wear respiratory protection and use work practices that minimize the generation of aerosols (16, 20).

COXIELLA BURNETII INFECTION (Q FEVER)

C. burnetii, the causative agent of Q fever, enters the laboratory animal facility mainly through sheep, goats, and cattle. Sheep have been the primary species associated with disease outbreaks, including those occurring in research animal facilities. Other cases of human infection have been linked to pregnant cats and wild rabbit exposures. *C. burnetii* organisms are shed in the urine, feces, milk and especially birth products of domestic ungulates exhibiting little or no signs of infection. The organism is highly infectious and is transmitted through infectious aerosols. It also produces a spore-like form that is resistant to desiccation and persists in the environment for a long time, contributing to the widespread dissemination of infectious aerosols. The importance of these factors was illustrated in outbreaks of the disease associated with the use of pregnant sheep in research facilities in the United States.

Q fever in humans varies in duration and severity often presenting as a flu-like illness with fever, headache, and chest pain with a nonproductive cough and pneumonia. However, serious heart, liver and kidney infections can also occur.

Sheep and other animals harboring Q fever infections should be maintained under Animal Biosafety Level (ABSL) 3 conditions to prevent the transmission of the organism in the research animal facility environment (20). In many institutions, ABSL 3 conditions would prove to be unachievable for sheep held under agricultural conditions for food and fiber production or for instructional exercises. Whenever possible, male or non-pregnant sheep should be used, and the use of personal protective equipment conforming to ABSL 3 practices should be implemented even when facilities may be deficient. Also, several commercial vendors now supply sheep from flocks without serological evidence of infection and which may be free of the disease.

CHLAMYDIOSIS (PSITTACOSIS, ORNITHOSIS OR PARROT FEVER)

Chlamydial agents are widely distributed among birds and mammals worldwide and occur naturally among many laboratory animal species including birds, mice, guinea pigs, hamsters, rabbits, ruminants, swine, cats, ferrets, muskrats, and frogs. Of these host species, birds have proven to be the most frequent source of virulent human infection. Ruminants and cats have also been involved in serious human cases of the disease.

The organism is spread to humans from infectious material present in exudates, secretions, or desiccated fecal material by direct contact or by the aerosol route. Most zoonotic infections in humans involve the respiratory tract or eyes but serious infections in other organs can also occur.

The use of birds (or other species) that are known to be free from chlamydia infection or that are appropriately treated with antibiotics can be used to eliminate this zoonosis in the research animal environment. Appropriate personal protective equipment should also be employed.

BARTONELLA HENSELAE INFECTION

B. henselae is the causative organism for cat scratch disease and bacillary angiomatosis in humans. Cats infected with this organism show little evidence of disease and can harbor the organism in the bloodstream for years. Cat fleas also spread the infection.

Following exposure, usually on an extremity, humans develop a small red papule at the site of inoculation followed several days later by vesicle and scab formation. Several weeks later, patients develop regional lymph node enlargement that can persist for months. Immunodeficient individuals are at risk for the development of severe vascular complications.

The incidence of this disease in cats from long-established, closed breeding colonies for research is not known but is likely to be low. Approaches to controlling this potential hazard in the research animal facility also involve training personnel in the proper handling of cats to prevent bites and scratches and implementing rigorous flea control programs for random source cats to prevent human infection from fleas infected with the organism.

RAT-BITE FEVER (*STREPTOBACILLUS MONILIFORMIS* OR *SPIRILLUM MINUS*)

S. moniliformis is the primary causative agent for rat-bite fever in the U.S.. It is present in the upper respiratory tract and oral cavities of asymptomatic rodents, especially rats. *S. moniliformis* has been involved in several cases of rat-bite fever in laboratory animal handlers but is now considered rare in the United States, and infection control efforts have largely eliminated this organism from commercially available laboratory rodents.

Most human cases result from rat bite incidents, but infection also has been transmitted by blood of an experimental animal and exposure to contaminated water. The infection is usually localized but can progress to regional involvement, polyarthritis, and the development of a rash on the extremities, palms, and soles. Serious complications involving other organs can also occur.

The avoidance of animal bites through proper animal handling techniques and barrier protection are key in the prevention of rat-bite fever, especially when dealing with wild-caught rodents or other rodents from unconventional sources.

Leptospirosis

Leptospirosis is distributed worldwide among domestic and wild animals. Rats, mice, field moles, hedgehogs, squirrels, gerbils, hamsters, rabbits, raccoons, dogs, domestic livestock, other mammals, amphibians, and reptiles are among the species that serve as reservoirs. The possibility of zoonotic transmission of leptospirosis from most animal species maintained in the laboratory would have to be considered, and wild-caught animals would warrant special attention. Several outbreaks of this zoonotic disease have been reported in research animal facilities in the past two decades, emphasizing the enduring importance of this problem.

Leptospires are shed in the urine of reservoir animals that often remain asymptomatic and carry the organism in the renal tubules for years. For example, mice infected with *Leptospira ballum* are believed to harbor the organism for life. Transmission occurs through skin abrasions and mucous membranes and is often related to direct contact with infected urine or tissues. Inhalation of infectious droplet aerosols and ingestion are also effective modes of transmission.

Humans frequently develop flu-like illness in leptospirosis, but the disease can range from asymptomatic infection to severe systemic illness with sudden onset, headache, chills, muscle pain, rash, skin and mucous membrane hemorrhage, anemia, lung involvement, and organ failure.

Efforts to prevent this zoonotic disease in the laboratory animal facility should focus upon effective control of this infection in laboratory animal populations and use of appropriate personal protective equipment particularly when wild-caught or random source animals are involved.

Intestinal Bacterial Infection (Campylobacteriosis, Salmonellosis, Shigellosis, and Yersiniosis)

Many laboratory animal species are potential reservoirs for the enteric bacterial zoonoses. Exposure to diarrheic animals is a significant risk factor for some of these infections; however, these organisms can also be contained in the feces of asymptomatic animals. Young animals, especially dogs, cats, nonhuman primates, pigs and other laboratory ruminants, may be particularly important to consider as sources due to the greater variability in their microbial floras in relation to the laboratory-bred rodents.

These organisms are transmitted by the fecal-oral route through contaminated food, water, or direct contact with infected animals and produce an acute gastrointestinal illness characterized by fever, nausea, abdominal pain, vomiting, and watery diarrhea laden with blood and mucous. The severity of the infection and the possibility for organ

involvement outside of the gastrointestinal tract varies with the causative agent. For example, *Campylobacter* and *Shigella* infections usually remain localized to the gastrointestinal tract, but *Shigella* infections
are more fulminant, rapidly debilitating and severe due to fluid and
electrolyte disturbances. In contrast, *Salmonella* and *Yersinia* infections
more often involve other organs, and therefore can mimic a variety of
other disease conditions.

Management practices that exclude the contamination of animals or
animal colonies with these agents are very important. Measures to
prevent the contamination of food, water, or other environmental sources
of infection should be implemented. Also, some institutions screen
individual animals or take representative samples of the animal populations periodically to determine if there are carriers of these organisms.
This is followed with appropriate quarantine, control, and treatment
efforts. The use of personal protective equipment readily eliminates the
zoonotic transmission of these organisms.

f. Protozoal Diseases

TOXOPLASMOSIS

Toxoplasma gondii is a parasite with a worldwide distribution among
warm-blooded animals (24). The definitive hosts for this organism are
wild and domestic felines who acquire the infection from one another or
by ingestion of an intermediate host. Felines support all phases of the *T.
gondii* life cycle in their intestinal tract resulting in infectious oocyst
production. Infected cats normally shed oocysts only once in their lifetime,
but oocysts are environmentally resistant, surviving up to a year, and they
may be mechanically transmitted to humans.

Intermediate hosts contract infection from oocysts in cat feces or
through the ingestion of infectious forms in the tissues of another
infected animal. This is why the possibility of acquiring the infection
from infected tissues of a variety of laboratory animal species serving
as intermediate hosts for *T. gondii* should be considered, particularly
when animals are known to be infected experimentally.

Toxoplasmosis generally produces an asymptomatic or mild infection,
but the infection of a pregnant woman can have serious consequences for
the fetus. In pregnant women, infection of the fetus across the placenta can
produce death of the fetus or eye deformities, brain damage, fever, jaun-
dice, rash, and neonatal convulsions. Primary infection in immunosuppressed individuals also can produce serious problems such as pneumonia,
central nervous system involvement, and death.

The use of personal protective equipment in combination with a
sound program of husbandry and sanitation providing the prompt removal cat feces and litter before oocysts sporulate and become infectious (24 hours) effectively control this hazard in the research animal

facility. However, pregnant women and women of childbearing age who might become pregnant and who lack antibody titers indicating that they are still susceptible to primary *T. gondii* infection should be advised of the risk associated with fetal infection and offered alternative work assignments.

INTESTINAL PROTOZOAL INFECTIONS (GIARDIASIS AND CRYPTOSPORIDIOSIS)

Of the potential intestinal protozoal infections of laboratory animals, giardiasis and cryptosporidiosis are the most important. Many wild, domestic, and laboratory animal species serve as reservoirs for these organisms, including dogs, cats, farm animals, and nonhuman primates. Rodents are a less likely, but not impossible, source for these infections. As with the intestinal bacterial infections, the prevalence of these organisms may be higher in young or infant animals.

The organisms are transmitted by the fecal-oral route chiefly through the transfer of cysts from an infected individual. The organisms reside in the gastrointestinal tract producing asymptomatic infection or disease characterized by anorexia, nausea, abdominal cramps, bloating, and chronic, intermittent diarrhea. The consequences of infection may be more severe in immunodeficient individuals. These infections are readily prevented through the use of appropriate personal protective equipment and sound work practices.

g. Fungal Diseases

DERMATOMYCOSIS

Dermatophytes occur worldwide and cause ringworm in humans and animals. In the United States, ringworm continues to be common among dogs, cats, and livestock animals, and several dermatophytes of animal origin are zoonotic. *Microsporum canis* is most prevalent in dogs, cats, and nonhuman primates, and in human infections acquired from these species, but it can also occur in laboratory rodents. *Trichophyton mentagrophytes* has been associated more commonly with ringworm in rodents and rabbits, and occurs among laboratory personnel working with these species and agricultural personnel working around granaries, barns, or other rodent habitats. *T. verrucosum* is restricted generally to cases of ringworm in the livestock species and in their agricultural attendants.

Dermatophyte transmission from animals to humans is by direct skin to skin contact with infected individuals or indirect through contact with contaminated equipment or materials. Infected animals may have no, few, or difficult-to-detect skin lesions resulting in transmission to unsuspecting individuals. Also, dermatophyte spores can become widely disseminated and persistent in the environment, thereby contaminating bedding, equipment, dust, surfaces and air (including building ventilation systems) and resulting in the infection of personnel who do not have direct animal contact. The clinical presentation of dermatophyte infection varies, usually producing focal, flat, spreading annular lesions that are clear centrally and crusted, scaly and inflamed in the periphery. Lesions often are located on the hands, arms, or other exposed areas. The control of dermatophyte infections in animal users should emphasize treatment of affected animals, sanitation to prevent environmental contamination, and the use of proper personal protective equipment.

2. Hazards from the Animal Facility Work Environment

a. *Ergonomic Hazards*

Anecdotal reports suggest that ergonomic hazards are emerging as the most important hazards in many animal care and use programs, although this awaits confirmation in published reports specifically on our industry. Animal facility personnel encounter physical trauma from lifting or pushing heavy loads such as equipment, supplies, or animals, and from repetitive small stresses from manipulating objects or working repeatedly outside of the normal movement comfort zone. The cumulative injuries from repetitive small stresses have been greatly exacerbated in many programs by the explosion in mouse populations and the adoption of microbarrier cages with rigid tops that require the animal caretakers to handle many more parts each day. The high bedding moisture content that can occur in these cages adds the problem of difficult bedding removal. Also, high density caging on large racks requires personnel to place cages at uncomfortable heights, and improper cage-changing designs that limit the range of motion of personnel result in additional musculoskeletal strain. These work conditions can produce a range of problems including carpal-tunnel syndrome, epicondylitis (tennis elbow), bursitis, and neck and back injury. There are innumerable other activities common in animal care that contribute to repetitive stress injury such as grasping (by hand or forceps) small animals during cage transfers, removing bottle stoppers, mopping floors, and operating a computer for extended periods. These problems can be addressed through the redesign of equipment or tools to minimize strain, varying the mix of tasks to break the repetition or re-engineering the task.

Personnel lifting heavy loads should be physically fit, assume a proper lifting position using a two-hand technique, and avoid sudden movements. As noted above, animal caretakers have many occasions to lift or move heavy materials and should be afforded the opportunity to try several strategies to ameliorate this recurring hazard. These include the use of lift equipment, automation of the lifting process, or splitting of the load.

The education and training of personnel in connection with the availability and proper use of engineering controls has the potential to reduce the injuries from these hazards. Personnel should be trained further as new tools to aid in an operation become available, and they should be periodically reminded of proper work techniques.

b.   Machinery and Equipment Hazards

Large equipment, such as cage washers of all types, conveyor belts, floor cleaners or polishers, sanders, and power wash equipment, has the potential to cause serious injury. Machine hazards are categorized by type and include in-running nip points, crush points, and pinch points that can be readily identified by an industrial hygienist if they are not readily apparent to supervisors and staff. Injuries can occur from any machine that has moving parts, and all machines should be examined to determine if they could entrap a worker's arm or hand during routine operation or ensnare clothing, creating a panic and uncontrolled movement in the worker. If such areas are identified, guards should be installed if possible even if workers indicate that they are aware of the hazard and know not to place their hands in the hazardous area. Entrapment within a cage (rack) washer if the chamber door is closed inadvertently is a recognized hazard that should be eliminated by the installation of an internal release mechanism.

c.   Heat, Steam, and Pressure Vessels

Hot water, steam, steam under high pressure, and compressed gas cylinders are other common animal facility hazards. Mechanical cage washers use water at very high temperature that can rapidly produce a severe burn injury. For example, the author is aware of one case where wastewater pooled in a cage wash particle trap flooded a worker's boot producing a severe "sock" burn on his foot. Cage washers and autoclaves also operate off pressurized steam lines, and the lines feeding these pieces of equipment as well as the autoclave chamber itself constitute steam and pressure hazards. Pinhole defects in steam lines can amputate fingers. Also, compressed gas cylinders should always be secured to prevent an explosive release of gas producing a dangerous projectile.

d.   Flammable Materials

Animal facilities contain many types of flammable materials. These materials are classified by type by the National Fire Protection Association to characterize the nature of the flammable or combustible material. Class A materials include animal bedding, paper gowns, paper towels, plastic cages, and other common combustible materials. Class B contains flammable solvents such as paints, solvents, materials used in facility cleaning, agents used for inhalant anesthesia in animals, and materials used in histologic tissue preparation. Class C materials are various types of electrical equipment. Explosive materials are rarely used in animal facilities with ether as a notable exception. This agent forms explosive peroxides and is highly volatile and flammable. Under conditions of room temperature (and even much colder) ether continues to vaporize, necessitating its storage under ventilation or in an explosion-proof refrigerator and away from flame or electrical spark hazard. Picric acid, an agent sometimes used to mark the coat of an animal for identification, can also be explosive when crystallized. Proper storage of Class B substances is dictated by their flashpoints: the lowest temperature needed by the liquid to produce a vapor that will propagate a flame. Facilities should review the MSDSs for all Class B substances to ensure their handling is in compliance with OSHA standards (25). Flammable and combustible liquids, although uncommon in animal housing areas, are often present in necropsy, surgery, and diagnostic laboratory areas that may be contiguous to animal housing. Hazardous chemicals can also be present during the construction and renovation of animal facilities. For example, the author had an experience with an explosion caused by the vapor from a freshly applied epoxy floor in an animal facility that was ignited by the spark of an iron pipe that was dropped on the floor.

e.　*Lighting, Electricity, and Electromagnetic Waves*

The lighting within an animal facility is rarely a source of hazard; however, fixtures can be hazardous to personnel if they are not properly installed or contain exposed bulbs susceptible to braking during room cleaning and sanitation procedures. The use of a red light or low-level light intensity (common in some research applications) may fatigue individuals working continuously in this environment and impair their safe navigation and task performance precision. Personnel working in these areas should acclimate to room conditions before beginning work and demonstrate the personal caution necessary to work safely in these areas. It is also important to check the room light cycles in animal facilities periodically to ensure that diurnal lighting is provided because animals kept under continuous light can become more agitated and fractious posing a hazard to personnel involved in their handling.

A variety of electrical fixtures in animal facilities and on the equipment used for animal care or studies can present hazards to personnel. These devices should be maintained in good repair, without frayed or exposed wires. Moisture-resistant switches, ground fault interrupted (GFI) outlets, and grounded (three-prong) plugs should also be used to protect personnel from electrical hazard.

Ultraviolet (UV) radiation has proven to be a relatively common hazard for animal facility personnel. UV is sometimes employed for infection control (or the control or elimination of environmental microbes) in areas such as biocontainment suites or isolation cubicles and in biosafety cabinets. Most of the devices used in animal facility applications emit UV-B or UV-C radiation, and these energies can be injurious to the skin and cornea of the eye. Depending upon the placement of the UV source in the room or biosafety cabinet and on the intensity and placement of room lights, the presence of UV radiation in the area may be undetected by personnel. The author is aware of several cases of UV-induced keratitis (corneal injury) and skin burns that personnel received in this manner. Accordingly, clear signage should be present to alert personnel to the UV hazard and personnel should be given instruction in the specific precautions they should follow to work safely in this environment.

Lasers are now used in a variety of experimental applications in animals and generally pose a hazard only to particular members of the animal care and use team involved in these specialized applications. Depending upon the power of the beam, lasers can cause burns, eye damage, skin lacerations or fires, and the generation of the beam entails the use of substantial electrical power posing an additional risk to personnel. Proper training of personnel who work with lasers about laser-associated hazards is essential for a laser safety program. The safety program should also include controlled access to the area of use to prevent inadvertent entry, proper signage, shielding devices and the control and elimination of the harmful by-products that might be generated by the laser (2).

f.   *Ionizing Radiation*

Ionizing radiation from the disintegration of particles of atomic origin (particulate radiation) or from high-energy electromagnetic waves (non-particulate radiation) has a long history of use and regulation in biomedical research involving laboratory animals. Most of the non-particulate radiation is encountered in imaging applications such as diagnostic x-ray machines or fluoroscopy or in treatment applications such as irradiators for tumor therapy or whole body irradiation for cell transfer studies. Personnel involved in the use of these non-particulate radiation devices must be properly trained in their safe use and should observe the personal protections specified. The specialized equipment used for these procedures requires a preventive maintenance program with periodic certification of proper function to ensure that it can be operated safely.

Particulate radiation results from the use of radionuclides that are unstable atoms that produce alpha particles, beta particles, neutrons, positrons, gamma rays or combinations of these upon disintegration depending upon the particular radionuclide involved. These decay particles or electromagnetic radiation inflict cellular damage as dictated by the route of exposure and the intrinsic ability of particle or electromagnetic wave to penetrate tissue. This type of radiation can be used in therapeutic applications such as the ^{131}I treatment for hyperthyroidism, imaging applications such as MRI (magnetic resonance imaging), PET (positron emission tomography), and gamma camera studies or in tracking cellular physiological and cellular events such as drug metabolism. The use of ^{131}I in the treatment of hyperthyroidism illustrates the fact that some radionuclides can become more concentrated in particular tissues requiring that these tissues be handled and disposed of differently to ensure radiation safety. Fortunately, radiation safety measures for the use of radionuclides have been long established due to the widespread use of these materials in biomedical research activities spanning many decades and federal oversight and control has been in place since 1971 under that U.S. Nuclear Regulatory Commission (2).

The safe handling of these materials depends on the appropriate use of shielding, personnel monitoring for exposure, screening, and documentation of tissues and bedding for radionuclide content to ensure safe handling and the proper disposal of contaminated materials according to established regulatory limits.

g.   *Sharps*

Skin and soft tissue wounds can occur from many of the materials used in an animal facility. As with an animal bite, skin trauma can potentially lead to local or systemic infections. This is the primary reason for suggesting that tetanus vaccination and prophylaxis should be provided to all personnel. Animal cages should be inspected routinely for possible safety hazards. Broken and bent wires on cages should be repaired and cages or equipment with serious deterioration should be discarded to ensure animal and human safety.

Sharps of many varieties are very common in the animal facility. These include needles and syringes, pipettes, scalpel blades, surgical needles, and glass. The control of these hazards is achieved through training workers in proper disposal techniques for sharps and ensuring that appropriate puncture-resistant, leak-proof receptacles are available in all areas where sharps are used. The improper disposal of sharps in a regular waste container has led to the injury of housekeeping and custodial staff in many institutions resulting in their potential exposure to infectious materials or chemical hazards. Recapping needles is prohibited in situations when bloodborne pathogens apply and should be discouraged under other circumstances. In this regard, many animal care and use programs have incorrectly made the assumption that it is appropriate to focus on the named disease entities and to narrowly interpret the OSHA Exposure to Bloodborne Pathogens to exclude animal pathogens (11). However, these regulations make it clear that other potentially infectious materials should be included, among them many common natural diseases of animals as well as various experimentally induced infectious diseases. Examples include leptospirosis, brucellosis, hantavirus, and B virus. Thus, if needle recapping must be performed (e.g., to safely transfer a drug for administration to an animal at some distant point), a one-handed technique should be used. In any use of a needle and syringe in animal procedures, the operator should be aware of exposed hands or arms that are unnecessarily in the area of action. Proper restraint and handling of animals receiving injections also reduces the risk of worker injury. Sedating the animal may also benefit risk reduction.

h.   Noise

Animals and the equipment used for their care in research facilities can produce sufficient noise to constitute a serious hearing hazard. Pigs, dogs, nonhuman primates, and large psittacine birds (e.g., parrots, macaws or cockatoos) can be particularly noisy during care procedures, and cage washers, pressure washers, vacuums, and other cleaning equipment present similar problems, especially when used in confined spaces. Personnel working in areas exceeding 85dBA should be covered by a hearing conservation program that includes monitoring, hearing tests, hearing protection, training, and record-keeping and controls must be implemented for personnel exposed to a time-weighted average (over 8 hours) of 90dBA or more (2, 26). A useful rule of thumb is that the noise level may be excessive if normal speech cannot be heard or if it is impossible to hold a phone conversation under prevailing conditions. These conditions should prompt the assessment of the area by a person knowledgeable about noise, noise measurement techniques, data interpretation, and abatement strategies. OSHA requires that engineering controls be implemented, if feasible, before the use of personal protective equipment is adopted as a primary means of noise control; however, earplugs, ear muffs, or other protective equipment may prove to be useful. Limiting the period of personnel exposure to the noise-hazard area is an administrative control method that should be pursued in concert with the use of personal protective equipment for control.

i.   Hazards Associated with Experimental Protocols

As emphasized above, the team approach is crucial to the safe conduct of animal studies that involve the use of experimental hazards. This team should include the investigator, institutional veterinarian, the animal care supervisors, and the health and safety professional. In addition, federal safeguards may also stipulate that the proposed studies receive review and approval by institutional committees (other than IACUC approval, which is always required) in some cases.

The hazards associated with an experimental protocol are influenced by two main factors: the **intrinsic qualities of the agent** and the **complexity of the procedures involving the hazard** in the project. Agent factors include toxicity, reactivity, corrosiveness, flammability, and explosiveness in the case of chemicals and virulence, pathogenicity, and communicability in the case of biological agents. The complexity of procedures involving hazards in animals impacts the potential for personnel exposure while conducting these studies. Careful study planning can often reduce the complexity of procedures and the opportunity for personnel exposures and sometimes agent substitutions can be exploited to reduce the intrinsic agent hazard. An example of the former might be that administration of a hazardous chemical agent by gavage rather than in the diet to reduce the dissemination of the agent in the environment. If the agent must be delivered in the diet, it may be preferable to purchase a diet premixed with the hazardous chemical rather than mixing the diet on-site in the animal facility.

Many organizations deal with chemicals of unknown toxicity warranting special attention in animal studies. Although it is usually always known whether a chemical agent is flammable or explosive, it may not be known whether or not it has a corrosive, toxic, mutagenic and/or carcinogenic capability. In institutions performing studies with such chemical unknowns, personnel are required to follow stringent personal protective equipment and personal hygiene practices (e.g., barrier protection for skin and mucous membranes, full-face respiratory protection, and showering upon exiting the facility) to prevent exposure. The reader should consult *Prudent Practices in the Laboratory: Handling and Disposal of Chemicals* for additional information on conducting studies of this nature (27).

In addition to the numerous zoonotic infectious agents already discussed, there are myriad infectious organisms that are transmissible to man that are used in animal studies in some institutions. These organisms are categorized according to the hazard they pose and the procedures required for safe handling into Animal Biosafety Levels 1–4 (ABSL 1–4). Animal Biosafety Level 1 organisms are ubiquitous and not associated with human disease, while ABSL 4 organisms are highly virulent for humans, spread by the aerosol route, and have no known vaccine or chemotherapeutic agents. Only a few, very specialized facilities are capable of conducting studies at ABSL 4 in the United States. Most research animal programs limit their studies at ABSL 2 or 3. Animal Biosafety Level 3 agents are also infectious for humans by the aerosol route, causing serious or lethal illness, but vaccination or treatments are available for these agents. Even ABSL 3 is beyond the reach of many research institutions because facilities must meet particular physical plant requirements (barrier controls) to preclude the airborne escape of the agent and permit all products to be sterilized prior to exiting the area. However, both the strain of the organism used and the host species being studied can influence the ABSL 2 or 3 categorization. For example, virulent strains of LCMV (mentioned above) are regarded as ABSL 3 whereas some mouse adapted strains are apparently less virulent for humans and can be handled at ABSL 2. Also, tuberculosis studies in an animal species that can cough generating organism aerosols such as the nonhuman primate is regarded as ABSL 3, but studies in mice are regarded as ABSL 2. Thus, studies involving experimental induction of infectious disease in animals should be carefully reviewed using available recommendations (20) and other pertinent literature before they are initiated.

Studies involving genetically modified organisms also must be reviewed by institutional committees (Institutional Biosafety Committees) by federal mandate according to the NIH *Guidelines for Research Involving Recombinant DNA Molecules* (17). These guidelines cover diverse organisms such as viruses, viral vectors, yeast, bacteria, and higher animals. The purpose of IBC review is to ensure that the planned genetic modifications are not expected to increase an organism's pathogenicity or virulence posing a risk to personnel or the environment. Also, genetic modifications of a host animal (e.g., transgenic mice) could make it acquire susceptibility to a human disease thereby serving as a new host for human infection. One such example is the poliovirus receptor transgenic mouse, allowing the use of the mouse to study human poliovirus infection. If these animals escaped and bred with wild or feral mouse populations, this could have serious implications for the control and spread of poliovirus at a time when we are moving closer to worldwide eradication of this disease. Cases such as this emphasize not only the importance of an effective IBC but also reiterate the important theme that there is a need for effective institutional cooperation among many areas of professional expertise to ensure a sound health and safety program for animal care and use activities.

III. CASE STUDIES FOR DISCUSSION

The following case studies are based roughly on incidents that the author has encountered over the past 20 years and are provided for the reader's analysis or classroom discussion. In each of the scenarios described, attempt to identify the factors (or sources of failure) within the institution that predisposed to the problem and suggest methods for correcting these problem areas.

A. CASE 1

An animal facility in an urban, academic institution became infested with a free-living rodent mite, *Ornithonyssus bacoti*. This mite is a recognized vector for a rickettsial disease that is zoonotic (transmissible to man) and is still reported in urban U.S. populations. The mites were present in all animal rooms and within many of the microbarrier cages housing mice. Cage changes were performed in a positive, horizontal flow, HEPA-filtered mass air displacement hood (tissue culture hood). Several animal caretakers had rashes from mite bites on their arms and were referred to occupational medicine for treatment.

The facility was treated with a pesticide for environmental decontamination. Cages were treated with dichlorvos strips placed in the cage. One of the veterinary technicians who cut the dichlorvos strips into pieces developed a severe dermatitis on her hands that appeared to be related to the handling of the strips, even though she had worn latex gloves during this process. Her treatment was overseen by occupational medicine; the condition was eventually resolved with a steroid-containing hand cream.

B. CASE 2

An experienced caretaker cut himself on a clean rabbit cage waste pan on a Friday afternoon and did not alert his supervisor or seek medical attention because he considered it to be only a minor scratch. Over the weekend, the scratch developed secondary infection requiring that the individual be hospitalized on Monday for intravenous antibiotic therapy.

C.   CASE 3

A laboratory animal facility supervisor with 20 years experience in the field climbed into a cabinet washer to remove and clean the trap screen. In the process, his protective rubber boot filled with scalding water, burning his foot. As a result, he missed two weeks of work because he had to keep his foot clean, dry, and elevated while the course of antibiotic therapy and local treatment of the injury was completed. There was no written record to indicate that this individual had received specific instruction to identify and avoid situations in the animal facility that might produce thermal injury.

D.   CASE 4

A technician crushed one of her fingers when the rack she was moving collided with another rack standing in the corridor. This was the third traumatic injury that she had incurred in 2 months; she had been cautioned shortly before the accident about exercising more attention and care in performing her duties, especially in areas of congestion and high activity. Hand protection through placement that prevents exposure had also been emphasized.

E.   CASE 5

A veterinary student trainee visiting another institution had his fingers crushed (bitten) while performing a dental exam on a sheep. Later, after returning to his "home" institution, large painful nodules appeared at the sites of the bite and he reported to the student health service for diagnosis and treatment. The surgical resident on call was baffled by the condition. After reviewing the patient's medical history, the surgeon assumed that these lesions might be abscesses and attempted to lance one. This proved to be a dismal failure, and the student was discharged with a prescribed course of antibiotic therapy and asked to return to see a dermatologist at a later date.

F.   CASE 6

A facility manager coping with an unusual level of staff absences elected to personally perform the animal care for a group of guinea pigs. He was aware of his significant allergy to the dander of this species. After 20 minutes in the room, he became flushed and experienced some wheezing and shortness of breath, and reported immediately to the hospital emergency room for treatment.

G.   CASE 7

An animal technician experienced a severe panic attack when she was working in a cubicle changing mouse cages and discovered a snake on the floor of the cubicle. Snakes were not housed in this facility as part of the institution's research programs; it was later determined that this snake was kept as a laboratory mascot elsewhere in the building. The animal technician coincidentally had a snake phobia from early childhood experiences in another country, and weeks of work rehabilitation were necessary to return this employee to her former level of performance.

H. CASE 8

A veterinary technician assisting in a research study was administering a systemic dye for bone to dogs used in a dental study. The dye turned the mucous membranes of the dogs bright red. Later that afternoon, the veterinary technician became alarmed when she too was noted to have bright red lips and oral mucous membranes by co-workers. She had handled these dogs (including their oral cavities) without gloves. These events prompted immediate review of the IACUC-approved protocol that mentioned that a bone marker would be used but provided no specifics or information about chemical safety review. Health and safety personnel and occupational medicine personnel were contacted immediately and treated and advised the patient according to the limited information they had available.

REFERENCES

1. **Committee to Revise the** *Guide for the Care and Use of Laboratory Animals, Guide for the Care and Use of Laboratory Animals,* National Research Council, National Academy Press, Washington, D.C., 1996.
2. **Committee on Occupational Safety and Health in Research Animal Facilities,** *Occupational Health and Safety in the Care and Use of Research Animals,* National Research Council, National Academy Press, Washington, D.C., 1997.
3. **Newcomer, C.E.,** General composition of the IACUC and specific roles of the IACUC members, in *The IACUC Handbook,* Silverman, J., Suckow, M.A., and Murthy, S., Eds., CRC Press, Boca Raton, FL, 2000, chap. 5.
4. **Fox, J.G., Newcomer, C.E., and Rozmiarek, H.,** Selected zoonoses and other health hazards, in *Laboratory Animal Medicine,* 2nd ed., Fox, J.G.,, Anderson, L.C., Loew, F.M., and Quimby, F.W., Eds., Academic Press, New York, in press.
5. **Newcomer, C.E.,** Zoonoses, in *Laboratory Safety: Principles and Practices,* 3rd ed., Fleming, D.O. and Hunt, D.L., Eds., American Society of Microbiology Press, Washington, D.C., chap. 9, in press.
6. **29 Code of Federal Regulations (CFR) Part 1910 [Docket No. S-777] [RIN No. 1218-AB36].** Ergonomics Program Occupational Safety and Health Administration.
7. **9th Annual Report on Carcinogens,** National Toxicology Program, 2000.
8. **U.S. Department of Health and Human Services,** Registry of Toxic Effects of Chemical Substances (RTECS, online database). National Toxicology Information Program, National Library of Medicine, Bethesda, MD, 1993.
9. **29 CFR 1910.1200,** Hazard Communication Standard, OSHA.

10. **29 CFR 1910.1450,** Occupational Exposure to Hazardous Chemicals in Laboratories, OSHA.

11. **29 CFR 1910.1030,** Occupational Exposure to Bloodborne Pathogens, OSHA Instruction CPL 2.103, Field Inspection Reference Manual.

12. **NIOSH Alert,** Preventing Allergic Reactions to Natural Rubber Latex in the Workplace. U.S. Department of Health and Human Services (NIOSH) Publication No. 97-135, 1997.

13. **Guidelines for Laser Safety and Hazard Assessment (Pub 8-1.7),** Occupational Safety and Health Administration, U.S. Department of Labor, Washington, D.C., July, 1991.

14. **National Research Council,** *Multiple Chemical Sensitivities: A Workshop*, National Academy Press, Washington, D.C., 1992.

15. **Interagency Workgroup on Multiple Chemical Sensitivity,** *A Report on Multiple Chemical Sensitivity (MCS)*, The American College of Occupational and Environmental Medicine (ACOEM), Arlington Heights, IL, 1998.

16. **29 CFR Part 1910 [Docket No. H-371] RIN 1218-AB46,** Occupational Exposure to Tuberculosis. Occupational Safety and Health Administration.

17. **NIH Guidelines for Research Involving Recombinant DNA Molecules** (NIH Guidelines), Federal Register, May 11, 1999 (64 FR 25361).

18. **10 CFR,** Energy. Department of Energy.

19. **Lipman, N.S. and Newcomer, C.E.,** Hazard control in the animal research facility, in *Biohazards Management Handbook*, Liberman, D.F. and Gordon, J.G., Eds., Marcel Dekker, Inc., New York, 1989, 107.

20. **Centers for Disease Control and Prevention — National Institutes of Health,** *Biosafety in Microbiological and Biomedical Laboratories*, 4th ed., HHS Publication No. (CDC) 93-8395, U.S. Government Printing Office, Washington, D.C., 1999.

21. **Centers for Disease Control and Prevention,** Fatal Cercopithecine herpesvirus 1 (B Virus) infection following a mucocutaneous exposure and interim recommendations for worker protection, *MMWR*, 47, 1073, 1998.

22. **Adams, S.R.,** Part B. Zoonoses, biohazards and other health risks, in *Nonhuman Primates in Biomedical Research*, Bennett, B.T., Abee, C.R., and Henrickson, R., Eds., Academic Press, San Diego, 1995, 391.

23. **Harmon, M.W. and Kendal, A.P.,** Influenza viruses, in *Diagnostic Procedures for Viral, Rickettsial and Chlamydial Infections*, 6th ed., Schmidt, N.J. and Emmons, R.D., Eds., American Public Health Association, Washington, D.C., 1989, 631.

24. **Rottman, J.B.,** Toxoplasmosis, in *The Merck Veterinary Manual*, Aiello, S.E., Ed., National Publishing, Inc., Philadelphia, 1999, 488.

25. **29 CFR Part 1910.106,** Flammable and Combustible Liquids, OSHA.

26. **29 CFR Part 1910.95,** Occupational Noise Exposure, OSHA.

27. **Committee on the Study of Prudent Practices for Handling, Storage and Disposal of Chemicals in Laboratories,** *Prudent Practices in the Laboratory: Handling and Disposal of Chemicals*, National Research Council, National Academy Press, Washington, D.C., 1995.

14 Emergency Response and Management

Catherine M. Vogelweid, D.V.M., Ph.D., Dipl. ACLAM

I. PURPOSE OF DISASTER PLANNING AND WHY THE COMMUNITY SHOULD INCLUDE RESEARCH ANIMALS IN ITS EMERGENCY/DISASTER RESPONSE PLAN

It is not unreasonable to pose the question "Why should you write an emergency/disaster response plan for your research animals?" On the most altruistic level, animals deserve protection because they enhance the quality of human life. Every society derives valuable benefits from its associations with animals, whether animals are used solely as sources of food and work, or whether they fulfill the desire of humans for companionship as pets. Research animals fulfill a very important role in society. They determine, in large part, the pace of progress in medical research that directly benefits human health. If a disaster causes the loss of unique animal models, the costs to society of the resulting delays in acquisition of knowledge and disruptions in research resulting from their demise cannot be calculated.

Research animals can also have a significant impact on the local economy of the community in which they reside. Many of the businesses and academic institutions that use research animals are among the largest employers within their communities. These employers need an educated, technology-conscious workforce. These types of businesses spur educational development, create well-paying jobs, and increase both economic development and cultural awareness in their communities. Following a disaster, the community needs to recover. Recovery is possible only when disaster survivors can return to their jobs and business functions resume. Because the operations of animal research businesses or academic institutions are critical to the economic health of their communities, plans to minimize losses and resume operations as quickly as possible following a disaster should be established.

Another aspect of planning to care for animals during disasters considers how the presence of animals at a disaster site influences human behavior. During the early, immediate response to a disaster, rescuers may experience fear if they encounter aggressive, wandering animals and/or intense conflict and psychological distress if they encounter injured animals that they must ignore because they are searching for human survivors. Many different interest groups that want to assist animals may emerge following a disaster, both from within and outside the stricken community. Outside interest groups, such as animal rights groups, may try to use the disaster to further their own agendas, including solicitation of contributions and visiting sites to gather information to support their political agendas (1). The activities of animal rights groups are of particular concern to the research community — we want our research animals to be rescued, not liberated. When animal research professionals participate in the development of response plans in their communities, they are setting in place a pre-determined organizational structure for the response at their facilities. The laboratory animal professionals can contribute their expertise to devise effective plans for capture and medical treatment of injured animals, and in return they can gain control of the types of volunteers who may be included, or more importantly, *who must be excluded*, from their facilities. To be effective during a disaster, this structure must be in place *before* a disaster happens.

Unfortunately, the involvement of the veterinary community in the development of emergency preparedness plans for animals has markedly lagged behind the plans developed for humans. The **Federal Emergency Management Agency (FEMA)** recently recognized this discrepancy, and in 1998 two courses were introduced (2, 3) to assist emergency planners in integrating response plans for animals into their existing community plans. The necessity of planning ahead for the needs of research animals was also recognized in the 1996 revision of the *Guide for the Care and Use of Laboratory Animals*, which included the recommendation for development of disaster plans for animal facilities (4).

II.   DISASTERS AND EMERGENCIES DEFINED — TERMS/CONCEPTS

When most of us think about the term "disaster," the images of widespread destruction caused by natural phenomena or terrorism and their resulting human casualties and suffering come to mind, usually via coverage by national news media. Most of us are correct in assuming that we will not be a part of any such large, chaotic event in our lifetime. However, many will experience a less-than-national-newsworthy disaster, and this we can plan to manage.

Disasters are classified in many different ways. They are often classified by their scope, rate of onset, and source. For example, an incident may affect several counties, a single community, or a single household. Thus, disasters may occur on catastrophic, local, or personal levels (1). Their source can be natural phenomena (fires, floods), technologic accident (toxic chemical spill), or biologic (disease epidemic) (1). The Federal Emergency Management Agency (FEMA) defines catastrophic disaster as "an event that results in a large number of deaths and injuries; causes extensive destruction of facilities that provide and sustain human needs; produces an overwhelming demand on state and local response resources and mechanisms; causes a severe long-term effect on general economic activity; and severely affects state, local and private sector capabilities to begin and sustain response activities" (1).

Sebastian Heath has very eloquently explained the differences between the terms "disaster" and "emergency" (1). In that author's opinion, "disaster" and "emergency" are at two ends of a scale of everyday events in which the size of the incident and the number of resources available are less important than how well they are matched. **Emergencies** result from incidents, regardless of their size, that are met by adequate resources. If resources to deal with the problem at hand are inadequate, the situation deteriorates and a state of disaster develops.

Consideration of the personal impact on the victims experiencing the adverse event is a very important reason to develop emergency response plans. For example, a lethal fire occurring within a research animal facility will not be a declared disaster if the local fire department response is adequate to contain it, but the outcome is certainly a disaster for the scientists whose research depended upon those models and the animal care staff who cared for the animals, as well as a real financial loss for the owners of the animals and the building. It is not relevant to these victims that they were not participants in a large-scale event; they have experienced a significant loss. For these reasons, the term "emergency management plan" is preferable to "disaster plan" for most facilities.

The cornerstone of effective emergency response planning is based on the idea that better preparation for predictable adverse events can make it more difficult for them to escalate into disasters. Most facilities have a past history in which occupants have experienced occasional failures of mechanical equipment or short-term interruptions in power supply. These are known adverse events that created problems that had to be addressed. Because it is likely that similar problems would occur during a larger-scale disaster, identifying and preparing to deal with these types of day-to-day problems is the foundation of effective planning. The information contained in a sound plan is largely based upon knowledge that has been gained from previous incidents or that can reasonably be predicted to occur during a specific emergency. Identifying and solving past problems allows one to anticipate future needs, formulate plans to minimize the impact of adverse conditions on the facilities, and even take steps to prevent some losses from occurring.

III. CONCEPTS OF EMERGENCY MANAGEMENT

Effective emergency management is based upon an **all-hazards approach**. Much of what will happen in an emergency or a disaster can be predicted. Most emergencies or disasters will cause a common set of problems, and emergency management plans should address these (2). Many of the same management strategies can be applied to all types of emergencies. For example, a summer tornado and a winter blizzard may seem like very different events because they occur during different seasons; but in reality, they both generate a similar list of problems for the manager of an animal resource — loss of power to the building, lack of temperature and ventilation control in the animal rooms, employees unable to get to work, and disruption of local telephone communication are some examples of problems that would likely occur in either scenario. Emergency response plans that effectively address how to provide common needs and services become flexible and responsive in *any* major emergency.

Effective emergency management requires a partnership between the public, voluntary organizations, industry, community businesses, and all levels of government (local, state, and federal). The people who reside and work in the community have the most at stake when a disaster strikes; therefore, they should be active contributors to emergency management planning in their communities. The development of local resource networks within the community is critical to effective response. The local resource networks will be the first lines of response activated after an incident occurs. Local preparedness requires identifying resources and expertise in advance, and planning how these could be used during an emergency. Local resources have the advantage of being immediately available at the site of a disaster. These area resources need to be identified and incorporated into the local government's emergency plan.

The function of local government in emergency response is to specify the chain-of-command during the emergency, as well as to link the citizens residing in the area to higher levels of government (i.e., state and federal emergency management agencies). The second line of assistance that will be activated following a disaster is from the state government via the state emergency management agency. The Governor will proclaim a state of disaster if the damages are severe enough to overwhelm local resources. This official declaration makes state resources available. If the combined local and state resources are insufficient to manage the damage, the Governor applies to the President for federal disaster assistance. Federal funds and resources become available if the President issues a major disaster declaration. The state emergency management agency fulfills the important role of linking the local emergency response of citizens to the more extensive resources available from the Federal government. When an effective partnership exists between the citizens in a community and their local, state and federal governments, the response to a disaster will be quicker, more efficient, and effective (5).

Another important concept to understand in emergency management is that most disasters have existed throughout time and have a life cycle of occurrence. Disasters do not just suddenly appear. Hazards exist in a community and some physical event or accident occurs that alters these hazards and produces a disaster (1). Some examples of this cyclical nature of physical events that cause disasters include a 5-year flood, a 500-year flood, or a 20-year blizzard. This cyclical nature of events that cause disasters to develop forms the basis for defining four phases of emergency management that reduce the impacts of a disaster. These phases are **preparedness, response, recovery,** and **mitigation** (1, 5).

A. **The preparedness phase** includes all activities that take place *before* an incident occurs that help a community prepare to handle it. Preparedness includes plans made to save lives and assist rescue and response operations. Preparedness is being ready to respond when an emergency cannot be avoided or prevented. Simple examples of preparedness activities include installing smoke detectors in your home, posting emergency telephone numbers in animal facilities, developing evacuation plans, and storing extra food and water (1, 5).

B. **The response phase** includes all activities that take place *during and immediately following* the emergency. Response activities are designed to provide emergency assistance to victims and reduce the likelihood of additional property damage or loss. The primary responders during this phase are the local fire departments, police, rescue squads, and emergency medical services personnel. Examples of response actions taken by citizens include seeking shelter when a tornado siren is heard, evacuating a building when a fire alarm is activated, and shutting off gas valves following an earthquake.

C. **The recovery phase** includes those actions taken to return to a normal or safer state that occur *after* the emergency. The recovery phase continues until all systems return to normal (or better). Short-term recovery returns vital life-support systems to minimum operating standards. Long-term recovery of a community may take several years. Once the immediate danger is over, the continued safety and well-being of people depends upon their ability to cope with the rearrangements in their lives and environments. Recovery phase activities include contacting one's insurance agent or getting financial assistance from the government to rebuild a home or business.

D. **The mitigation phase** includes actions that prevent or minimize the effects of an emergency. This phase occurs *both before and after* an emergency (1, 5, 6). Mitigation is a very important phase of emergency management because its goals are to prevent emergencies or reduce the damaging effects if an emergency is unavoidable. All mitigation is local, and it should be based upon hazard identification and risk assessment. Mitigation is the most cost-effective intervention in disasters. Examples of mitigation activities include purchasing flood insurance, enforcing building codes in earthquake-prone areas, installing tie-downs on mobile homes, backing up computer databases, and passing zoning ordinances that restrict residential development in flood plains. The National Governors Emergency Preparedness Study found that mitigation activities were a relatively minor part of state and local emergency planning efforts. This study recommends that mitigation activities become a more important part of emergency management planning (1).

In summary, local disaster preparedness should be the top priority of animal research facilities because disasters occur most frequently at the local level and the problems that occur in small-scale disasters are the same problems that occur in large-scale disasters. The only functional animal facilities that exist following a disaster will be those that had good contingency plans before the disaster occurred.

IV. INCIDENT MANAGEMENT/INCIDENT COMMAND SYSTEM

When a disaster occurs within a community, the local emergency operations plan is activated. The **emergency operations center (EOC)** is opened. This center is usually a permanent, fixed facility from which the response to the incident is activated. It is organized in such a way that department heads, government officials, and disaster agencies can gather to coordinate their response. The role of the emergency operations center during the response to a disaster is to make certain that the policies and procedures stated in the community's plan are implemented (5). Groups that have not been included during prior development of the community's emergency operations plan will likely not be allowed access to the emergency operations center during the emergency. This means that a perfect response plan for an animal facility can be worthless if the plan is unknown to the Emergency Managers in the community at the time the disaster strikes. This is the basis for the recommendation in the *Guide* that a responsible manager or veterinarian from the facility be a member of the appropriate safety committee and an "official responder" (4). Without this connection, the facility's plan is not officially recognized and may not be supported during the emergency.

The response to emergencies is coordinated through the **Incident Management System (IMS)**, also called the **Incident Command System (ICS)**. This system is designed to operate from the time the incident occurs until it is resolved. The objectives of using the incident management system are to save lives, protect property and the environment, coordinate resources so that duplication of effort is avoided, enable multi-jurisdictional activities so that hazards can be managed more effectively, and integrate support with state and federal emergency management agencies. An important concept to understand about the incident management system is that it is based upon unity of command. This means that the lines of authority and decision making are pre-determined and rigid. When conflicts arise, only one person is in charge. This individual is designated in the emergency operations plan. The incident management system uses existing resources and agency procedures when directing its response to the emergency. It is best if the responders during a disaster perform functions that are similar to those that they perform in everyday life. For example, firemen extinguish fires and police secure buildings and arrest looters, not vice versa. Trained animal care professionals should capture and remove animals. The structure of an effective IMS is modular, allowing it to be easily expanded as the complexity of an incident increases, and to allow recruitment of only those units in the community that are required for the response. Modular design allows the IMS to maintain an effective span of control by keeping the functions of units focused on their objectives, and not allowing the size of any single unit to become too large to be effectively supervised and directed (5, 6).

The **Incident Command Post** is set up near the location of the incident. From this location, all response to the incident will be coordinated and directed. The **Incident Manager** is assigned responsibility for resolution of the incident. In most cases, the Incident Manager is the first trained representative of the primary response unit that reports to the scene. For example, the fire chief would be designated as incident manager if a fire were the primary incident, while a police officer would assume the role of incident manager if the incident involved a crime or an accident. Other important individuals at the incident command post include the **Safety Officer**, who is responsible for protecting response personnel, and the **Information Officer**, who interfaces between the incident manager and the media. The interaction between the EOC and IMS is shown in Figure 1.

It is important to understand that a gap commonly exists in integration of response for animals because emergency managers are unaware of the size and complexity of the animal care industries within their communities, and animal health care providers are uninformed and do not understand the definitive authority and responsibility of emergency management over all operations during disasters. To ensure the welfare of animals during an emergency or disaster, only veterinarians and professional animal care providers should perform supervisory functions at the incident command post.

The steps that need to be taken to stabilize an emergency are briefly summarized in Figure 2.

V.   EMERGENCY OPERATIONS PLAN

An **Emergency Operations Plan (EOP)** is developed to provide systematic response to an emergency. There are three important concepts to keep in mind when developing an EOP (1, 5):

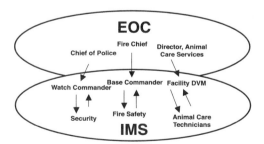

Figure 1. The interaction between the Emergency Operations Center (EOC) and the Incident Management System (IMS).

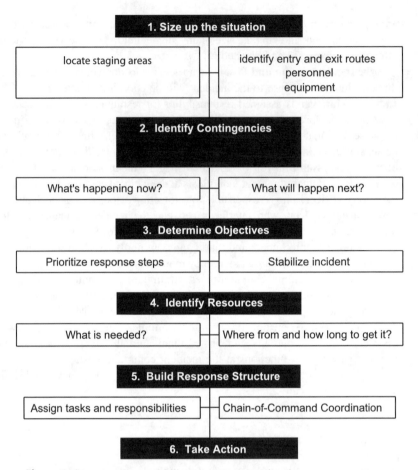

Figure 2. Steps to take to stabilize an emergency situation.

A. **The plan should rely on existing structures of organizations that are responsive in non-emergency situations**. Veterinarians and skilled animal care professionals should determine the needs of animals following a disaster. Local veterinary services, animal control agencies, humane shelters and permanent businesses, including research facilities, should be participants.

B. **Crises should be met at the lowest and most immediate level of government**. The local response capabilities within the community must be identified and recruited first. Effective response for animals can only occur if veterinarians and professional animal care providers are represented in the emergency operations center, the emergency operations plan and the incident management system.

C. **Voluntary response and involvement of the private sector must be emphasized.**

Emergency operations plans are living documents. Good plans share several characteristics. First, they are based on facts or valid assumptions. The quality of decision that an incident manager makes during an emergency is largely determined by the accuracy of the information being received about the incident and the correctness of the response capabilities outlined in the plan. The plan should address common threats to the community. Second, the plan must be based on the inventory of resources present within the community. To effectively draw upon local resources from the private sector, these businesses and organizations must be identified and included in the plan. Third, the plan must provide the necessary organizational structure and define the chain-of-command. Finally, the elements of the plan must be coordinated together so that multiple groups are not working at cross-purposes. Emergency operations plans must be reviewed and updated frequently so that the information contained within them is current. It is common for information that changes frequently, such as names and telephone numbers, to be included as an appendix to the basic plan so that extensive editing is not necessary (1, 5, 6).

VI. TRAINING AND TESTING AN EMERGENCY OPERATIONS PLAN

In order to be reasonably certain that the plan and emergency response procedures will work, it should be tested before a real emergency occurs. Testing is usually done in four separate phases, with each phase acting as a building block for the more complicated training exercises that follow it (5). The phases are outlined below.

PHASE 1: ORIENTATION

In this phase of training, key responders of the animal facility's staff meet with official first-responders from their institution to review the proposed plan. Contacts with the appropriate county and/or state emergency planners should be initiated by the first-responders at the institution/company during this phase. Meetings are scheduled between the managers/veterinarians and the technicians to inform them about the plan and seek their input in revising it. The initial methods proposed in the plan for moving animals and cages are tested by technicians to make certain that they work, and they are revised accordingly as problems are uncovered. At this stage, living animals are not needed for practice. A lot can be learned about potential evacuation problems by moving empty racks. Proposed evacuation routes can be walked off, and obstacles to evacuation, such as narrow doorways and egress-only doors can be identified along the routes. At this stage, the incident command system is not practiced. This is a very low key, low stress phase of training.

Phase 2: Tabletop Exercise

In this phase of training, the plan has already been reviewed at least once and revised. The focus of a tabletop exercise is to familiarize the participants in the plan with their roles, responsibilities, and the procedures they will follow during emergency response. During this phase of training, a scenario is created, and individuals are required to make decisions and respond just as they would in a real emergency. During this phase, animal facility managers/veterinarians interact with the official first-responders at their institution. The managers/ veterinarians gain training and experience with the incident command system. The stress level is slightly higher during this training phase because facility managers/veterinarians must respond to a threatening situation with a decision. After our facility managers were comfortable with the incident command system, we went back into our facility and taught it to our technicians. At this stage of training, no animals or equipment were actually moved. The major purpose of the tabletop exercise was to emphasize how coordination among the various responding agencies would occur during a real emergency.

Phase 3: Walk-Through Drill

In this exercise, the emergency management group and the response teams actually perform their emergency functions. In this phase, the IMS system is practiced, and equipment and animals are moved in the same manner that they would be moved in a real emergency situation or evacuation. An Incident Manager is placed in charge, an Incident Command Post is set up, and the key responders for the animal facility report to it. Call-up procedures for technicians are tested. Animals are evacuated from the facility. At the author's facility, we moved only a few racks of animals, and we did not subject rodents on research studies to the additional stress of evacuation; rather, we practiced with rodents that were being culled from breeding colonies, and used large animals that were already accustomed to traveling between facilities. Gaps in the assignment of tasks became obvious during this stage of testing. Whether the functional exercise runs smoothly or poorly, information is gained that can be used to further modify the plan and strengthen it. At this stage, we invited representatives from county and state emergency management agencies to view our exercise and evaluate it. The goal of every animal resource's emergency plan should be to conduct this type of exercise at regular intervals.

Phase 4: Functional Drill

This exercise is very similar to the walk-through drill, but focuses on evaluating a specific function or component of the plan. For example, you may have uncovered problems with security during a previous walk-through drill, and revised your plan accordingly. You now wish to test these improvements. You would run an exercise and have the security aspects re-evaluated by trained emergency management professionals.

PHASE 5: FULL-SCALE EXERCISE

This phase is a test of the complete emergency management system, including activation of the **Emergency Operations Center**. This exercise combines the functional drill, in which all components of the animal facility's plan are tested, with the coordination of outside agencies, such as county and state emergency management agencies. Because full-scale exercises require multi-agency participation, they are the largest training exercises and they are not conducted very frequently. The testing of full interagency coordination is the goal of this exercise.

It is important that advanced exercises not be attempted until the easier exercises and drills are running well. The surest way to have the emergency response plan fail is to try to manage a large-scale exercise without having the basic training of the staff completed first.

VII. STEPS IN WRITING AN EMERGENCY RESPONSE PLAN FOR AN ANIMAL FACILITY

The steps in writing a plan are briefly outlined below. These steps have already been described in detail elsewhere (6, 7).

A. ESTABLISH A PLANNING TEAM

The members of the planning team should include the first-responders at the company or institution, representatives from upper management, veterinarians, technicians, members from the public relations office, and members from the health and safety office, legal and financial areas. The group should be authorized by the C.E.O. of the company or institution to develop the plan. A mission statement should be developed that defines the purpose of the plan. A tentative schedule and budget should be developed at this stage.

B. ANALYZE CAPABILITIES AND HAZARDS

In this step, information about current response capabilities and potential hazards is gathered. Existing policies and plans such as evacuation procedures, fire protection plans, security procedures, and environmental practices are reviewed. A vulnerability analysis is done to determine how well a given facility could handle a given type of emergency. Critical functions of the animal facility are identified at this stage, and multiple methods for ensuring these functions are developed. Examples of critical functions in an animal resource include providing shelter and safe confinement, feed, water, veterinary care, humane euthanasia, and clean caging. Some of the methods the manager might choose to use to accomplish these vital functions are summarized in Table 1 below.

It is important that the plan include how to create back-up systems for loss of lifeline services such as electrical power, water, and telecommunications. Portable generators can be used to power fans to keep animals from overheating. Back-up sources of light include flashlights, light sticks, and lanterns. Head-mounted flashlights are useful because they provide illumination while enabling a person to have full use of both hands. This is very important if work must be performed in the dark. Back-up sources of water include clean water contained in pipe chases, stills, and soft water tanks. Many research buildings have soft water supplied throughout the building. Huge tanks hold and condition this water. These tanks could be tapped to provide drinking water for animals in an emergency. Many research laboratories throughout the building may make their own water by using stills or filtering systems. It might be possible to get small quantities of clean, drinkable water from these sources, too. An additional source that should not be forgotten for rodents includes the gel-packs that are commonly placed inside of shipping boxes. These gel packs provide a safe, non-spillable source of moisture that could sustain a cage of rats or mice for up to a week. Depending upon the size and type of emergency, the local fire department may also be able to bring large quantities of clean drinking water. Back-up sources for telecommunications include walkie-talkies, radios, and cellular phones.

External resources that might be needed in an emergency are also identified at this stage. This would include finding alternative locations where animals could be housed if an evacuation was mandatory. The author has found that many members of our local American Association of Laboratory Animal Science (AALAS) branch are very cooperative in volunteering to assist with emergency sheltering of research animals.

C.   DEVELOP THE PLAN

The following basic components should be included in every plan: **Executive Summary, Emergency Management Elements, Emergency Response Procedures and Support Documents**. The executive summary gives management an overview of the purpose of the plan, the authority and responsibility of key personnel, and where response operations will be managed (6).

TABLE 1. Examples of Addressing Critical Functions in an Emergency

Critical Function	Usual Method That Accomplishes Critical Function	Alternate Method That Might Be Used to Accomplish Function
House a dog	Stainless steel pen inside facility	Plastic airline transport crate from pet store
Sanitize dirty caging	Mechanical washer in facility	Dip in 1:10 solution of water and bleach
Euthanize rodents	Carbon dioxide gas tank	Veterinary euthanasia solution

The emergency management elements include a description of the incident command system, the location of the EOC, how security will be maintained, and how response will be coordinated with outside units. Communications procedures that will be followed during the emergency are described, as well as the notification and warning procedures for employees at the time the emergency occurs. Evacuation routes, areas where evacuating personnel should assemble, and how they will be accounted for are detailed. Shutdown procedures that minimize damage inside the facility and methods for preserving vital records should be included in the response plan. Contacts with community groups, such as local emergency program managers, and contact persons at regulatory agencies need to be stated. The procedure for dealing with media during the emergency should be clearly defined in the response plan, and the public information officer should be designated. The plan should also be appended with important logistical information, such as names and phone numbers, maps, resource inventories, and contact persons who repair critical equipment.

D.   IMPLEMENT THE PLAN

This is the final step. It includes increasing awareness among employees of the importance of the plan and the procedures that will be followed, and training them to execute the plan.

VIII. CONCLUSION

Developing an emergency response plan for an animal facility is not difficult. When an emergency or disaster occurs, advanced planning is the key to mobilizing resources quickly. By tying the plan for an animal facility into the existing response structure of the institution and the community, the plan becomes properly authorized and it can be promptly enacted when an emergency occurs. With a basic understanding of the structure of the incident management system and knowledge of the basic needs of the animals, anyone can write an effective plan. A properly developed response plan allows the manager of an animal facility to maintain responsibility and control over activities that might affect his or her animals. As the national trend for including animals in community disaster plans grows, members of the animal research community should participate.

REFERENCES

1. **Heath, S.E.**, *Animal Management in Disasters*, Mosby, Inc., St. Louis, 1999.
2. **Federal Emergency Management Agency**, *Animals in Disaster: Module A: Awareness and Preparedness*, Course No. IS-010, Emergency Management Institute, Emmitsburg, MD, May, 1998.

3. **Federal Emergency Management Agency**, *Animals in Disaster: Module B: Community Planning*, Course No. IS-011, Emergency Management Institute, Emmitsburg, MD, May, 1998.

4. **Committee to Revise the *Guide for the Care and Use of Laboratory Animals***, *Guide for the Care and Use of Laboratory Animals*, National Research Council, National Academy Press, Washington, D.C., 1996.

5. **Federal Emergency Management Agency**, *The Emergency Program Manager*, Course No. IS-1, Emergency Management Institute, Emmitsburg, MD, September, 1993.

6. **American Red Cross**, *Emergency Management Guide for Business and Industry. A Step-by-Step Approach to Emergency Planning, Response and Recovery for Companies of All Sizes*. American Red Cross Publication No. ARC 5025, American National Red Cross, Washington, D.C., November, 1993.

7. **Vogelweid, C.M.**, Developing emergency management plans for university laboratory animal programs and facilities, *Contemp. Top. Lab. Anim. Sci.*, 37, 52, 1998.

15 Animal Resource Security

DeWayne H. Walker, D.V.M., Dipl. ACLAM

Facility security is often viewed as "someone else's job," and is often an incidental component in an animal care and use program. While this is partially true in that many institutions have on-site or consulting security experts, the job of securing an institution should be the job of everyone within the program. Facility managers in particular must assume the role of seeing security from virtually every aspect but most importantly they must appreciate the "big picture," Effective security measures are vital to protect the integrity, quality, and worth of the research as well as to protect researchers, animal care staff, animal colonies, and physical structures. A well-managed security program needs to be obvious and visible to those seeking to invade or disrupt an animal care and use program while being as transparent as possible to those legitimately working within the program. **The objective of security is to develop a balanced program with prevention and protection of assets while providing a work environment where innovation and mobility are not hampered by a "bunker mentality."**

This chapter will view the issue of security from an initial broad perspective down to individual details that may be of benefit in a given program. The "big picture" commences with a risk analysis of each facility and its activities so as to project the potential risks involved. This is followed up with development of plans, policies and procedures for securing the facilities, strategies to protect resources, and crisis action plans should a security incident take place. This chapter will then examine "hard" security, those pieces of security equipment that can increase the level of protection. These range from standard locks to more sophisticated sensor detection systems. Finally, this chapter will discuss "soft" security, the need to address personnel whether they be visitors, animal care staff, investigators, maintenance staff, etc. There is typically a need for continuing education and a large dose of common sense when dealing with personnel.

I. RISK ASSESSMENT, RISK REDUCTION, AND CRISIS RESPONSE

A. THE NEED FOR A RISK ASSESSMENT

The objective of an animal care and use program risk assessment includes an assessment of the physical security needs of the program and an evaluation of risk for the types of research being conducted in the program. One has to generally assume that individuals who invade or disrupt animal care and use programs are not doing so for financial gain (theft of valued property) or casual vandalism. Instead, it is more likely that they are pursing an animal activist cause with purposeful vandalism, disruption of business, harassment of personnel and/or potential bodily harm in mind. Therefore, one of the first assessments to be made is the program's susceptibility to attack in terms of location and access, and the types of research or activity involved in the program. The most desired targets for animal activists are those that are easily penetrated while having a high value for sensationalism. Those facilities that conduct work with companion animals or nonhuman primates and/or conduct work in areas that are considered more sensitive, such as toxicity testing, trauma and burn studies or invasive surgeries, are inherently preferred targets (1). Even when the animal use efforts are fully justified and are necessary research procedures, these species and procedures are likely to elicit public concern and, therefore, provide the activists with an opportunity for maximizing the emotional play following a security breach. A risk analysis of all of the research or animal holding areas may reveal that potential weaknesses do exist in areas of sensitive research or specific species of animals thereby warranting consideration for fortifying these critical areas.

B.   THE RISK ASSESSMENT TEAM

Although a risk assessment can often be conducted satisfactorily by animal care management staff, the best approach to securing a program is by establishing a representative team. In addition to management/administration, the team should have representation from the research staff, the animal care staff, security, and public relations. A team has the advantage of assessing risk from each member's viewpoint and should include awareness and support of top management given the potential need for investment. A research staff member can provide input on trends in research efforts toward a higher or lower state of sensitivity as previously described. They can also help discuss the potential impact of security initiatives on research innovation and logistics. The animal care staff is best represented by an individual(s) with a working knowledge of the institution's day-to-day operation and an appreciation of animal activism tactics and current activities. The security team member brings to the table the experience and knowledge of the technology available for securing sites and a good understanding of crisis response management. Finally, the public relations representative brings to the table the philosophy of the institution in addressing major issues and the strategy and practices currently in place to interact with the public regarding such issues. Although other individuals can undoubtedly bring added value to the project, the above team would represent a good starting point.

C.   PLANNING RISK REDUCTION

The risk assessment team should approach security from all of the perspectives of the diverse team. The research investigator and animal care staff should categorize all ongoing projects using animals to provide the team with an overview of the physical location of various species and projects that carry a higher risk because of potential controversy (e.g., invasive work as previously noted). Animal activist organizations frequently obtain regulatory inspection information on institutions through the Freedom of Information Act; therefore, the animal care representative should review the institution's history with regulatory bodies and any cited infractions that could be a source for activist attention. The research investigator might provide an opinion on the attitudes of other investigators and students on animal activism, the perceived level of loyalty to the institution and the emotional climate of the institution. The security representative would be called upon to apprise the team of the type of security system in place, component advantages and disadvantages, history of security issues pertinent to the animal care and use program, and functional status of the security system. Additionally, this individual might wish to also assess the general layout and location of animal facilities, laboratories conducting animal research and accessibility of non-research/animal care personnel to these vulnerable areas. Finally, the public relations representative should provide current information on local risks from animal activist organizations, particularly noting any shifts in their priorities and strategies and providing updating of local events such as rallies. Based upon a concern that everyone may be too familiar with the institution's mode of operation, it may be an option, approved through the public relations representative, to contract with a knowledgeable outsider to review the institution's animal care and use program. This could provide a useful, candid, third-party impression of the program. All members of the team should also be encouraged to tactfully network with peer institutions in order to share respective information and benchmark similar security efforts.

The initial risk assessment of an animal care and use program should not be viewed as a one-time event. Meetings should be held on a regular basis for updates by all of the members of the risk assessment team. Security deficiencies from any perspective should be identified, discussed, timely correction dates established and audited for completeness. In periods of apparent low risk activity, consideration should be given to developing various crisis scenarios (break-ins, demonstrations, personnel threats, etc.) to allow the team to evaluate various contingency responses. As a final preparatory note, a clearly defined chain of command arrangement and team responsibilities, according to job function, should be identified in preparation for any crisis.

D.   RESPONDING TO A CRISIS

Although risk assessment, including regular team risk assessment meetings, is invaluable in reducing or lessening the impact of a security breach, a security crisis may still arise. A security crisis differs from all of the prevention efforts that have been undertaken by a risk assessment team up to this point. Risk assessments and pre-crisis preparation will be implemented but must be augmented by additional institutional resources. Depending on the crisis situation, the administration and additional public relations experts are likely to have a more prominent role in communicating appropriate information to the media (refer to Chapter 16). Much of this up-to-date information on research projects, animal care program regulatory records and institutional policies and procedures should be assembled and refined into position statements with the help of the risk assessment team. Additionally, this should bring into action the institution's disaster plan. The animal facility manager should have readied a document that not only addresses natural disasters but also manmade threats. This document should include not only the evacuation plans for animal facility personnel but also the short and long term fate of the housed animals. The key to successful crisis management of any issue or situation is preparation, which will reduce the actual emergency response to systematic mechanics.

II. HARD SECURITY: EQUIPMENT AND SYSTEMS

A. General Considerations

Several general statements can be made regarding physical security.

First, equipment does not stand alone in providing a security system. Security personnel and individuals working within an animal care and use program are as critical, if not more so, to the success of a security system. Personnel will be addressed in the next section.

Second, physical security should be viewed as having a layered configuration. That is, no single piece of security equipment can be the ultimate deterrent to intruders. An effective security system is multi-layered for redundancy not only in case one layer is disabled by an intruder but also to provide time delays so that other system components can be activated to handle the situation.

Third, physical security can be very expensive. It is important to conduct a financial assessment of the benefits of various additions or upgrades to a system. A security expert should always be included in any system assessment; however, remember that from that expert's perspective, security is the number one issue and budget is not the top priority. Security advice should be taken seriously, although the animal resource manager should have considerable say in the final decision of system equipment and financial costs.

Fourth, it is important to take the time to be actively involved with the design of any new animal care and use building or the refurbishment of an existing animal care and use building. The manager should think "big picture" vs. more or bigger locks. During the design stage, one should discuss equipment options with security experts and urge that access points to critical areas be minimized. Minimizing access points where feasible can result in cost savings and reduce vulnerability.

Finally, the manager should remember to periodically test for equipment failures and personnel intervention. For example, it is not uncommon for maintenance personnel working in restricted areas to deactivate alarms for convenience reasons and not reconnect them when their work is finished. Even security personnel have been known to turn alarms off following episodes of frequent false alarms. The system should be tested both during the day and at night if a response by security personnel is required. It is important to communicate regularly with the security department to learn of any changes in personnel that may cause delays in response or monitoring.

B. EXTERNAL LAYERING

To evaluate security systems, it is worthwhile to re-emphasize the importance of layering. Layering can ideally commence at the extreme borders of the institution's property line. Natural barriers, such as rivers, lakes, cliffs, rock formations, and difficult terrain, can be used as a part of a facility's first layer of security. However, natural barriers alone are rarely available to the average institution so the first layer is often a fence. Although warning signs and fences can be intimidating to casual trespassers, fences are typically easily breached in minutes by anyone intent on serious invasion of the property. Fences often give an institution a false sense of security and can be compromised by factors such as landscaping. To make a fence less intrusive to the general public, landscaping is commonly used to camouflage the fence. Although an aesthetic improvement, the downside is that addition of bushes, high plants, and other structures provide excellent hiding places for potential intruders. When assessing landscaping along fence lines, preference should be given to locating the landscaping a reasonable distance outside of the perimeter fence. Low foliage or beautification structures are generally acceptable around a building structure but they should also be placed several feet away from the building structure. Most importantly, there should be a large expanse of open space between the perimeter fence and the building. Closed circuit television (CCTV) cameras to scan the open space and building perimeter provide a good level of deterrence. When properly configured, it is estimated that an intruder should require at least 10 minutes from initially breaching the security fence to reaching the target building while triggering multiple alarm systems. This is calculated in most instances to give security personnel and local police adequate time to respond (2). However, the theme of layering must continue within the building in case response time is delayed.

C. INTERNAL LAYERING

Physical security systems within a given building must be designed with layering that provides both diversity and redundancy. Diversity provides cross-checking on a situation while redundancy ensures that every component is backed up in case of failure. Security systems for layering within a building include, but are not limited to, warning signs, secured doors, lock systems, alarm systems, CCTV, and electronic access systems.

1.   Warning Signs

Warning signs are part of the first layer of control in a physical security system. They provide information to the legitimate visitors and personnel within a facility. Although they are not a direct deterrent for an actual break-in, they can indirectly be a deterrent to a mole (a person who infiltrates the organization by stealth) who is gathering information on the facility. Warning signs indicating restricted entry and/or noting an area protected by a security system (e.g., alarm, CCTV) may result in the individual electing not to enter the area, and therefore not giving themselves away if challenged. However, it is important that warning signs be legitimate in having a functional security component and not be a false notice that cannot be delivered.

2.   Secured Doors

Doors can be a component of the second layer of deterrence. Doors to secured areas should be of commercial or industrial grade materials and construction. The doors should be equipped with a detection device and monitored to ensure that they return to a closed and locked position after being opened. If equipped with magnetic door contacts, the mechanism should be tested regularly. Traditionally, access control is weak in areas that contain dock doors for transfer of feed, bedding, waste, etc. Dock doors should be evaluated for complete closure and alarmed after hours. Dock doors should lock from the inside and be inaccessible from the outside. Emergency doors also present a problem in weighing safety vs. security. As an example, in 1999 a major break-in at a university animal facility was accomplished when the intruders scaled the building's exterior wall and entered through an unlocked roof entry door (3). Given the multiple scenarios associated with safety codes, no common solution can be proposed. However, given the potential for emergency doors to be a weak link in the security program, the issue should be thoroughly considered. Finally, it is prudent to have all doors numbered and coded for easy identification. A door code numbering system enables employees and security staff to identify a specific door quickly. This is especially valuable in a large decentralized facility.

3.   Lock Systems

Locks are the most essential component of many physical security systems. They must, however, be suited to the security expectations with an understanding that they all have inherent weaknesses. Combination locks are one of the least secure methods for controlling access as there is frequently a failure to follow the procedures for purging and updating combinations. Combinations should be changed periodically, at least every 3 months, to minimize the risk of compromised and unauthorized access. Keys are effective, but require considerable oversight in terms of accountability. As a manager, one should have considerable input into who is authorized to have a key. A single individual should manage assignment of keys; maintain master keys that never leave the facility; periodically conduct key validation reviews; and be prepared to re-key critical entry points if assigned keys are lost. Mechanical key-pads provide a low level of security and are generally not recommended unless the area already has very restricted traffic and individuals have passed through multiple security checks to this entry point. The three- to five-digit code must be frequently changed, minimally every 3 months, in order for this system to have any security value since codes are easily exchanged between individuals and there is no means of auditing.

4.   Alarm Systems

Alarm systems come in multiple combinations with increasing levels of sophistication. However, their main function of signaling the presence of a situation that requires immediate attention is the same regardless of type. In fulfilling this function, they must be 100% reliable and not be prone to false alarms, which create complacency among staff responsive to the alarm. Appropriate signage should accompany alarms to prevent individuals from accidentally tripping an alarm. Alarms that annunciate locally are used to deter unauthorized activity by alerting personnel in the area. These types of local alarms are not expensive and can be effective if supported by periodic assessment. However, they can be easily dismantled and depend upon the life of battery(s). Hard-wired systems that also transmit signals to a central location are preferred, albeit considerably more expensive.

Alarm sensors can be of several types, but the most common are magnetic contact switches and motion detection devices. Magnetic contact switches are located on a hinged or sliding door or on a window where they will signal an alarm when the magnetic switches lose contact. If these devices are used, it is recommended to recess the switches to reduce potential tampering and to use balanced switches. Regular magnetic switches can be disabled with an external magnet, whereas a balanced magnetic switch operates by creating a balanced magnetic field that detects increases and decreases in the sensor's magnetic field strength. Motion detectors are a part of most modern alarm systems and can have a variety of technologies: ultrasonic waves, infrared light waves, microwave fields, and passive infrared. All of the technologies are reasonably good; however, consideration should be given to a dual element sensor system. By using two of the technologies, many false alarms caused by such anomalies as an outside vibration, temperature fluctuations, or even flying insects can overcome the limitations of a single element sensor.

In addition to the hardware, it is important that a call list be agreed upon for response to an alarm condition. The list should be prioritized with the animal resource manager near the top of the list. Name, address, and telephone number should be on the list. In addition, there should be a requirement for creating a written report to provide an audit trail for each alarm. The report documents the alarm date and time, the cause of the alarm, the name of the person from the call list who was contacted, and the date and time of the contact.

5.　CCTV Systems

Closed Circuit Television (CCTV) is an excellent tool for general surveillance, assessment, and verification; however, it is still only a part of a layered security system and not a first response component. The display of cameras can have a deterrent effect for general security issues, but will not deter serious security threats. There are four components to a CCTV system: cameras, monitors, recorders, and switches. In the selection of cameras, preference should be given to solid-state chip units for providing optimum image quality and minimal maintenance costs. For interior and daytime exterior applications, color cameras are preferable to black and white as they provide superior identification and verification of subjects; however, the color units require more light and may not be suited to night-time applications. Cameras that can pan, tilt, and zoom are suited only to general surveillance as they can create "dead zones" of non-continuous coverage. Fixed position cameras are, therefore, preferable for most applications. Color monitors with a viewing screen of 12 to 15 inches are the preferred norm. If security personnel must monitor several screens continuously one may wish to encourage using motion detection to send alarm signals to the security station to identify activity in the monitored area. Given the potential for fatigue from the continuous viewing of multiple screens, the motion detection system increases the attendant's effectiveness by providing alerts to real-time events. Commercial grade recorders should be used to continuously record images of the monitored area and to provide an audit trail of all activity. Video switches are an option for multiple camera systems but are best suited for general surveillance only. They basically provide a 10-second snapshot of an area then rotate to one or more additional areas creating dead zones of up to 30 seconds before returning to a scan of the original site. Additionally, video motion detection is not an option when switches are employed. Thus, switches are generally not recommended in applications that require continuous video coverage.

6.　Electronic Access Systems

Electronic access systems, or card and personal identification number (PIN) access systems, are used to control access into and out of an area. There are multiple commercial systems available, and the card or PIN may be used alone or in combination with an electronically controlled access system. All electronic access systems must be equipped for the possibility of losing the primary power source. A battery backup must be designed into the overall system since door locks may become inoperative with power loss, thus trapping personnel. Given the need for year-round coverage by animal care personnel, such entrapment could be a serious safety concern over a weekend shift. In extremely secure areas such as surgery or containment areas, consideration might be given to a dual validation system that offers a higher level of access control. This might be a system of a card reader combined with a requirement to enter a unique PIN on the numeric keypad. Both card and PIN systems have their shortcomings although both systems are becoming commonplace in animal facilities. Lost or stolen cards should be reported immediately to security personnel so that access privileges can be removed from the system. The PIN system is generally secure, but in a large institution there is a concern that a failure to delete old PINS from the system or to update PINS can cause vulnerability in the system. Both card and PIN systems have the capability to provide an audit trail.

III. THE HUMAN COMPONENT TO SECURITY

Institutional personnel are the cornerstone and collective strength of a security system, as neither sophisticated hardware nor dedicated security personnel alone or together can guarantee a fail-safe system without willing participants. It is critical that personnel are made aware of the security risks associated with their work and their responsibilities for maintaining a safe and secure workplace.

A. TRAINING AND EDUCATION

Training and education programs keep people informed about potential security risks, teach them physical security procedures and techniques, show them how to respond in case an incident occurs, and ensure that everyone knows what resources are available. The following is a collection of suggested training topics related to security for animal facility personnel.

1. Response to Local Alarms

A quick, consistent response to every local alarm situation shows that the institution is serious about enforcing security procedures. Personnel should be trained to immediately communicate any alarm to the facility manager. In turn, an immediate assessment can be made as to any problem with the system or the need for immediate follow-up should the alarm reflect a real intrusion.

2. Validation Testing

All systems should be periodically tested to verify functionality and performance. Although the majority of this effort lies with the security experts, it provides the opportunity for assessing staff action to an alarm situation.

3.   Reminding Staff of Bad Practices

Staff should not prop doors open or shut off alarms on weekends. Staff should not allow delivery personnel inside the facility. Staff should not allow piggy-backing (potential unauthorized person following an authorized person) or tailgating (potential unauthorized person entering as an authorized person leaves) through a control point such as a card reader. Staff should be instructed never to give out to unconfirmed requesters the home address or telephone number of a coworker.

4.   Reminding Staff of Responsible Practices

The staff should be instructed to challenge anyone not displaying proper credentials (badge system). Further, the staff should be made aware of temporary situations that may put their facility at risk. Examples include the presence of contract workers in the animal facility who might accidentally disconnect local alarms being disconnected for the convenience of their work or the exposure of these temporary workers to sensitive areas without proper training in the unit's mission. Also, on-site construction can result in unfenced scaffolding running up the side of the building to roof entry points, as well as an opportunity for accidental power loss consequential to any wiring work. The manager should teach the staff to be constantly on guard for infiltrators. For example, past incidents have shown that persons who never eat with other workers might be scribbling notes or phoning a contact, or those who never change out of work clothes in anyone else's presence might be concealing a camera. At the same time, however, one should remind staff that they are not vigilantes and that they should share security concerns with the manager and security personnel (2).

B.   Hiring Personnel and Keeping Them Satisfied

A vast majority of institution security breaches of a physical break-in or public relations nature have come about through either the careless hiring of an infiltrator or consequential to information being leaked to activists by a disgruntled employee. Photographs or videotape and eyewitness accounts by infiltrators or disgruntled employees enable activists to attract media attention and convince the public and authorities of their alleged charges. As a result, security of a research program involves a broad, multifaceted plan to discourage or eliminate infiltration and to inhibit, or at the very least identify, disgruntled employees.

1.   Hiring Animal Care Staff

Conducting background checks to identify infiltrators or those with excessive sensitivity on animal use issues is an essential preventive measure. It is not enough to verify the professional credentials of an applicant. Before permitting an employee to enter the research facility, the institution should be assured of the true identity and purpose of each applicant, and how he or she will handle the issue of animal research. A comprehensive background check would generally include calls to all listed references with appropriate questions about animal research issues. It is also helpful to obtain additional references from listed references and to ask those additional references questions about the applicant's views on animal research issues. Additional references could include educators (i.e., instructors from animal technician programs) and minimally the last employer from the animal care field. In the United Kingdom the issue is so serious that there is a database called the Animal Rights National Index which is provided by Scotland Yard as an employer hiring reference (4). In the United States this measure is not available; however, pending the acceptance by the institution's department of human resources, you may request applicants to supply information on prior arrests and convictions. Perhaps more subtle and equally effective is to network as a manager, talking with your peers about their knowledge of a given candidate. It is increasingly common that new hires come from technical programs or transfer from peer institutions as opposed to being hired off the street. Finally, to avoid discrimination charges in hiring personnel that meet security requirements, institutions should document all actions carefully, be consistent, and forewarn all applicants that background checks are conducted (5).

2.   Disgruntled Employees

Factors that may be completely out of a manager's control such as cutbacks in personnel or the freezing of promotions, wages, bonuses, or benefits, may convert an otherwise loyal employee into an individual on a quest to get even. Although this is generally rare, it is nevertheless something managers and supervisors should be aware of and seek early guidance from their institution's human resources department. Another cause for an employee to become disgruntled is the existence of animal welfare concerns leading to an employee's disclosure to the animal activist community. This is a situation in which the manager can and should have knowledge and involvement. The opportunity to be an animal welfare "whistle-blower" without fear of reprisal by the institution is mandated within the Animal Welfare Act Regulations and needs to be honored (6). However, "whistle-blowing" implies that something improper is going on within the institution and if it is within the animal facility, it should be identified and immediately remedied. If it is outside of the animal facility, perhaps in a given investigators laboratory, a good manager should show empathy and intervene on behalf of the concerned employee. The manager should work with the employee to investigate misunderstandings, misconceptions, or to support the individual through the proper Institutional Animal Care and Use Committee mechanisms for investigating animal welfare concerns.

Finally, a good manager should be aware of the status of morale of the staff and be sensitive at all times to the good work of personnel in jobs that may be erroneously perceived by others as low level or only semi-skilled.

C.   INTERNAL COMMUNICATION

Communication is very important within an institution. Everyone within the institution should feel comfortable with the animal care and use program, and should feel secure with the way they and their resources are being protected. It should be understood that security measures are not meant to be punitive to employees but are based upon sound risk assessment of vulnerable areas. Animal resource managers should feel comfortable that everyone in the institution has an understanding of, albeit not always in complete agreement with, why and how animals are used in the institution. Individual institutions need to decide how this is achieved, perhaps by a pamphlet or perhaps by meetings. Regardless of the method employed, it goes a long way when the personnel within the institution have awareness and acceptance of the program and, therefore, assume an enhanced level of responsibility in keeping it secure.

D.   EXTERNAL COMMUNICATION

Communication outside of the institution can also provide great value, although the extent of the communication may vary among institutions, based on need and resources to support such an effort. It is essential to interact with groups, such as the local fire and police departments, that may require access to the facility. It is well worth the time to invite representatives of these agencies to the facility to discuss not only the physical layout of the unit, but also to discuss such issues as restricted access areas (e.g., hazard containment areas). This will also provide the manager the opportunity to sensitize outsiders to the "whys" and "hows" of using animals in the institution. The next level of communication would be to establish rapport with the local media and politicians who can intervene on the institutions's behalf should a crisis develop. Finally, based upon the philosophy of the institution and with guidance and acceptance by the institution's public relations group, scheduled presentations to community groups and clubs will keep the lines of communication open. In doing so, one will have contacts in key segments of the community who can be informed and supportive allies in a time of crisis.

IV.   SUMMARY

The issue of security is far more complex than bricks and mortar and the occasional lock.

Animal facility security needs to be orchestrated with many components of an institution from the top management down to the animal care staff. This chapter describes some recommendations for enhancing security at the specialized level; however, the message should be that security needs a "big picture" approach. It should begin with the institution's risk assessment followed by strategies and plans to address the identified risks. Hardware is important but the human element is critical in the total security program. Managers must be proactive in encouraging individual responsibility among their staff towards security needs and in being a major player in communicating the value of animal use inside and outside of the institution.

REFERENCES

1. *Animal Research Crisis Management Manual*, National Association for Biomedical Research, Section IV-Risk Assessment, Reston, VA, 3, 1989.
2. **Gips, M.A.**, A pharmacopoeia of protection, *Sec. Mgmt.*, 43, 3, 1999.
3. ALF hits University of Minnesota, *Natl. Assn. Biomed. Res. Update*, 20, 8, 1999.
4. *Animal Care and Research: Challenges and Changes for the Institutional Animal Care and Use Committee*, Proceedings of a conference sponsored by Public Responsibility in Medicine and Research, Office for Protection from Research Risk, and Tufts University of Veterinary Medicine. Panel II — Safety Issues: Security, Occupational Health, and Biosafety, March 13–14, 1995, 51–57.
5. *Security Conference Summary*, National Association for Biomedical Research, Reston, VA, September 19–20, 1985, 1–18.
6. **CFR Code of Federal Registration, Title 9, Subchapter A, Section 2.32(c)(4)**, 1989.

Other Resources Used as Background Information for This Chapter and Suggested for Review:

- *Protecting Researchers and Their Work*, National Association for Biomedical Research Conference, November 7–9, 1990.
- Security Web site, www.securitymanagement.com, generic updated security information.
- *When Civility Ends: The Escalation of Animal Rights Extremism and Its Threat to Biomedical Research,* National Association for Biomedical Research Conference, April 2–4, 2000.

16 Public Affairs

Lynn C. Anderson, D.V.M., Dipl. ACLAM,
Jacquie Calnan, M.P.A., and Janet Skidmore, M.A.

The power of public perception cannot be overestimated. As Abraham Lincoln once stated, "Public sentiment is everything. With public sentiment, nothing can fail; without it, nothing can succeed."

For biomedical progress to continue, the public needs to understand science and support research with laboratory animals. Fortunately, most people will support the humane use of animals in the quest for treatments and cures if they are given an honest portrayal of biomedical research. The key is to reach the public with accurate information on the necessity, value, and humane nature of animal-based studies.

There are many opportunities for managers of laboratory animal resource programs to play a role in this process of public education. The shape of that role depends largely on the size and nature of one's facility; for example, the options open to a manager of a large pharmaceutical facility may be different from that of a director of a small university vivarium.

The goals of this chapter are to (1) provide an understanding of how animal activists are using the news media and other means to erode public support for animal research; (2) suggest proactive public affairs approaches that may be taken by both facilities and individuals to bolster the public's support of research; and (3) outline a crisis communication strategy.

I. THE ANTI-ANIMAL RESEARCH MESSAGE AND TACTICS

Animal rights activism follows a two-pronged strategy. While the movement's leaders and celebrity spokespeople are working to build the animal rights philosophy in the public's mind, others are willing to use threats of violence, break-ins, sabotage, theft, and arson to achieve their goal of stopping research (see Table 1).

Animal rights groups have tremendous resources to bring to bear on the campaign against laboratory animal research. In 1998, the top ten animal rights groups reported budgets totaling $143 million, and it is estimated that in all more than $300 million was donated to animal activist groups that year. By comparison, the combined budgets for the main national support groups — Americans for Medical Progress, Foundation for Biomedical Research and National Association for Biomedical Research reached just over $2 million in 1998.

TABLE 1. Examples of Tactics Used to Target People, Property, Programs, and Perceptions

- **Demonstrations**, often aimed at disrupting a key meeting of a company, university, or trade organization (e.g., an annual meeting, analyst briefing, or opening ceremony for a new facility).
- **Picketing** of a company, university, biomedical conference, or medical meeting at which the findings of research involving animals are presented and discussed.
- **Phone or fax blockades** in which an institution is bombarded with hundreds of nuisance phone calls or faxes in an effort to disrupt normal activities.
- **Phone, letter, or in-person threats** to staff or property, including physical violence or death.
- **Break-ins and burglaries**, the most devastating and costly incursions, usually cloaked in darkness and aided by "insiders," with impact ranging from theft of animals to destruction of equipment, defacement of property, and arson.
- **Vandalism**, defacement and destruction of property, including broken windows, graffiti, posters, stickers, or banners decrying animal research and "blood" smeared on buildings where research is conducted.
- **Letters, hoax and incendiary devices**, including envelopes filled with razor blades, letter bombs, and nail bombs that can maim or even kill.
- **Infiltrators and whistle-blowers**, who surreptitiously shoot photos allegedly showing mistreated and fearful laboratory animals, which the activists provide to the media and enlarge to poster size and post on Web sites.
- **Contamination** of experiments and resources.
- **Hunger strikes** by activists, in which extremist groups pledge to kill a number of scientists if the hunger striker dies.
- **Home visits and harassment** of staff and their families, as well as writing to neighbors alleging that an individual is an animal abuser.
- **Personal attacks** on staff, vendors, or shareholders.
- **Destruction** of personal property (e.g., homes, cars) belonging to staff.
- **Publishing** names, addresses, and phone numbers of staff in animal rights groups' publications/Web sites.
- **Sending** unwanted businesses or materials to staff homes and answering advertisements in the name of staff members. One laboratory staff member arrived home to find a mountain of manure on his lawn, the result of an order placed in his name by an animal activist.
- **Animal releases**, including the release of animals born into captivity and incapable of surviving in the wild.
- **Boycotts** of businesses or products, often including long-term demonstrations.
- **Legal actions**, including civil suits, or filing complaints with federal regulatory bodies such as USDA or FDA.
- **Cybercrimes**, such as altering a company's Web site with false and destructive messages, or attempting to render a computer server inoperable by flooding it with junk e-mail messages.

A.   HOW ACTIVISTS MANIPULATE PUBLIC OPINION

Public support for animal-based research is vital — and animal activists know this! That is why many of their campaigns, demonstrations, articles, newspaper letters, billboards, and other tactics are designed not so much to persuade scientists to stop working with animals as to compel the public to withdraw its support for animal-based research. If public support wanes, activists correctly reason, so, too, will political endorsement and funding. The activists' ultimate goal, then, is a total ban on all animal-based research.

Over the last 20 years, leaders of the animal rights movement have shown their mastery at manipulating public opinion. The widespread use of the term "animal rights" by activists, the public, the news media, and even the research community itself, represents a victory for the movement.

The activists have skillfully created a warm, friendly, fuzzy media image for themselves while mounting their assault on biomedical research. One reason they have been able to obtain a strong foothold in the media and popular culture is because the research community has failed to respond to the threat in a timely or adequate way. Many institutions have preferred not to become involved in the debate. Others did not see the assault on public opinion as a serious challenge. The activists were able to fill the public affairs void.

The media demands strong messages and the activists provide them: Animal research is cruel; animal research is unnecessary; animal research does not work and diverts limited resources from "legitimate" research. Those involved in research are portrayed by the activists as mad scientists and sadistic animal torturers, greedy for grant money/profits, and too corrupt/lazy/insensitive to seek alternatives to animal use.

Activists seek out research targets that carry emotional weight with the public. Typically, these include research projects involving nonhuman primates, cats and dogs, as well as behavioral and substance abuse research. These are all high on the activists' radar as potential targets. So, too, are programs funded by health charities or those conducted at publicly funded institutions.

Another demand of the media is for vivid images. Activists often use pictures to misrepresent the nature of animal research. For example, some depict animals in distress. Many of them are dated, staged, or edited out of context. Certainly these have a strong impact on audiences. One of the most powerful images in the activists' arsenal is that of a closed, locked laboratory door. The activists can then pose the question, "What is going on behind those doors?" This image allows activists to prey on the public's fears, apprehensions, lack of information, and misconceptions about animal-based research.

B.   THREATS TO PROGRAMS, PROPERTY, AND PEOPLE

Highly publicized attacks against research institutions have grown increasingly more frequent, destructive, and violent in the last decade: "There is no such thing as a company that is impenetrable," said Colin Wiggins, a former chief of Scotland Yard, who spent much of his law enforcement career tracking the activities of the U.K.'s most aggressive and successful animal rights extremists. Current targets include pharmaceutical companies, biotech companies, universities, and contract research laboratories, as well as laboratory animal suppliers and other vendors. Even charities that support animal-based research are targets of the activists' furor.

Attacks against institutions are often assisted by 'insiders,' some of whom infiltrate the institution for the express purpose of obtaining information and launching an attack. One of the greatest vulnerabilities is an institution's own employees, one or more of whom may be sympathetic to an animal activist group or may be influenced by friends or family members.

Individuals are also targeted. Many receive death threats, harassing phone calls, and "home visits" from activists. Leaders of the movement have said that anyone connected with laboratory animal research in any way — veterinarians, technicians, patient advocates, vendors, office staff — may become a target.

Examples abound of the means animal activists use to tirelessly drive their agenda:

- The Animal Liberation Front (ALF) claimed responsibility for breaking into laboratories in two campus buildings, where they vandalized, destroyed, and stole laboratory equipment, research data, and 116 animals. The 1999 attack damaged research being conducted on Alzheimer's and Parkinson's diseases and brain cancer studies. University officials estimated monetary damage at $1 million. One scientist estimated that her research, which was praised as a promising step toward development of treatments for Alzheimer's disease, was set back 2 years. The perpetrators apparently entered one of the buildings through an unlocked rooftop maintenance door.
- Several months later, animal activists took to the highways for the "1999 Primate Freedom Tour," another highly publicized initiative that targeted facilities in 24 U.S. cities, including Pittsburgh, San Francisco, Atlanta, Portland, San Antonio, Phoenix, Chicago, Madison, Boston, Philadelphia, Baltimore and Washington, D.C. Activists traveling in buses, vans, and trucks used sit-ins, office takeovers, night-time visits to scientists' homes, picketing, and banners on freeway overpasses to decry the use of nonhuman primates in research. The 3-month campaign led to 48 arrests.
- Also in 1999, an extremist faction of the animal rights movement that calls itself the "Justice Department" warned through an e-mail posting that it had mailed envelopes containing razor blades to 86 researchers working with nonhuman primates to find vaccines and treatments for AIDS, cancer, and other diseases. The group previously targeted the fur industry, declaring the mail initiative to be the start of a "millennium" campaign of terror to end the fur trade. It encouraged other animal rights activists to participate and even advocated coating some razor blades with rat poison.

C. LONG-TERM EFFECTS OF ANIMAL EXTREMISM

Experts on animal extremism in the law enforcement and biomedical research communities say these activities are certain to continue, increasingly targeting people as well as property. The real damage from such attacks — to an institution's public image — frequently lasts beyond the physical clean-up and the departure of the media.

The repercussions may lead to political intervention and diminished ability to conduct animal research. For individual institutions, they can have a devastating effect on an institution's long-term reputation and create public relations problems that last for years. The may also demoralize employees, diminish confidence among key external audiences, and impede cooperation from contractors or suppliers. Other adverse effects on industrial research institutions may be manifested as decreased support by investors and customers. In the case of a university, student admissions or support by funding agencies may be adversely impacted, which could profoundly damage the institution's fiscal health. Finally, administrative and management attention diverted to address animal activism may draw leadership away from more productive endeavors, potentially weakening the institution.

II. PRO-ANIMAL RESEARCH STRATEGIES

A. EDUCATING THE PUBLIC

The encouraging news is that the public is receptive to the pro-research message. Polls indicate three out of four Americans do support necessary animal studies done under humane conditions.

Two separate surveys by Americans for Medical Progress (September 1998) and by *New Scientist Magazine* (May 1999) demonstrated that support increases as the public learns more about the true nature and importance of animal research.

In the AMP poll, when audiences heard research advocacy statements contrasted with animal rights messages, support for research increased dramatically and backing for the animal rights position declined. The *New Scientist* poll demonstrated that just a few introductory words about the importance of animals to biomedical research had a significant effect on increasing public support.

B. WORKING THROUGH THE NEWS MEDIA

The most effective way to reach the public is through the news media. National and local T.V. news anchors are welcomed into tens of millions of homes every night as trusted friends. The morning newspaper remains a ritual. Radio and T.V. talk shows are constant companions for many. What is reported through these outlets gains an immediate validity and currency.

Especially in television, there is a growing demand for the new, different, and latest. CNN, MSNBC, and Fox News run 24-hour cable news networks. Local news programming can run up to 6 to 8 hours a day. Therefore, competition among media outlets is fierce. There is unrelenting pressure to be first on all stories, no matter what it takes. In this environment, truth often takes a backseat to conflict, entertaining personalities, and powerful video. There is little wonder, then, that the bizarre campaigns by People for the Ethical Treatment of Animals (PETA) and other animal rights groups receive widespread coverage.

De Tocqueville's oft-quoted admonition that "The public will believe a simple lie rather than a complex truth" has new currency in this media age. The average television news soundbite today is less than 8 seconds. Thus, tremendous skill is required to deliver a message to viewers. In 1992, rather than a complex explanation of his policy on tax reform, viewers heard George Bush say "Read my lips, no new taxes." Animal activists' claims against research are framed to fit into similar tight sound bites. A charge that "Scientists are animal torturers" is an easy sound bite; an explanation of the regulatory process that ensures humane animal care is not as easy to articulate.

Timing is nearly everything in journalism. It is a profession ruled by deadlines, and this works against facilities facing animal rights claims. Scientists are trained to be deliberate and to gather evidence, think, review, and think again before offering a position. This is counter to the workings of the media. No matter how meticulously crafted a facility's response to an animal rights protest may be, it is useless if it reaches the reporter after the news story airs or the newspaper article is printed.

The media is not a monolith, and it is a mistake to prepare a communications strategy without an understanding of the differences among the forms of media, and the individual outlets and reporters. Some reporters may be cynical, shallow and untrustworthy. They may report inaccurate information, oversimplify and sensationalize the issues. Yet most journalists are hardworking and honest. They are simply looking for a news story that will interest their viewers/readers. They are not approaching the animal research issue with a bias. It is likely they have never thought about the issue before. They are as open to hearing the scientific community's case as they are the activists' claims. Most will do their homework and present the issue as fairly as possible.

C.   TELL YOUR STORY BEFORE YOUR CRITICS DO

Paul Watson, an animal rights leader, once stated "You are who the media defines you to be." Like it or not, these words are true. No matter what a biomedical research institution has achieved or what it stands for, it is the media that determines how that institution is perceived by society at large.

Animal rights activists understand this, and are using their considerable media skills in campaigns to discredit animal-based medical research. It is vital for those responsible for managing laboratory animal resource programs to understand the impact of the media and how to work with it.

An effective media strategy for an animal research program is a comprehensive approach aimed at developing and nurturing relationships with key journalists that will see the institution through good times and bad.

The manager should help the institution reach out to the news media before the activists do. It is useful to brief news editors, relevant reporters, and editorial page editors, either as a single institution or as part of a local, state, or industry consortium, about the kinds of ongoing research involving animals. In addition, one should highlight the contributions of animals in basic research and the development of new medicines, and the threat posed by animal rights activists. Media support, through news and editorial coverage, can be invaluable if and when animal extremists target an institution. The manager might selectively use letters to the editor to correct misinformation and communicate the institution's position if the media carry negative stories or cover the activities of animal rights groups.

Inoculation of journalists against animal rights rhetoric is the single most important step one can take in debunking activists' claims. Institutional representatives, including the laboratory animal resource manager, might get to know the relevant reporters in his/her community. This is not as daunting as it sounds: good reporters are always interested in talking with someone who may provide a fascinating news story. One should identify those who frequently write on health and science issues, as well as general assignment reporters who have covered animal or health stories in the past. Business reporters can also be good prospects, especially if the biomedical research facility is an important economic resource for its community.

Most reporters have not given much, if any, thought to the role animal research has played in the development of treatments and cures throughout this century. There are many ways to raise their awareness level.

Advance media work is a vital part of your facility's crisis planning. Relationships with key reporters, built on trust, honesty, and mutual respect, are the coinage on which one can draw in times of animal rights crises. As positive media coverage for the institution's animal-based research develops, an effort should also be made to help the public understand the importance of such work.

Several universities and other institutions prepare regular "tip sheets" for reporters: news leads about ongoing research programs. The laboratory animal resource manager should work with the public relations/public affairs department to ensure that news about animal-based research is included. Whenever an important research breakthrough is announced, it is important to make sure the news release mentions the role animals played in the discovery. If video is being provided to television stations, one might include some tape of the species studied, so the reporter can say "mice like these led scientists to understand..." Incrementally, this will help the public connect animal research to the health benefits they enjoy.

The manager should be on the lookout for related news leads outside of the facility that would also interest reporters. When actor Michael J. Fox revealed that he had Parkinson's disease, several institutions opened their doors to reporters to discuss promising animal research. Similarly, when actor Christopher Reeve was paralyzed as the result of a severe spinal cord injury, reporters were invited in to see rats that had recovered some function due to experimental therapies after their spines were severed.

Note the phrases "opened their doors," and "invited" in the previous paragraph. Activists often raise the specter of "mad science going on behind locked doors" to trigger horrific, albeit false, images in the public's mind. A facility that is unnecessarily secretive in the conduct of its research helps activists foster this image.

Of course, animal research laboratories are not and never can be public spaces, and for many safety and proprietary reasons, layers of security must be added. However, there are ways in which research can be made more accessible to the public via the news media. With adequate notice and precautions, reporters can often suit up for a tour. Laboratory personnel can take videotape and still pictures of animals for distribution to the media, or, with appropriate planning, news photographers can be allowed in to obtain their own pictures. The amount of media access that can be permitted will vary from facility to facility. The point is not to create artificial barriers that will damage relationships with reporters or make it look like the facility has something to hide.

The size of the media market in which the facility is located will also influence strategy. In a small town, there may be only two or three reporters likely to cover the animal research issue. In larger cities, there are greater numbers of journalists, possibly including some for national media outlets such as TV networks and news magazines. The manager might keep a simple database of the reporters with whom he/she has worked, the subjects in which they are interested, the times the manager has been contacted, and whether the reporter prefers to communicate by phone, fax, e-mail, or snail mail. Often, reporters will gladly receive information when it represents a good story about research for their audiences.

The manager might consider working with other research interests in his/her area. For example, one can join forces with others to hold an informal media briefing or to meet with the editorial board of the local newspaper. The aim of both editorial board meetings and reporters' briefings is not to create headlines in the paper the next day, but to provide background materials and context for future coverage of the animal research issue and to identify information resources that will be available to a reporter as he or she develops a story.

Establishing solid relationships with reporters before the institution is targeted by animal activists enables the manager to develop a reputation for honesty and accuracy in the media that will serve him/her well in a crisis. Institutions with the best media relations are straightforward with reporters, providing appropriate spokespeople who will answer questions as frankly as possible, within a reporter's deadline, rather than brushing them aside or stonewalling. Reasonable journalists will respect honest boundaries such as a straight, "I can't talk about that," or "I just don't know," but their radar detectors are sensitive to evasions and bluffs. Above all, one should never lie to a reporter. It may be tempting to do so in the short run, but it will destroy any chance for a positive relationship with that journalist. Even as a private citizen, without drawing on one's institutional affiliation, the manager can do much to shape the coverage animal-based research receives in the media (see Table 2).

For example, one might send a note to a reporter, or a letter to the editor of a newspaper (see Table 3), concerning a recent story. Reporters and editors are responsive to feedback. They want to know that they are doing everything

TABLE 2. Steps the Manager Can Take to Make a Difference

- **Stay informed** about issues related to animal research
- **Connect** with local and national research support organizations
- **Send** letters and commentaries of newspapers
- **Reach out** to schools, senior citizens, and other public forums
- **Support** those who are targeted by activists

TABLE 3. Tips on How to Write a Letter to the Editor (2)

- **Make one point** (or at most two) in the letter or fax.
- **Be timely.** Either address a specific article, editorial, or letter that recently appeared in the paper or tie the issue being addressed to a recent event.
- **Become familiar** with the coverage and editorial position of the paper to which the letter is being written. Refute or support specific statements, address relevant facts that have been ignored, but **do not** engage in blanket attacks on the media in general or the specific newspaper in particular.
- **Check the letter specifications** of the newspaper to which the letter is being written. In general, two **short paragraphs** are ideal. The letter writer should also include his/her name, signature, address, and phone number since most newspapers will not publish a letter without confirming that it came from the person who signed it.
- **Read** the letters that appear in local and national newspapers. It is interesting to note if a certain type of letter is favored for publication.
- **Support the letter with facts.** If the topic being addressed is controversial, one might consider sending documentation along with the letter; however, one should be careful not to overload the editor with too much information.
- **Encourage others** to write letters when possible. This will demonstrate that others in the community are concerned with the topic.
- **Monitor the newspaper for the letter.** If a letter has not appeared within a week or two, one might follow up with a call to the editorial department of the newspaper.
- **Write to different sections of the newspaper.** Sometimes the issue one wishes to address is relevant to the lifestyle, book review or other sections of the newspaper.
- **Consider approaching other media.** An increasing number of broadcast news programs (e.g., 60 Minutes, All Things Considered, etc.) solicit and broadcast "letters to the editor." One may wish to consider such an outlet in addition to newspapers.

possible to present balanced coverage. Recently, an editor of the *Seattle Post Intelligencer* observed that most newspaper articles about animal research were focused on the claims of animal rights groups and were nearly uniformly negative. He asked the Washington State Association for Biomedical Research to prepare a five-part series of articles to educate readers about the value of animal research. The articles, which were written by physicians, veterinarians, a patient, and an ethicist, generated many responses and discussion from people on both sides of the issue.

Table 4 outlines how to write an op-ed. Op-eds are longer than letters to the editor, and there is more competition for space. It is advisable to call the paper for length requirements (usually 600 to 800 words).

Remember, the worst image activists can show is a locked laboratory door. It is important to demystify the work!

III. CRISIS COMMUNICATION: PREPARATION IS THE KEY

Without knowing when, where or how animal activists may strike next, having a crisis communications plan in place can minimize the damage to an institution's image if media coverage contains misinformation, is sympathetic to activists or does not reflect the institution's side of the story. It is critical to know exactly what to say and do should a crisis occurs. The time to decide is not when animal activists

---

TABLE 4. Tips on How to Write an Op-Ed (2)

- **Try to write on a controversial issue** being covered at that time. If possible, one should use a professional title that suggests authority. In particular, it can be valuable to get permission to sign the op-ed as a representative of your institution.
- **Send the op-ed piece to local as well as distant newspapers**. It is advisable to avoid sending the piece to two newspapers in the same market (e.g., sending it to the *San Francisco Examiner* and the *Seattle Times* is acceptable, but not to the *Examiner* and the *San Francisco Chronicle*). National newspapers such as the *New York Times*, *Los Angeles Times*, *Washington Post*, *Christian Science Monitor,* and *USA Today* generally do not accept op-eds that are also being offered to other newspapers.
- **Submit the same piece to several local dailies in different regions** to increase the chances of publication.
- **Assure the op-ed editor that the piece has not been submitted to any other paper in his/her market**. This should be stated in the cover letter; on the other hand, if the piece is being submitted to only one newspaper, one may wish to let the editor know that he/she is being offered an exclusive.
- **Avoid excessive rhetoric**. It is important to state the subject under controversy very clearly. It is important to remember that it is the middle-of-the-road readership that one is trying to persuade. If facts not commonly found in the mainstream media are used, sources (particularly those that are "respectable") should be cited.
- **Use a catchy title**, otherwise the newspaper might run its own title which may not emphasize the intended central message.
- **Be prepared to shorten and re-submit** the article as a letter to the editor if it is not accepted as an op-ed.

— and the news media — are pounding on the institution's door. Specific points that the manager of the animal research resource should consider include:

A. **First and foremost, establish a crisis response team —** *now*. It is valuable to assemble an internal team whose role is to coordinate efforts before, during, and after a crisis. The team should include representatives from management/administration, research/animal care, security, legal, and public/government relations. Other functions can be added according to the institution's needs.

B. **Develop action plans.** The group should develop an action plan to reduce risks, with each member assessing the institution's vulnerability from his or her viewpoint. In addition, the group will determine how and what to communicate about animal research in both crisis and non-crisis situations. [Note: Keep in mind that animal activism is merely one type of crisis. The response team should also consider other types of crises as described in Chapter 14.] Table 5 summarizes efforts which should be undertaken to prepare for communications in the event of a public affairs crisis.

TABLE 5. A Checklist for Crisis Communications (4)

- **Mobilize** the crisis response team.
- **Identify:**
  - Type of crisis
  - Location
  - Project(s) targeted
  - Number of people involved and whether individual safety is at risk.
  - Specifics of location, e.g., near employee entrance, exit, laboratory, etc.
- **Analyze** the situation as quickly as possible. Determine what information still needs to be collected and obtain it.
- **Decide on response** to specifics of allegations.
- **Decide on timing, content and format** of public release of information.
- **Advise** auxiliary members of crisis response team, i.e., institutional spokesperson, government relations, legal counsel.
- **From your risk assessment and pre-crisis planning**, you already have the following established and ready:
  - Up-to-date information on research projects and institutional policies and procedures ready to distribute.
  - Designated spokespersons who can address the situation from the point of view of the institution.
  - Lines of communication with key audiences.
- **Determine the principle messages** you wish to communicate and the order of priority for delivering them. It is key not to leave important audiences waiting and wondering what the institution did to fall into the current situation. On the other hand, one should not go public with any communications until all the relevant facts have been established.

C. **Be well informed.** The manager should ensure that up-to-date information on research projects and institutional policies and procedures, including policies on humane animal care and standards of animal care, on hand and ready to be distributed as needed. The materials should also include the accreditation of the institution and statements of assurance or compliance from regulatory agencies. It is important to be familiar also with the number of ongoing projects that do not use animals. In addition, the manager should stay up to date on existing and proposed legislation that may affect animal research.

D. **Develop key messages.** One should develop four to five essential points of information that communicate what key audiences need to know about the institution and its animal research. These points should be short, concise, succinct kernels of information. Try this: Imagine yourself at a social gathering where a guest asks about your institution's research with animals. What facts do you want this person to remember at the end of the evening? Those are your key messages.

E. **Identify and train media spokespersons.** It is preferable to have one individual designated to speak on behalf of the institution, but several potential spokespersons should be identified and prepared in the event that the primary spokesperson is unavailable. All spokespersons should be prepared to respond appropriately on the animal research issue in both non-crisis and crisis situations (see Table 6).

F. **Know the animal rights activists and how they operate**. It is important to gather as much information as possible about local groups and their leadership, as well as major groups such as PETA. The institution may wish to keep a list of names, addresses, and phone numbers of local groups and individuals involved in animal activism, including those who write letters to the editor. In addition, one might monitor activist hotlines and Web sites and track activities that could be trend setting in other areas of the country. Such activities, usually driven by well-funded major groups, present the institution with serious response imperatives. One should keep in mind that activist stories may involve celebrities, which can inflate and prolong media coverage, as well as generate articles in the lifestyle or entertainment sections of publications, making them harder to balance. Finally, issues involving controversial studies and/or larger animals (dogs, cats, and primates) will generate more public interest.

G. **Know the media and what they are reporting**. It is important to determine which media outlets and journalists are reporting news concerning biomedical research and testing as an issue and in the context of medicine, health and science news. Establishing relationships with these journalists by contacting them and providing access to information and spokespersons for either background or attribution can be valuable. One should keep in mind that building relationships with key media on this issue takes time.

TABLE 6. News Media Interview Tips (3)

- **Be accessible and responsive.** In the case of a demonstration by activists, one should let the reporters know that he/she is available to deliver an appropriate response, but insist on being interviewed away from the protesters.
- **Always tell the truth.** One should not be afraid to say, "I don't know." Never try to bluff through a response and assume that everything is on the record.
- **Prepare** before the interview. Anticipate likely questions. Develop three key points that need to be made. These should be written down and memorized. Stick to these points during the interview.
- **Don't wait for the reporter to ask the right questions.** One should bridge from undesirable questions to key messages: "I can understand why you are asking that, but the real issue is...".
- **Repetition works.** The basic rule of television news is to tell them that you are going to tell them; tell them; and then tell them that you told them. One must stay "on message" since the interview may be edited.
- **Be brief.** The average television news soundbite is between 8 and 14 seconds. One may recall the success of "Read my lips: no new taxes." It is worthwhile to prepare some soundbites in advance. Even with print interviews, lengthy monologues should be avoided and short sentences used. If the reporter wants more, let him or her ask.
- **Don't fear silences.** One should not feel the need to fill every moment of the interview with talk.
- **Never repeat a negative.** For example, one should not say, "We are not torturing animals."
- **Be as positive and upbeat as appropriate to the circumstances**.
- **Avoid exaggerations and "no comment."** If one cannot discuss a subject, he/she should explain why. It is important not to speculate or answer hypothetical questions.
- **Speak calmly, clearly, in a conversational style.** One should talk slowly for television; regular pace is best for radio.
- **Don't forget to breathe.** Unless there is some disaster to which one is responding, the interview should begin with a warm, friendly, relaxed smile.
- **Avoid scientific terminology or jargon.** The majority of Americans have the equivalent of an eighth grade science education. It is useful to speak plainly and use examples and illustrations where possible.
- **Don't assume that the audience or the reporter knows the vital role of animals in medical breakthroughs**. Most people have never given this issue a thought, and the interviewee should emphasize concern for animal welfare.
- **Keep the message simple.** The mission is to communicate, not impress. It is vital that the reporter has a clear understanding of the issue as the result of the interview — if the reporter does not, the audience will not.
- **Challenge incorrect assumptions.** If a reporter uses inaccurate information during the interview, he/she should be corrected, but without repeating a negative.
- **Respect media deadlines** and be on time for scheduled interviews. Television and radio time is often split-second critical. If you promise to get back to a print reporter, find out his/her deadline.
- **Maintain eye contact.** On television, the interviewee should look at the reporter, not the camera. This enhances credibility. If there is no interviewer and you are in a TV studio at some remote location listening to questions by earpiece, look squarely into the camera at all times, even when you are not talking. Don't let your eyes wander.
- **Don't worry if you are nervous** when you talk to a reporter. Being a little nervous will keep you alert. One is not expected to be perfectly poised and slick. It is far better that honesty, sincerity, and conviction come through. It is important to be human, be yourself, and to deliver the key messages.

H. Invite the media. Some institutions have found bringing reporters together with spokespersons to discuss animal research issues in the animal research facility to be a valuable exercise. The institution might consider providing an escorted tour. However, one should never allow a journalist, with or without a camera, to tour the facility without an escort who can discuss the purpose of the research, the policies and procedures of the institution, and the care and treatment of lab animals. If cameras are allowed into the facility, the manager should discourage photographers from shooting into cages, since the bright light may make the animals recoil and appear fearful to viewers. It is useful to prepare an orientation for journalists before they tour the facility so they are prepared for what they will see. Video footage generated internally, known as b-roll, is often used for this purpose. Facility staff should always be alerted that the media will be on site. The manager is wise to ask for the staff's help in presenting the most professional image of the facility. Finally, before arranging to escort a journalist through the facility, the manager should tour it. A valuable exercise is for the manager to put him/herself in the place of the reporter and imagine he/she is seeing the facility for the first time. This helps to ensure that everything is in order.

I. Have print and video materials on hand. Providing the media with background materials in the form of press releases, fact sheets, and media backgrounders about animal research in the facility can be a valuable approach. For broadcast media, it is worthwhile to provide b-roll footage as well.

J. Communicate with key audiences. The manager should keep staff, employees, and other key internal and external audiences abreast about what is happening if animal activists target the facility and/or institution. It is important to communicate the benefits of animal research in advance to keep them abreast of the issues and help them understand the institution's position.

K. Conduct a crisis simulation. An especially valuable approach is to develop scenarios for various contingencies — break-ins, demonstrations, staff threats, negative media coverage, etc. This allows one to plan in advance the steps to be taken for each situation, then test the response team's performance through a mock crisis drill. The more realistic the drill is made, the more valuable the exercise will be.

L. Debrief thoroughly. After a crisis simulation has been conducted, one should thoroughly analyze the experience and determine if and where improvement is needed. When identified, problems should be fixed. It is better to find out what is not working in a simulation than in a real crisis.

REFERENCES

1. **Aldhous, P.**, *New Scientist*, 2187, 26–31, May 22, 1999.
2. FAIR — Fairness & Accuracy in Reporting, http://www.fair.org/activism/communicate.html.
3. Americans for Medical Progress, http://www.amprogress.org.
4. *Crisis Management Manual*, National Association for Biomedical Research, Washington, D.C., 1997.

Index